Leong's Manual of Diagnostic Biomarkers for Immunohistology

Fourth Edition

Leong's Manual of Diagnostic Biomarkers for Immunohistology

Fourth Edition

Edited by

Runjan Chetty
University of Toronto

Kumarasen Cooper
University of Pennsylvania

Carol Cheung
University of Toronto

Srinivas Mandavilli
Hartford Hospital, Connecticut

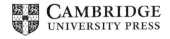
CAMBRIDGE
UNIVERSITY PRESS

CAMBRIDGE
UNIVERSITY PRESS

University Printing House, Cambridge CB2 8BS, United Kingdom

One Liberty Plaza, 20th Floor, New York, NY 10006, USA

477 Williamstown Road, Port Melbourne, VIC 3207, Australia

314–321, 3rd Floor, Plot 3, Splendor Forum, Jasola District Centre, New Delhi – 110025, India

103 Penang Road, #05–06/07, Visioncrest Commercial, Singapore 238467

Cambridge University Press is part of the University of Cambridge.

It furthers the University's mission by disseminating knowledge in the pursuit of education, learning, and research at the highest international levels of excellence.

www.cambridge.org
Information on this title: www.cambridge.org/9781108491570
DOI: 10.1017/9781108863797

First and second editions © Greenwich Medical Media Limited, 1999, 2002

Third and fourth editions © Cambridge University Press 2016, 2022

First published 1999

Second edition 2002

Third edition 2016

Fourth edition 2022

Printed in the United Kingdom by TJ Books Limited, Padstow Cornwall

A catalogue record for this publication is available from the British Library.

ISBN 978-1-108-49157-0 Hardback

It is with much nostalgia that we dedicate the fourth edition of this book to Professor Anthony S.-Y. Leong, BBS, MD, FRCPA, who passed away in 2011. In honor of Professor Leong's memory, we have decided to entitle the book *Leong's Manual of Diagnostic Biomarkers for Immunohistology*. This is a fitting tribute to Tony's brainchild, which was first published in 1999. More importantly, we are deeply indebted to his wife Wendy and children Joel and Trishe for their unconditional support for publishing this fourth edition.

Contents

Color plates can be found after page 504

Contributors

Sandra D. Bohling, MD
Pathologist and Associate Director of Hematopathology and Clinical PCR Services, PhenoPath Laboratories, Seattle, WA, USA

Runjan Chetty, MBBCh, FFPath, FRCPA, FRCPath, FRCPC, DPhil
Interim Medical Director, Laboratory Medicine Program, University Health Network, Professor, University of Toronto, Toronto, Canada

Carol Cheung, MD, PhD, JD, FRCPC
Medical Director, Immunopathology Laboratory, Laboratory Medicine Program, University Health Network, Assistant Professor, University of Toronto, Toronto, Canada

Kumarasen Cooper, MBChB, FFPath, FRCPath, DPhil
Professor, University of Pennsylvania Hospital, Philadelphia, PA, USA

Kossivi E. Dantey, MD
Bone and Soft Tissue Pathology Fellow, Department of Pathology, University of Pittsburgh Medical Center, Pittsburgh, PA, USA

Jan Delabie, MD
Division of Hematopathology, Laboratory Medicine Program, University Health Network and University of Toronto, Toronto, Canada

Charuhas Deshpande, MD
Associate Professor at the Pennsylvania Hospital, Department of Pathology and Laboratory Medicine, University of Pennsylvania Health System, Philadelphia, PA, USA

Allen M. Gown, MD
Director, PhenoPath Laboratories, Seattle, Washington, USA, and University of British Columbia, Vancouver, BC, Canada

Jui-Han Huang, MD, PhD
Assistant Professor at the Pennsylvania Hospital, Department of Pathology and Laboratory Medicine, University of Pennsylvania Health System, Philadelphia, PA, USA

Harry Hwang, MD
Director, Molecular Pathology, PhenoPath Laboratories, Seattle, WA, USA

Steven J. Kussick, MD, PhD
Associate Medical Director and Director, Hematopathology and Flow Cytometry, PhenoPath Laboratories, Seattle, WA, USA

Priti Lal, MD, FCAP
Associate Professor, Pathology, Perelman School of Medicine, and Director of the GU subdivision at the Department of Pathology, University of Pennsylvania Hospital, Philadelphia, PA, USA

Srinivas Mandavilli
Vice Chief of Pathology, Hartford Hospital, CT, USA

Maria Martinez-Lage, MD
Assistant Professor in Neuropathology and Surgical Pathology, Department of Pathology and Laboratory Medicine, Perelman School of Medicine, University of Pennsylvania, Philadelphia, PA, USA

David Ng, MD
Hematopathologist, PhenoPath Laboratories, Seattle, WA, USA

Karen Pinto, MD
Department of Pathology, Kuwait Centre for Cancer Control, Kuwait for the infograms

M. Carolina Reyes, MD
Assistant Professor, Department of Pathology,
University of Pennsylvania Hospital, Philadelphia,
PA, USA

Stefano Serra, MD
University Health Network, Assistant Professor of Pathology,
University of Toronto, Toronto, Canada

Stuti G. Shroff, MD, PhD
Assistant Professor of Anatomic Pathology, Department
of Pathology and Laboratory Medicine, University of
Pennsylvania Hospital, Philadelphia, PA, USA

Kristen M. Stashek, MD
Assistant Professor of Clinical Pathology and Laboratory
Medicine, Perelman School of Medicine, University of
Pennsylvania, Philadelphia, PA, USA

Preface

The fourth edition of Leong's Manual of Diagnostic Biomarkers for Immunohistology sees a slight change in title to reflect the role of antibodies also as biomarkers as more and more of them inform therapeutic practice.

In addition, we have pared the content quite dramatically with omission of tables and appendices. Instead we have introduced infograms which contain more condensed and easy to read offerings on a selection of biomarkers and antibodies. It is hoped that this format will become the mainstay of presentation in the future.

Immunohistochemistry and immunohistology are rapidly evolving fields and new biomarkers appear on a daily basis. As such, we have endeavoured to capture most of the mainstream markers, and those that have been omitted will be covered in forthcoming editions.

I would like to thank all contributors and co-editors for all their help in assembling this fourth edition.

Runjan Chetty

α-1-antitrypsin

Background

α-1-antitrypsin (AAT), a 51 kD glycoprotein, is mainly synthesized in the liver, where a pair of at least 24 possible codominant alleles, which belong to the protease inhibitor (Pi) locus on chromosome 2, determine production. It functions as an inhibitor of proteases, especially elastase, collagenase, and chymotrypsin. Individuals homozygous for Pi M produce normal quantities of functionally normal AAT, whereas individuals with abnormal Pi genes, such as those designated ZZ, SZ, and PS, have serum concentrations of AAT that are 40% of normal. Such individuals are at risk for hepatic cirrhosis in childhood or pulmonary emphysema as young adults.

Applications

AAT, AACT, and lysozyme can still provide useful diagnostic information, but they have to be used in the context of a panel of antibodies directed to the diagnostic entities considered in differential diagnosis.

1. In pleomorphic tumors of the skin, these markers are useful for the separation of atypical fibroxanthoma from its mimics, although other markers can provide more relevant information to separate such entities, and in identifying tumors rich in phagolysosomes, such as granular cell tumors.
2. Immunolabelling for AAT remains an important way of demonstrating the presence of accumulated enzyme within hepatocytes in AAT deficiency. Hepatocyte globules characteristically associated with AAT deficiency may be mimicked by AACT deficiency, and the distinction can only be made by immunolabelling.

Selected references

Dictor M. Alpha-1-antitrypsin in a malignant mixed mesodermal tumor of the ovary. *Am J Surg Pathol* 1981;5:543–50.

Isaacson PG, Jones DB, Millward-Sadler GH, et al. Alpha-1-antitrypsin in human macrophages. *J Clin Pathol* 1981;34:982–90.

Kindblom LG, Jacobsen GK, Jacobsen M. Immunohistochemical investigations of tumors of supposed fibroblastic-histiocytic origin. *Hum Pathol* 1982;13:834–40.

Leong AS-Y, Milios J. Atypical fibroxanthoma of the skin: A clinicopathological and immunohistochemical study and a discussion of its histogenesis. *Histopathology* 1987;11:463–75.

Marshall RJ, Braye SG. Alpha-1-antitrypsin, alpha-1-antichymotrypsin, actin and myosin in uterine sarcomas. *Int J Gynecol Pathol* 1985;4:346–54.

Palmer PE, Wolfe HJ, Dayal Y, Gang DL. Immunocytochemical diagnosis of alpha-1-antitrypsin deficiency. *Am J Surg Pathol* 1978;2:275–81.

Poblete MT, Nualart F, del Pozo M, et al. Alpha-1-antitrypsin expression in human thyroid papillary carcinoma. *Am J Surg Pathol* 1996;20:956–63.

α-Fetoprotein (AFP)

Background

α-Fetoprotein (AFP) is a glycoprotein composed of 590 amino acid residues. Cells of the embryonic yolk sac, fetal liver, and intestinal tract synthesize this glycoprotein. By immunostaining, the antigen is detectable in hepatocellular carcinoma and in gonadal and extragonadal germ cell tumors, including yolk sac tumors. It is otherwise not present in adult tissues.

Applications

Staining for AFP is largely used for the identification of the glycoprotein in germ cell tumors and in the separation of hepatocellular carcinoma (HCC) from its mimics such as cholangiocarcinoma and metastatic carcinoma. AFP is of low sensitivity and estimated to be present in no more than 44% of HCCs.

Selected references

Chedid A, Chejfec G, Eichorst M, et al. Antigenic markers for hepatocellular carcinoma. *Cancer* 1990;65:84–7.

Fucich LF, Cheles MK, Thung SN, et al. Primary versus metastatic hepatic carcinoma: An immunohistochemical study of 34 cases. *Arch Pathol Lab Med* 1994;118:927–30.

Guindi M. Yazdi HM, Gilliatt MA. Fine needle aspiration biopsy of hepatocellular carcinoma: Value of immunocytochemical and ultrastructural studies. *Acta Cytol* 1994;38:385–91.

Leong AS-Y, Sormunen RT, Tsui WM-S, Liew CT. Immunostaining for liver cancers. *Histopathology* 1998;33:318–24.

Alpha-1-antichymotrypsin

Background

α-1-antichymotrypsin (AACT), a 68 kD glycoprotein, is a serum protease inhibitor that is synthesized mainly by cells of the mononuclear phagocytic system. AACT was initially employed as a marker of histiocytes (monocytes/ macrophages), but the demonstration of this enzyme in a large variety of normal and neoplastic tissues of both epithelial and mesenchymal derivation has resulted in only restricted use in diagnostic immunohistology. It most likely identifies cells that are rich in phagolysosomes and has no tissue specificity. Within restricted settings, AACT can be of value in diagnostic immunohistology, although, to a large extent, more specific markers of histiocytes/macrophages have replaced this marker.

(*See discussion on* α-1-antitrypsin.)

Alpha methyl acyl CoA racemase (AMACR)

Background

AMACR, also called P504S, is a mitochondrial and peroxisomal enzyme involved in the metabolism of branched chain fatty acid and bile acid intermediates. It catalyzes the racemization of alpha methyl branched carboxylic coenzyme A thioesters. Deficiency of AMACR is associated with certain adult onset sensory motor neuropathies. Variable levels of AMACR protein expression are seen in a wide range of tissues and cancers, including colorectal, prostate, ovarian, breast, bladder, lung, and renal cell carcinomas. Additionally, AMACR is also expressed in lymphoma and melanoma. AMACR is thus considered a common abnormality and thought to participate in the early stages of cancer development. Prostate and colorectal carcinomas show the highest expression at 92% and 83%, respectively.

AMACR has also emerged as a putative therapeutic target in cancer treatment. While overexpression of AMACR is seen in a high percentage of the cancers named in the previous paragraph, it is either negative or minimally expressed in the adjacent normal tissue. This property makes it a potential candidate for targeted therapy either as an antibody or as an enzyme inhibitor.

Applications

Prostate carcinoma

AMACR is a sensitive (82–100%) and relatively specific (70–100%) marker for prostate cancer. It is most specific if circumferential luminal to subluminal and diffuse cytoplasmic staining is noted. It is a commonly used tool in the diagnosis of morphologically difficult prostatic adenocarcinomas in combination with basal cell markers including p63 and 34BE12 (CK903). AMACR staining is not uniform in prostate carcinoma. Approximately 25% of carcinomas are weakly positive, 40% moderately positive, and 35% strongly positive. Histologically benign prostate tissue can sometimes be positive (5–8% of cases). Additionally, premalignant and

benign entities that are known to lose basal cell markers may also be positive for AMACR, such as atypical adenomatous hyperplasia (15% of the cases), atrophy, partial atrophy, and crowded benign glands.

It is also important to note that unusual morphologic variants, including foamy gland, pseudo-hyperplastic and atrophic prostate cancers, are less frequently positive for AMACR expression, with only 69–80% of cases staining positive. The diagnostic implications of these findings are that while AMACR is a great addition to the armamentarium of stains for the work up of atypical small acinar proliferation (ASAP), it has its limitations. About 20% of cases considered to be carcinoma on hematoxylin and eosin (H&E) may be negative for AMACR and basal cell markers. So, while the initial studies indicated that AMACR was uniformly and strongly positive in 97% to 100% of prostate cancers, only about 80–85% of cancers are positive on needle biopsies.

Minimal prostatic adenocarcinoma and atypical proliferations

A cocktail stain containing racemase along with p63 and CK903 is becoming increasingly common in the work up of atypical small acinar proliferations and to support the diagnosis of small foci of prostatic adenocarcinomas. Approximately 10% of cases thought to be atypical can be diagnosed as carcinoma after addition of AMACR to the basal cell marker cocktail. Approximately 45% of atypical diagnoses were converted to a definitive diagnosis of carcinoma on the basis of a positive AMACR.

Prostatic "pseudo-neoplasms"

Mimics of prostatic adenocarcinoma include atypical adenomatous hyperplasia (AAH), adenosis, atrophy, post-atrophic hyperplasia, basal cell metaplasia, and seminal vesicles or ejaculatory duct epithelium. Only a small number of AAH cases reveal focal staining. Atrophic glands and post-atrophic hyperplasia have also been shown to be positive for AMACR in a very small number of cases.

Post-treatment prostate carcinoma

Radiation therapy has no effect on the AMACR staining of prostatic adenocarcinoma in needle biopsies, TURP (transurethral resection of prostate) chips, or salvage radical prostatectomies. Benign glands with radiation atypia are negative. A significant decrease in the intensity of AMACR staining is noted in hormone refractory prostatic adenocarcinoma when compared with clinically localized cancer. To assess residual, post-treatment prostatic adenocarcinoma, a panel of stains containing AMACR is useful.

Renal tumors

AMACR has been found to be strongly expressed in papillary renal cell carcinomas (RCC), mucinous tubular and spindle cell carcinoma, Xp11 translocation RCC, and acquired cystic disease associated RCC.

Clear cell (CC) RCC and CC papillary RCC are negative for AMACR.

In a poorly differentiated RCC, or in cases with overlapping histological appearances, AMACR forms a useful adjunct to diagnosis.

Other sites

A. In the gastrointestinal (GI) tract:
  i) Colon adenomas with high-grade dysplasia stain positive for AMACR.
  ii) Barrett-related dysplasia is found to be positive; 95% of cases with high-grade dysplasia and 45% of cases with low-grade dysplasia have been reported positive.
  iii) Stomach adenocarcinoma may also show positivity for AMACR in approximately 25% of cases.
B. Extramammary Paget disease: 70% of cases are reportedly positive.

Selected references

Dabir PD, Ottosen P, Hoyer S, Hamilton-Dutoit S. Comparative analysis of three- and two-antibody cocktails to AMACR and basal cell markers for the immunohistochemical diagnosis of prostate carcinoma. *Diagn Pathol* 2012;7:81.

Hameed O, Humphrey PA. p63/AMACR antibody cocktail restaining of prostate needle biopsy tissues after transfer to charged slides: A viable approach in the diagnosis of small atypical foci that are lost on block sectioning. *Am J Clin Pathol* 2005;124:708–15.

Jiang Z, Woda BA, Rock KL, et al. P504S: A new molecular marker for the detection of prostate carcinoma. *Am J Surg Pathol* 2001;25:1397–404.

Rubin MA, Zhou M, Dhanasekaran SM, et al. Alpha-Methylacyl coenzyme A racemase as a tissue biomarker for prostate cancer. *JAMA* 2002;287:1662–70.

Shi XY, Bhagwandeen B, Leong AS. p16, cyclin D1, Ki-67, and AMACR as markers for dysplasia in Barrett esophagus. *Appl Immunohistochem Mol Morphol* 2008;16:447–52.

Zhou M, Aydin H, Kanane H, Epstein JI. How often does alpha-methylacyl-CoA-racemase contribute to resolving an atypical diagnosis on prostate needle biopsy beyond that provided by basal cell markers? *Am J Surg Pathol* 2004;28:239–43.

Zhou M, Chinnaiyan AM, Kleer CG, Lucas PC, Rubin MA. Alpha-Methylacyl-CoA racemase: A novel tumor marker over-expressed in several human cancers and their precursor lesions. *Am J Surg Pathol* 2002;26:926–31.

Amyloid

Background

The amyloidoses are characterized by local, organ-limited, or generalized proteinaceous deposits of autologous origin. The pattern of distribution, progress of disease, and complications are dependent on the fibril protein. Amyloid is characterized by the following: (i) a typical green birefringence with polarized light after Congo red staining, (ii) non-branching linear fibrils with a diameter of 10–12 nm, and (iii) an X-ray diffraction pattern that is consistent with Pauling's model of a cross-β fibril. Apart from the rare familial syndromes, localized forms of amyloid affect certain organs or lesions (Aβ in brain; calcitonin in medullary carcinoma; islet amyloid polypeptide in insulinomas or islets of Langerhans). The five major different fibril proteins are usually associated with the most common generalized amyloid syndromes: amyloid A (AA), amyloid of λ– (Aλ) and κ– (Aκ) light chains, and of transthyretin (ATTR) and β2-microglobulin origin. These fibril proteins may be deposited in a wide variety of tissues and organs.

Applications

1. AA-amyloidosis is commonly associated with chronic inflammatory disorders. AL-amyloidosis (either λ– or κ– light chain origin) is linked mainly to the plasma cell dyscrasias or interpreted as being idiopathic.
2. ATTR-amyloidosis is found in cases with familial amyloidosis.
3. Aβ2microglobulin-amyloidosis is associated with long-term hemodialysis.

Interpretation

Occasionally, more than one antibody may show immunostaining of amyloid deposits. Immunohistochemistry detects any associated contaminating component in the amyloid deposit (amyloid P component, apolipoprotein E, and glycosaminoglycans) and not merely the currently known obligate fibril proteins. Further, the five syndromic fibril proteins originate from plasma proteins, which may themselves "contaminate" amyloid deposits. The most critical of these are the immunoglobulin light chains.

Another problem area is the false negative detection of amyloid. This can be avoided by increasing the sensitivity of detection by using both immuno- and Congo red staining methods. Long-term hemodialysis–associated β2-microglobulin amyloid may also involve the gastrointestinal and reproductive systems, in addition to osteoarticular involvement.

The distinction and classification of amyloidosis has major therapeutic implications, as studies have recommended that AL-amyloidosis be treated with cytotoxic drugs (melphalan and prednisolone), whilst AA-amyloidosis responds better to colchicine and dimethylsulphoxide.

The role of antibodies against amyloid β precursor protein has assisted in the diagnosis of Alzheimer's disease and early detection of axonal injury in the brain. Antibodies to transthyretin amyloid protein are useful in the diagnosis of cardiac amyloidosis and familial amyloidotic polyneuropathy.

Selected references

Iwamoto N, Nishiyama E, Ohwada J, Arai H. Distribution of amyloid deposits in the cerebral white matter of the Alzheimer's disease brain: Relationship to blood vessels. *Acta Neuropathol (Berlin)* 1997;93:334–40.

Jacobson DR, Pastore RD, Yaghoubian R, et al. Variant-sequence transthyretin (isoleucine 122) in late-onset cardiac amyloidosis in Black Americans. *N Engl J Med* 1997;336:466–73.

Lansbury PT Jr. In pursuit of the molecular structure of amyloid plaque: New technology provides unexpected and critical information. *Biochemistry* 1992;31:6865–70.

Ravid M, Shapiro J, Lang R, et al. Prolonged dimethylsulphoxide treatment in 13 patients with systemic amyloidosis. *Ann Rheum Dis* 1982;41:587–92.

Sherriff FE, Bridges LR, Sivaloganathan S. Early detection of axonal injury after human head trauma using immunocytochemistry for beta-amyloid precursor protein. *Acta Neuropathol (Berlin)* 1994;87:55–62.

Shimizu M, Manabe T, Matsumoto T, et al. β_2 Microglobulin haemodialysis related amyloidosis: Distinctive gross features of gastrointestinal involvement. *J Clin Pathol* 1997;50:873–5.

Sousa MM, Cardoso I, Fernandes R, et al. Deposition of transthyretin in early stages of familial amyloidotic polyneuropathy: Evidence for toxicity of nonfibrillar aggregates. *Am J Pathol* 2001;159:1993–2000.

Anaplastic lymphoma kinase (ALK)

Background

Anaplastic lymphoma kinase (ALK), also known as ALK tyrosine kinase receptor or CD246 (cluster of differentiation 246), is an enzyme that in humans is encoded by the *ALK* gene. The *ALK* gene is located on chromosome 2p23 and codes for a protein that is expressed in some cells of the central nervous system but in virtually no other normal human cells. ALK plays an important role in the development of the brain and exerts its effects on specific neurons in the nervous system. ALK shows the greatest sequence similarity to LTK (leukocyte tyrosine kinase). Interest in this protein among diagnostic pathologists has been related to its utility in recognizing a subset of CD30+ anaplastic large-cell lymphomas (ALCLs) with the characteristic t(2;5)(p23;q35) translocation. This translocation results in an abnormal fusion gene involving the *ALK* gene and the nucleophosmin (*NPM*) gene (located on chromosome 5q35), which codes for a ubiquitously expressed nucleolar phosphoprotein that functions in transporting components of ribosomes between the cytoplasm and nucleolus during the final stages of ribosome assembly. Transcription of this abnormal *NPM-ALK* fusion gene results in the production of an abnormal protein (called p80) that functions as a protein tyrosine kinase. The ALK antibody recognizes this abnormal human protein.

Applications

1. Antibodies to ALK have diagnostic, prognostic, and predictive usefulness in different situations. These include CD30+ anaplastic large-cell lymphoma, where ALK positivity is associated with better prognosis.
2. ALK lung cancer adenocarcinomas (unlike the standard ALK antibodies, the new generation of ALK antibodies are sensitive enough to demonstrate the expression of ALK in lung adenocarcinoma), where patients have been found to respond to an ALK inhibitor (crizotinib).
3. *ALK-TPM3* translocated renal cell carcinomas will show immunohistochemistry (IHC) expression of ALK protein.
4. Metastatic melanomas with the novel *ALK-ATI* fusion can also be ALK positive. About 1% of Spitzoid melanomas also have an ALK fusion, and 5–10% of Spitz nevi and atypical Spitz tumors have an *ALK* fusion.
5. Inflammatory myofibroblastic tumor (IMT) is a soft tissue tumor of intermediate malignant potential and has been shown to have gene fusions involving *ALK*, *ROS1*, *RET*, and *NTRK3*. Many partner genes have been described, resulting in ALK expression. *ALK* gene rearrangements are found in 50–60% of IMTs, leading to ALK detection by IHC (half of these cases show strong positivity). IMTs in younger patients are more frequently ALK positive than in adults. Diffuse cytoplasmic staining is seen in tumors associated with *TPM3-ALK*, granular cytoplasmic staining with *CLTC-ALK*, and nuclear membrane positivity with *RANBP2-ALK* fusions. *RANBP2* fusion has been associated with epithelioid/round cell morphology in IMT, and such tumors pursue a more aggressive clinical course. ALK expression is seen in 45% of pulmonary, 60% of digestive tract, and all cases of peritoneal IMT. Spindle cell tumors in differential diagnosis of IMT, such as desmoid tumors, gastrointestinal stromal tumor (GIST), and nodular fasciitis, are all negative for ALK.
6. Almost 90% of epithelioid fibrous histiocytomas show both ALK immunoexpression (cytoplasmic) and *ALK* rearrangement.
7. Approximately 2% of papillary thyroid cancers show ALK protein expression and rearrangements.
8. Neuroblastomas may harbor *ALK* fusions and express ALK protein.
9. Non-*ALK* rearranged tumors such as malignant peripheral nerve sheath tumors (40%), rhabdomyosarcoma (particularly alveolar rhabdomyosarcoma: 60%), epithelioid sarcoma, and leiomyosarcomas can show ALK expression.

Interpretation

Four clones are used for non-small-cell lung cancer (NSCLC): ALK1, 5A4, D5F3, and anti-ALK. ALK fluorescence in situ hybridization (FISH) may miss cases of ALK+ adenocarcinoma (30%), especially with EML4-ALK fusion.

It is worth mentioning that the neoplasms harboring the characteristic t(2;5) (p23;q35) typically show both nuclear and cytoplasmic staining with ALK antibody, whereas those with variant translocations often only show cytoplasmic staining.

Given the expression of ALK IHC in tumors that show *ALK* rearrangement, *ALK* FISH should be interpreted in the appropriate morphologic context as well. Since there are other partners to ALK, negative ALK FISH does not exclude the diagnosis of IMT. The recognition of such IMT becomes more important with the possibility of treatment with tyrosine kinase inhibitors.

Selected references

Antonescu CR, Suurmeijer AJH, Zhang L, et al. Molecular characterization of inflammatory myofibroblastic tumors with frequent ALK and ROS1 fusions and rare novel RET gene rearrangement. *Am J Surg Pathol* 2015;39:957–67.

Telugu RB, Prabhu AJ, Kalappurayil NB, et al. Clinicopathological study of 18 cases of inflammatory myofibroblastic tumors with reference to ALK-1 expression: 5-Year experience in a tertiary care center. *J Pathol Translational Med* 2017;51:255–63.

Yoshida A, Shibata T, Wakai S, et al. Anaplastic lymphoma kinase status in rhabdomyosarcomas. *Mod Pathol* 2013;26:772–81.

Androgen receptor

Background

The intracellular action of androgens is mediated by the androgen receptor, which is a key element in the superfamily of ligand responsive transcription regulators. The gene is located on X q11 – q12. Qualitative and quantitative alterations of androgen receptor expression in prostatic carcinomas and their possible implications for tumor progression and treatment are therefore of diagnostic and research interest. Findings in prostatic tumor cell lines of rat and human origin suggest that reduction of androgen receptor protein expression is accompanied by an increase in tumor aggressiveness. However, immunohistochemical analysis and binding assays have demonstrated the presence of androgen receptors in all histological types of prostatic carcinoma and in both therapy-responsive as well as therapy-unresponsive tumors.

Applications

1. Many of the immunohistochemical studies of androgen receptors have been related to prostatic carcinoma. The androgen receptor content of prostatic carcinoma has been inversely correlated to Gleason grade in stage D2 carcinomas. Activation of mutant androgen receptors by estrogen and weak androgens could confer on prostate cancer cells an ability to survive testicular androgen ablation through the activation of the androgen receptor by adrenal androgens or exogenous estrogen. Thus, mutated androgen receptors that occur prior to therapy may characterize a more aggressive disease.
2. In triple negative breast cancer, luminal androgen subtype.
3. It is an apocrine cell marker.
4. It stains sebaceous carcinomas and is useful in separating these from squamous and basal cell carcinomas.
5. Immunostaining also seen in endometrium, genital melanocytes, meningiomas, most bone marrow cells other than erythroid and lymphoid cells, and urinary bladder carcinomas.
6. Salivary duct carcinoma shows frequent staining for androgen receptor. Androgen receptor immunohistochemistry has been used in other salivary gland tumors that show potential apocrine differentiation, such as pleomorphic adenomas.
7. Androgen receptor staining has been demonstrated in 45% of adenocarcinomas and 21% of squamous carcinomas of the esophagus.
8. Androgen receptor positivity has also been noted in spindle cell lipoma.

Interpretation

The receptor is intra-nuclear in location. A cut-off of 10% androgen receptor-positive cells has been suggested to maximize prognostic interpretation.

Selected references

Carroll RS, Zhang J, Dashmner K, et al. Androgen receptor expression in meningiomas. *J Neurosurg* 1995;82:453–60.

Hakimi JM, Rondinelli RH, Schoenberg MP, et al. Androgen-receptor gene structure and function in prostate cancer. *World J Urol* 1996;14:329–37.

Hoang MP, Callender DL, Sola Gallego JJ, et al. Molecular and biomarker analyses of salivary duct carcinomas: Comparison with mammary duct carcinoma. *Int J Oncol* 2001;19:865–71.

Mertens HJ, Heineman MJ, Koudstaal J, et al. Androgen receptor content in human endometrium. *Eur J Obstet Gynecol Reprod Biol* 1996;70:11–13.

Moriki T, Ueta S, Takashi T, et al. Salivary duct carcinoma: Cytologic characteristics and application of androgen receptor immunostaining for diagnosis. *Cancer* 2001;93:344–50.

Syed S, Martin AM, Haupt H, et al. Frequent detection of androgen receptors in spindle cell lipomas: An explanation of this lesion's male predominance? *Arch Pathol Lab Med* 2008;132:81–3.

Tihan T, Harmon JW, Wan X, et al. Evidence of androgen receptor expression in squamous and adenocarcinoma of the esophagus. *Anticancer Res* 2001;21:3107–14.

Zhuang YH, Blauer M, Tammela T, et al. Immunodetection of androgen receptor in human urinary bladder cancer. *Histopathology* 1997;30:556–62.

Anti-apoptosis

Background

Cell death may occur by necrosis or apoptosis. Necrosis results from direct physical or chemical damage to the plasma membrane or disturbances in the osmotic balance of a cell. With the entrance of extracellular fluid into the cell, resultant cell swelling and lysis precede a subsequent inflammatory response. Furthermore, necrosis affects groups of cells, with consequent disruption of normal tissue architecture. In contrast to necrosis, apoptotic cell death is a highly regulated physiologic process. The BM-1 antibody is directed to the Lewis^y antigen, which has been identified phenotypically as a marker of specific types of cells and possibly specific stages of differentiation. Lewis^y is totally absent at the morula stage but is highly expressed on the blastocyst surface and has been shown to play a role in the implantation process. Recently, Lewis^y has been identified as a characteristic of cells undergoing apoptosis. In Lewis^y positive areas of tissue sections, typical apoptotic morphological changes and DNA fragmentation were frequently observed in certain loci, although not all Lewis^y positive cells showed such signs of apoptosis. Although the BM-1 antibody against the Lewis^y antigen is reputed to detect apoptotic cells, further studies to test its efficacy, including a comparative analysis with the in situ end labeling techniques, is awaited.

Another method of detection of apoptotic bodies is the use of Annexin V, which is a 35–36 kD Ca^{2+}-dependent phospholipid-binding protein that has a high affinity for the membrane phospholipid phosphatidylserine (PS). In apoptotic cells, PS is translocated from the inner to the outer leaflet of the plasma membrane, thereby exposing PS to the external cellular environment and allowing its binding to Annexin V. Binding to a signal system such as fluorescein isothiocyanate allows the easy identification of apoptotic cells (in frozen sections and cell preparations). Annexin V is thought to identify cells at an earlier stage of apoptosis than assays based on DNA fragmentation because externalization of PS occurs earlier than the nuclear changes associated with apoptosis.

Several other methods of assessing apoptosis in paraffin-embedded sections are available, and they include cyclin Dl, bcl-2, MDM2, p53, Fas (CD95), c-kit (CD117), and CD40 L, some of these being of relevance as prognostic markers. Antibodies to all these proteins are separately discussed under their respective headings. In addition, antibodies to Bcl-X, Bax, and Bak can also be used to study apoptosis.

Applications

BM-1 antibody may be applied to neoplasms in general to assess the apoptotic index.

Interpretation

Strong BM-1 immunoreactivity is observed in the apical surface of tubular urothelium and basal cells (glandular foveoli) of gastric and esophageal mucosa, and these tissues may be employed as controls.

The application of multiple methods, each based on a different feature of the apoptotic process, may provide more information about the cell population than any one method would give alone.

Selected references

Arends MJ, Wyllie AH. Apoptosis: Mechanism and roles in pathology. *Int Rev Exp Pathol* 1991;32:223–54.

Bukholm IR, Bukholm G, Nesland JM. Reduced expression of both Bax and Bcl-2 is independently associated with lymph node metastasis in human breast carcinomas. *APMIS* 2002;110:214–20.

Evans JD, Cornford PA, Dodson A, et al. Detailed tissue expression of bcl-2, bax, bak, and bcl-x in the normal human pancreas and in chronic pancreatitis, ampullary and pancreatic ductal adenocarcinomas. *Pancreatology* 2001;1:254–62.

Raynal P, Pollard HB. Annexins. The problem of assessing the biological role for a gene family of multifunctional calcium and phospholipid-binding proteins. *J Biol Chem* 1994;265:4923–8.

Schelwies K, Sturm I, Grabowski P, et al. Analysis of p53/BAX in primary colorectal carcinoma: Low BAX protein expression is a negative prognostic factor in UICC stage III tumors. *Int J Cancer* 2002;99:589–96.

Sjostrom J, Blomqvist C, von Boguslawski K, et al. The predictive value of bcl-2, bax, bcl-xL, bag–1, fas, and fasL for chemotherapy response in advanced breast cancer. *Clin Cancer Res* 2002;8:811–16.

Wyllie AH, Kerr JFR, Currie AR. Cell death: The significance of apoptosis. *Int Rev Cytol* 1980;68:251–306.

Arginase-1

Background

Arginase-1 is a binuclear manganese metalloenzyme that catalyzes the hydrolysis of arginine to ornithine and urea. Arginase-1 is expressed in the periportal hepatocytes and is a sensitive and specific marker of benign and malignant hepatocytes in human formalin-fixed paraffin-embedded tissue.

Applications

1. Arginase-1 is a sensitive and specific marker of hepatocytes and demonstrates diffuse cytoplasmic expression in both normal liver samples and hepatocellular neoplasms. It can be used to distinguish HCCs from metastatic tumors in the liver with superior sensitivity to that of HepPar-1 within each grade of HCC. Arginase-1 has been shown to be highly specific compared with other hepatocellular markers such as HepPar-1 and Glypican-3 in cytology specimens and should be used as part of a panel of these three markers for the diagnosis of HCC. Its expression is specific to HCC with no expression of arginase-1 noted in tumors mimicking an HCC in the liver, such as, for example, RCCs, melanomas, neuroendocrine tumors, adrenocortical carcinomas, and gastric adenocarcinomas.

2. Expression of arginase-1 has rarely been noted in metastatic carcinomas and cholangiocarcinoma in the liver.
3. Occasional expression of arginase-1 has been noted in pancreatic ductal adenocarcinoma.

Interpretation

It is a cytoplasmic stain with sometimes patchy nuclear reactivity.

Selected references

Fatima N, Cohen C, Siddiqui MT. Arginase-1: A highly specific marker separating pancreatic adenocarcinoma from hepatocellular carcinoma. *Acta Cytol* 2014;58:83–8.

Radwan NA, Ahmed NS. The diagnostic value of arginase-1 immunostaining in differentiating hepatocellular carcinoma from metastatic carcinoma and cholangiocarcinoma as compared to HepPar-1. *Diagnostic Pathol* 2012;7:149.

Yan BC, Gong C, Song J, et al. Arginase-1: A new immunohistochemical marker of hepatocytes and hepatocellular neoplasms. *Am J Surg Pathol* 2010;34:1147–54.

ATRX (alpha-thalassemia/mental retardation syndrome X-linked)

Background

The *ATRX* gene is located on Xp21.1, and ATRX protein is part of the chromatin remodeling complex that plays a role in the telomere maintenance mechanism. A proportion of tumors use *ATRX* mutations causing "alternating lengthening of telomeres (ALT)" to overcome senescence. There is loss of immunohistochemical expression due to inactivating mutations, and such testing can be used to evaluate for *ATRX* mutations. The ATRX syndrome is characterized by mental retardation, intellectual impairment, and skeletal deformities.

Applications

1. *ATRX* mutations are common (80%) in *IDH*-mutant astrocytomas (which represent about 80% of astrocytomas) but not seen or rare in *IDH*- mutant cases of oligodendroglioma with 10/19q codeletion. However, 20% of IDH-mutant gliomas can lack *ATRX* alterations. So most gliomas with ATRX IHC loss cases have *IDH* mutations (90–95%). It should be remembered that ATRX IHC positive cases are ATRX wild-type in 85% of cases, and ATRX IHC negative cases show a mutation in 80% of cases. So the correlation between IHC and mutation is not perfect.

ATRX mutation and 1p/19q codeletion are mutually exclusive but wild-type ATRX does not necessarily indicate a codeletion. Rare (fewer than 1%) ATRX-negative tumors can show 1p/19q codeletion.

Also, 67–90% of Grade II astrocytomas and 75–90% of Grade 3 astrocytomas show ATRX IHC loss/*ATRX* mutations.

In glioblastoma, ATRX loss is seen in 10–20% of cases. There are some glioblastomas with ATRX loss without *IDH* mutation, and these have shown similarities to pediatric glioblastoma (with *H3HFA* mutations).

3. Rare astrocytomas without *IDH* mutation or ATRX loss could represent a rare variant or possibly glioblastoma (with *H3FA* mutation; or 7p gain/10q loss).

4. Pancreatic neuroendocrine tumors: loss of ATRX immunoexpression identifies those tumors with chromosomal instability and is associated with a poor prognosis.

Selected references

Ikemura M, Shibahara J, Mukasa A, et al. Utility of ATRX immunohistochemistry in diagnosis of adult diffuse gliomas. *Histopathology* 2016;69(2):260–7.

Liu X, Gerges N, Korshunov A, et al. Frequent ATRX mutations and loss of expression in adult diffuse astrocytic tumors carrying IDH1/IDH2 and TP53 mutations. *Acta Neuropathol* 2012;124(5):615–25.

Reuss DE, Sahm F, Schrimpf D, et al. ATRX and IDH1-R132 H immunohistochemistry with subsequent copy number analysis and IDH sequencing as a basis for an "integrated" diagnostic approach for adult astrocytoma, oligodendroglioma and glioblastoma. *Acta Neuropathol* 2015;129(1):133–46.

Rodriguez FJ, Vizcaino M, Lin M-T. Recent advances on the molecular pathology of glial neoplasms in children and adults. *J Mol Diagn* 2016;18(5):620–34.

Yamamichi A., Ohka F, Aoki K, et al. Immunohistochemical ATRX expression is not a surrogate for 1p19q codeletion. *Brain Tumor Pathol* 2018;35(2):106–13.

NOTES

β-hCG (human chorionic gonadotropin)

Background

Human chorionic gonadotropin (hCG) is a glycoprotein (40 kD) comprising a protein core and a carbohydrate side chain. The molecule is composed of two dissimilar subunits, α and β. The α subunit is indistinguishable immunologically from the α subunit of pituitary glycoprotein hormones: luteinizing hormone (LH), follicle stimulating hormone (FSH), and thyroid stimulating hormone (TSH). The β subunits are different from each other and confer specificity. hCG, secreted in large quantities by the placenta, normally circulates at readily detectable levels only during gestation.

The monoclonal antibody (IgG[1]) to βhCG was produced by immunization with pure chorionic gonadotropin beta subunit. βhCG is demonstrable in syncytiotrophoblasts of normal human placenta.

Applications

1. βhCG is the most important marker of gestational trophoblastic cells, being present in syncytiotrophoblastic cells and cells of the intermediate trophoblast but absent in cytotrophoblast. In syncytiotrophoblast cells, hCG is demonstrable from the 12th day of gestation, reaches a peak at six weeks, and decreases thereafter; at term hCG is present only focally in these cells. In choriocarcinoma strong diffuse immunostaining for βhCG occurs in syncytiotrophoblastic cells (and focal immunostaining for human placental lactogen). In contrast, placental site trophoblastic tumor shows focal βhCG immunopositivity but diffuse human placental lactogen immunoreaction.

2. βhCG expression in non-trophoblastic tumors may indicate aggressive behavior of the tumor. βhCG may be demonstrated in 14% of hepatocellular carcinoma and in the trophoblast-like cells that develop in undifferentiated carcinoma of the endometrium.

   βhCG has also been demonstrated in poorly differentiated areas with cells resembling syncytiotrophoblasts in serous papillary or mucinous adenocarcinomas of the ovary. In 6–8% of dysgerminomas, there are individual or collections of syncytiotrophoblastic giant cells that contain/produce hCG.

4. βhCG staining is seen in gastric (60%) and pancreatic (55%) carcinomas and extrahepatic cholangiocarcinomas (40%).

Interpretation

Polyclonal antibody shows a higher frequency of positivity.

Selected references

Bellisario R, Carlsen RB, Bahl OP. Human chorionic gonadotropin: Linear amino acid sequence of the α subunit. *J Biol Chem* 1973;248:6796–809.

bcl-2

Background

The bcl-2 gene was identified more than a decade ago with the discovery and analysis of the t(14; 18) (q32; q21) translocation. This translocation occurs in 70–80% of follicular lymphoma, comprising juxtaposition of the bcl-2 gene with the immunoglobulin heavy chain (IgH) gene on chromosome 14q32. This results in an overexpression of the translocated bcl-2 allele induced by enhancers in the IgH region; although the translocation is not a prerequisite for bcl-2 protein expression, since this occurs in many cases without this rearrangement. The bcl-2 polypeptide is a 26 kD protein that is found on intracellular (mitochondrial and nuclear) membranes and in the cytosol (on the smooth endoplasmic reticulum) rather than on the cell surface. bcl-2 is not an oncogene and has no effect on cell replication; bcl-2 protein does, however, prevent cells from undergoing apoptosis, conferring a survival advantage on cell harboring the t(14; 18) translocation. In normal lymphoid tissue, bcl-2 antibody reacts with small B lymphocytes in the mantle zone and many cells within T-cell areas. In the thymus, many cells in the medulla are stained, with weak/negative reaction in the cortex.

Applications

1. The initial diagnostic application of bcl-2 immunostaining was for the distinction of reactive follicular lymphoid hyperplasia from follicular lymphoma. Positive staining is cytoplasmic in location. Follicular lymphomas show striking bcl-2 expression in neoplastic follicles, whilst only isolated individual cells within the reactive follicle centers are positive (mostly T cells). This difference in staining pattern is due to a post-translational mechanism that results in decreased protein levels. Furthermore, bcl-2 protein expression is demonstrated in all grades of follicle center cell lymphomas in both small and large cells. Strongly bcl-2-positive lymphoid aggregates in the bone marrow of patients previously diagnosed with nodal follicular lymphoma are indicative of lymphoma involvement. However, there is no practical value of applying the bcl-2 antibody for classification of a malignant lymphoid infiltrate, since many different lymphoma types (both non-Hodgkin's and Hodgkin's lymphomas) can be bcl-2 positive. Nevertheless, it has been demonstrated that non-Hodgkin's lymphoma with bcl-2 expression had a significantly higher relapse rate and a lower cause-specific survival than non-Hodgkin's lymphoma without bcl-2 expression.

2. Expression of bcl-2 has been noted in many epithelial neoplasms and attempts have been made to correlate bcl-2 expression with survival. In general, better prognoses accompany bcl-2 positive neoplasms than negative ones, with some prostatic cancers being the exception to the rule. A reciprocal relationship has been demonstrated between bcl-2 reactivity and p53 overexpression in 65% of colorectal neoplasia, with a bcl-2 +ve/p53 −ve subgroup showing a strong correlation with negative lymph node status, implying a less aggressive pathway of neoplastic transformation. A similar reciprocal relationship was shown in acute leukemias. bcl-2 protein was also detected in all grades of cervical intraepithelial neoplasia (CIN), with a striking increase in the number of positive cells with increasing severity of CIN, in combination with a mild increase in staining intensity.

3. bcl-2 expression has been demonstrated in 80% of synovial sarcomas but is usually negative in leiomyosarcomas, malignant peripheral nerve sheath tumors, and fibrosarcomas.

4. bcl-2 is expressed in solitary fibrous tumor, sclerosing epithelioid fibrosarcoma, giant cell angiofibroma, myofibroblastoma, and spindle cell epithelioma of vagina.

Selected references

Chetty R, Dada MA, Gatter KC. bcl-2: Longevity personified. *Adv Anat Pathol* 1997;4:134–8.

bcl-6

Background

The *bcl-6* gene was identified from translocations involving the 3q27 locus in diffuse large B-cell lymphomas. The *bcl-6* gene product is a 92–98 kD nuclear phosphoprotein that is highly expressed in germinal center B cells and their neoplastic counterparts. bcl-6 protein is thought to be anti-apoptotic and is expressed exclusively by follicular center B cells in reactive lymphoid tissue and lymphomas that are thought to arise from follicular center cells.

Applications

1. bcl-6 is used for follicular lymphoma, Burkitt's lymphoma, some diffuse large B-cell lymphomas, angioimmunoblastic T-cell lymphoma, and nodular lymphocyte-predominant Hodgkin's disease (NLPHD). bcl-6 protein is expressed in the L&H cells of NLPHD in the majority of cases. Half of cases of classic Hodgkin's disease were also immunopositive for bcl-6. Cases of primary cutaneous follicular lymphoma also express bcl-6. In follicular lymphoma, bcl-6 is expressed in both follicular and interfollicular neoplastic B cells. bcl-6 provides a distinction between pseudo-growth centers and entrapped germinal centers, which are bcl-6− and bcl-6+, respectively. Marginal zone/MALT lymphomas and mantle cell lymphomas are negative.

2. Among high-grade MALT lymphomas, 50% demonstrate bcl-6 immunoreaction similar to systemic diffuse large B-cell lymphoma.
3. All primary mediastinal large B-cell lymphomas have been demonstrated to express bcl-6 protein, supporting a germinal center derivation.
4. Only 40% of T-cell rich B-cell lymphomas are immunoreactive with bcl-6. Diffuse large B-cell cutaneous and plasmablastic lymphomas that are AIDS-related have also been shown to express bcl-6 in 50% of cases.

Interpretation

Nuclear staining.

Selected references

Onizuka T, Moriyama M, Yamochi T, et al. BCL-6 gene product, a 92-to 98-kD nuclear phosphoprotein, is highly expressed in germinal center B cells and their neoplastic counterparts. *Blood* 1995;86:28–37.

Ye BH, Rao PH, Chaganti RS, et al. Cloning of BCL-6, the locus involved in chromosome translocations affecting band 3q27 in B-cell lymphoma. *Cancer Res* 1993;53:2732–5.

B

BCOR (bcl-6 interacting
corepressor) and CIC-
DUX4

BCOR (bcl-6 interacting corepressor) and CIC-DUX4

Background

Within the family of small round cell sarcomas (prototypic of which is Ewing sarcoma), BCOR and CIC rearranged sarcomas have recently been described that lack EWSR1 fusions (with either the ETS family or another rare non-ETS family of genes). There are potential biologic behavioral differences (sarcomas with CIC-DUX4 fusion are aggressive, often showing rapid progression of disease), making it important to recognize some of these entities. Hence, BCOR and CIC rearranged sarcomas are classified separately and not referred to as "Ewing-like sarcoma."

CIC rearranged sarcomas represent almost up to 70% of EWSR1/FUS negative tumors. CIC-DUX4 and CIC-FOX04 (t(4:19) or t(10;19)) rearranged and NUTM2A-CIC tumors have been described in children and young adults, often with heterogeneous nuclear morphology, including size variation, prominent nucleoli, and abundant eosinophilic or clear cytoplasm with a high mitotic index. Unlike Ewing sarcoma, CD99 is not diffusely expressed (or is variably expressed) in these tumors.

BCOR is a transcriptional repressor encoded by the *BCOR* gene at Xp11.4 that acts as a silencing of gene expression. BCOR IHC expression in adult human tissues was identified in testis and germinal centers of tonsil. Tumors with BCOR genetic alterations include a subset of small round cell sarcoma (involving *BCOR-CCNB3*, *BCOR-MAML3*, and *ZC3H7B-BCOR*), endometrial stromal sarcoma (ESS) (*ZC3H7B-BCOR*), clear cell sarcoma of kidney (BCOR ITD [in tandem duplications]), and ossifying fibromyxoid tumor (*ZC3H7B-BCOR*). Soft tissue round cell sarcomas with BCOR fusion tend to occur as mainly bone and soft tissue tumors in young males (older children and adolescents) and are comprised of mainly round cells but some spindle cells in a myxoid or collagenous background, accounting for 4% to 13% of EWSR1-negative sarcomas.

Within high-grade (HG) ESS, *YWHAE-NUTM2B* fusion and *BCOR ITD* have been described. More recently,

ZC3H7B-BCOR fusion has been described in a variant of HG ESS that morphologically can resemble myxoid leiomyosarcoma.

Applications

Soft tissue sarcomas

It has been shown that the majority, if not all, of round cell sarcomas with *BCOR-CCNB3*, *BCOR ITD*, or *BCOR-MAML3* fusion rearrangements show strong and diffuse immunohistochemical (IHC) expression of BCOR (nuclear staining). With the exception of synovial sarcoma (49% positive for BCOR but showing variable positivity instead of strong diffuse staining), other sarcomas without *BCOR* gene alterations are only rarely positive (myxofibrosarcoma, Ewing sarcoma, and rhabdomyosarcoma can show BCOR IHC expression in rare cases). So BCOR IHC appears to be a sensitive marker but not entirely specific to identifying round cell sarcomas with *BCOR* rearrangement. Hence, such a tumor diagnosis should likely be confirmed by molecular methodology. The sarcomas with *CCNB3* fusion also show CCNB3 IHC expression, unlike Ewing sarcoma. But other tumors with *BCOR* (*ZC3H7B-BCOR*) fusions, such as ossifying fibromyxoid tumor, are negative for BCOR IHC.

CCNB3 IHC has been less useful as it is not expressed in all *BCOR-CCNB3* sarcomas and has rarely been described in Ewing sarcoma, solitary fibrous tumor, and fibrosarcoma (although the staining has been described as focal and/or weak). CIC:DUX4-positive tumors have been classified as Ewing sarcoma–like tumors because of the overlap with ES both morphologically and by IHC results.

Typically, CIC:DUX4 tumors are positive for WT1 (N-terminus), ETV4, and FLI1. While the majority (86%) show CD99 positivity, the staining is variable; only seldom (24%) is CD99 positivity diffuse and membranous as in ES. ERG is also positive in 18% of cases. These tumors are usually

NKX2.2 negative and BCOR negative. DUX4 IHC shows distinctive nuclear positivity in such tumors.

Endometrial stromal sarcoma

BCOR IHC is a sensitive marker, being positive with strong, diffuse positivity in all cases of HG ESS with *YWHAE-NUTM2* rearrangements and a subset of HG ESS with *BCOR* rearrangement and ITD. In HG ESS with BCOR rearrangement (involving *ZC3H7B*), BCOR is usually also positive (although not 100%; likely in half of such tumors) and typically weak in any associated fibromyxoid component. BCOR IHC shows no positivity in LG ESS, esthesioneuroblastoma (ESN), or LMS (although rare weak positivity has been described in a minority of these cases). BCOR IHC positivity should be followed by molecular confirmation of YWHAE and BCOR rearrangements or sequencing for BCOR ITD.

Interpretation

Pattern of staining:
Nuclear: WT1, ETV4, CCNB3, Fli-1, TLE-1, SATB2
Cytoplasmic: CD99

BCOR-CCNB3 sarcomas have also been seen to express immunohistochemical markers typically seen in synovial sarcoma, including TLE-1, CD99, bcl2, and CD56 or osteosarcoma (SATB2). Such tumors are typically NKX2.2 negative and ETV4 negative (ETV4 expression has also been described rarely in SMARCA-4 deficient sarcoma).

CD99 shows a typically diffuse membranous staining pattern in ES, unlike BCOR-CCNB3 and CIC-DUX4 tumors, which show focal/patchy/variable CD99 reactivity.

ES shows the following profile: positive CD99, NKX2.2; negative ETV4; and usually BCOR negative (although BCOR can rarely be positive in ES). A new variant with EWSR1-NFATC2 fusion and EWSR1 amplification has been described.

Selected references

Chiang, S., Lee, C-H, Stewart, C. J. R., et al. (2017). BCOR is a robust diagnostic immunohistochemical marker of genetically diverse high-grade endometrial stromal sarcoma, including tumors exhibiting variant morphology. *Mod Pathol* 30: 1251.

Hoang, L. N., Aneja, A., Conlon, N., et al. (2017). Novel high-grade endometrial stromal sarcoma: A morphologic mimicker of myxoid leiomyosarcoma. *Am J Surg Pathol* 41(1): 12–24.

Hung, Y. P., Fletcher, C. D. M., Hornick, J. L. (2016). Evaluation of NKX2-2 expression in round cell sarcomas and other tumors with EWSR1 rearrangement: Imperfect specificity for Ewing sarcoma. *Mod Pathol* 29(4): 370–80.

Lewis, N., Soslow, R. A., Delair, D. F., et al. (2017). ZC3H7B-BCOR high-grade endometrial stromal sarcomas: A report of 17 cases of a newly defined entity. *Mod Pathol* 31: 674.

Machado, I., Yoshida, A., Morales, M. G. N., et al. (2018). Review with novel markers facilitates precise categorization of 41 cases of diagnostically challenging, "undifferentiated small round cell tumors": A clinicopathologic, immunophenotypic and molecular analysis. *Ann Diagn Pathol* 34: 1–12.

Matsuyama, A., Shiba, E., Umekita, Y., et al. (2017). Clinicopathologic diversity of undifferentiated sarcoma with BCOR-CCNB3 fusion: Analysis of 11 cases with a reappraisal of the utility of immunohistochemistry for BCOR and CCNB3. *Am J Surg Pathol* 41(12): 1713–21.

Ber-EP4

Background

Ber-EP4 was raised against MCF-7 cells and is directed against two glycoproteins of 34 and 49 kD present on the surface and in the cytoplasm of all epithelial cells with the exception of the superficial layers of squamous epithelia, hepatocytes, and parietal cells. A positive reaction is seen in epithelial cells known to contain large amounts of the Ber-EP4 antigen, e.g., epithelial cells in the bile ducts and ducts of the epididymis.

Applications

Ber-EP4 shows a broad pattern of reactivity with human epithelial tissues from simple epithelia to basal layers of stratified non-keratinized squamous epithelium and epidermis.

1. Most adenocarcinomas demonstrate immunoreaction. The only adenocarcinomas that fail to react consistently are breast and renal cell cancers.
2. Mesothelioma is negative for BerEP4 and this helps in separation from adenocarcinoma.
3. Synovial sarcomas (biphasic) show BerEP4 positivity.

Interpretation

The use of Ber-EP4 to help distinguish epithelial mesothelioma from adenocarcinoma should be accompanied by a panel of antibodies.

Selected references

Latza U, Niedobitek G, Schwarting R, et al. Ber-EP4: New monoclonal antibody which distinguishes epithelia from mesothelia. *J Clin Pathol* 1990;43:213–19.

BOB-1

Background

The B-cell-specific octamer-binding protein-1 (BOB-1), also known as OBF-1 or OCA-B, is a B-lymphocyte-specific transcriptional coactivator that interacts with the Oct-1 and Oct-2 transcription factors in B cells to transactivate immunoglobulin genes. As a transcription factor, BOB-1 is predominantly expressed in the nucleus, although in strongly BOB-1-expressing cell populations, such as plasma cells, there is frequently detectable BOB-1 protein at a low level in the cytoplasm. BOB-1 is expressed in a similar distribution to its partner gene Oct-2, in all mature B-lymphoid cells from naïve B cells through plasma cells. While Oct-2 appears to be lymphoid specific, it is not B-cell specific, and expression has been described in thymic T cells as well as cases of anaplastic large cell lymphoma.

Applications

Unlike Oct-2, which is normally expressed in neuronal tissue and some histiocytes as well as aberrantly expressed in some large T-cell lymphomas, definitive BOB-1 expression in non-B-lineage tissues of either benign or neoplastic type has not been reported, although expression has been induced by various external means in several neoplastic cell lines. Because of its relative B-cell specificity, BOB-1 can be a useful marker of B-lineage in poorly differentiated B-cell non-Hodgkin lymphomas (B-NHL) such as plasmablastic lymphomas and primary effusion lymphomas (PEL). In such specimens, detection of convincing BOB-1 expression often will go along with polymerase chain reaction identification of a clonal immunoglobulin gene rearrangement, which may be sufficient to confirm B-lineage, although it should be noted that these transcriptional factors and clonal immunoglobulin gene rearrangements have also been reported in acute myeloid leukemias/myeloid sarcomas.

In addition to its application to confirm B-lineage in B-NHL and plasma cell neoplasms (PCN), BOB-1 immunohistochemistry plays an important role in the diagnosis of Hodgkin lymphoma. Specifically, nearly all cases of classical Hodgkin lymphoma (CHL) express either no nuclear BOB-1 or extremely weak BOB-1, in contrast to all other B-lymphoid neoplasms, including B-NHL, PCN, and nodular lymphocyte-predominant Hodgkin lymphoma (NLPHL, the major morphologic differential with CHL). In those CHL cases in which nuclear BOB-1 is expressed, its coactivating factor Oct-2 should be either negative or minimally expressed.

Selected references

Advani, A.S., Lim, K., Gibson, S., et al. OCT-2 expression and OCT-2/BOB.1 co-expression predict prognosis in patients with newly diagnosed acute myeloid leukemia. *Leuk Lymphoma* 2010;51(4):606–12.

Kim, U., et al. The B-cell-specific transcription coactivator OCA-B/OBF-1/Bob-1 is essential for normal production of immunoglobulin isotypes. *Nature* 1996;383(6600):542–7.

Brachyury

Brachyury is a 47 kDa embryonic transcription factor encoded by the *T* gene. It binds to specific DNA regions near the palindromic sequence TCACACCT (T-site) through the T-box in its N-terminus. Brachyury functions during embryogenesis to regulate midline development by establishing the anterior–posterior axis through the regulation of genes involved in mesoderm and notochord formation. It is expressed in notochord-derived cells. Variations in the *T* gene in humans are associated with neural tube defects and chordomas.

Chordomas are slow-growing malignant neoplasms with epithelioid and chondroid morphology that arise in the central axial skeleton, thought to derive from notochordal remnants. These tumors harbor a variety of chromosomal aberrations that result in gain of the T locus and overexpression of brachyury, which plays a major role in tumorigenesis and proliferation.

Expression of brachyury has also been identified in some epithelial tumors and in cancer-derived stem cells. Brachyury IHC expression has been described occasionally in spermatogonia of normal testis and focally in some cases of testicular germ cell tumors.

Applications

1. Brachyury nuclear expression is seen in virtually all cases of chordomas and is not expressed in chondrosarcoma. This is an extremely useful marker in this setting. Other tumors in the differential diagnosis of chordoma, such as chordoid meningioma, mucinous adenocarcinoma, and gliomas, are negative for brachyury. Poorly differentiated chordomas can show weak expression or loss of expression of brachyury.
2. Brachyury expression has also been described in extra-axial chordomas (a rare entity) and as a marker helps to differentiate chordoma from other differential considerations, including myoepithelioma/parachordoma, extra-skeletal myxoid chondrosarcoma, and mucinous adenocarcinoma.
3. Others showing brachyury expression include testicular seminoma (45%), embryonal carcinoma (74%), and pulmonary small cell carcinoma (41%). However, this is an interesting observation rather than a practical utility for this marker.
4. Brachyury expression is also described in stromal cells of hemangioblastomas (91%) and not expressed in clear cell renal cell carcinoma (which can be a differential diagnostic consideration for hemangioblastoma).
5. Only rare/isolated cases of malignant melanoma, malignant peripheral nerve sheath tumor, rhabdomyosarcoma, and synovial sarcomas have been shown to have nuclear expression.

Comments

Chordomas can show loss of SMARCA4 (INI 1) loss, especially in poorly differentiated cases and in some pediatric cases. In such a scenario (cranial location), atypical teratoid rhabdoid tumor is a differential diagnostic consideration, since it also shows loss of SMARCA4. Brachyury is a useful marker in making this distinction.

Selected references

Barresi V, Vitarelli E, Branca G, et al. Expression of brachyury in hemangioblastoma: Potential use in differential diagnosis. *Am J Surg Pathol* 2012; 36:1052–7.

Lauer SR, Edgar MA, Gardner JM, et al. Soft tissue chordomas: A clinicopathologic analysis of 11 cases. *Am J Surg Pathol* 2013; 37:719–26.

CA125

Background

CA125 was discovered in a monoclonal screen for tumor-specific antigens of hybridomas derived from mouse lymphocytes immunized to an ovarian cell culture line, OVCA433. CA125 is a high-molecular-weight mucin-like glycoprotein complex that can be resolved to a 200–250 kDa species on gel electrophoresis. The antigen is located on the surface of ovarian tumor cells with essentially no expression in normal adult ovarian tissue. Significantly, CA125 is also found in sera of patients with ovarian, pancreatic (about 50%), liver, colon, and other (30%) adenocarcinomas. Although CA125 is not specific for ovarian carcinoma, it nevertheless does correlate directly with disease status. Similarly to other tumor markers, CA125 is also expressed normally in fetal development: the antigen has been localized to the amnion celomic epithelium and derivatives of Mullerian epithelium. In adult tissue, the monoclonal antibody OC125 reacted with the epithelium of the fallopian tube, endometrium, endocervix, apocrine sweat glands, and mammary glands.

Applications

1. The utility of CA125 in workup of tumors is rather limited with availability of more specific markers for tumors of Mullerian origin. It is commonly expressed in ovarian carcinomas with the exception of mucinous tumors of the ovary (where the expression is seen in limited cases). In addition to the ovary, other gynecologic tumors, including endometrial and cervical carcinomas, commonly express CA125.
2. However, as several other carcinomas, including colon, breast, thyroid, and urinary bladder, also express CA125,

its utility as an immunohistochemical (IHC) marker is fairly limited.
3. One potential and limited role for CA125 as an IHC marker is in the differential diagnosis of workup of metastatic carcinoma with clear cell features in which both renal cell carcinoma and Mullerian carcinoma are in the differential diagnosis. The specific Mullerian marker PAX8 is expressed consistently in both of these tumors, while clear cell renal cell carcinoma is negative for CA125.

Interpretation

The major role of CA125 in immunohistology is in the identification of metastatic serous carcinoma of the ovary. Primary serous cystadenocarcinoma of the ovary is the recommended positive control tissue for optimization of CA125. However, CA125 cannot reliably establish an origin of cancer.

Selected references

Bast RC Jr, Feeney M, Lazarus H, et al. Reactivity of a monoclonal antibody with human ovarian carcinoma. *J Clin Invest* 1981;68:1331–7.

Davis AM, Zurawski VR, Bast RC, et al. Characterization of the CA 125 antigen associated with human epithelial ovarian carcinomas. *Cancer Res* 1986;46:6143–8.

Kuzuya K, Nozaki M, Chihara T. Evaluation of CA 125 as a circulating tumor marker for ovarian cancer. *Acta Obstet Gynecol Jpn* 1986;38:949–57.

O'Brien TJ, Raymond LM, Bannon GA, et al. New monoclonal antibodies identify the glycoprotein carrying the CA 125 epitope. *Am J Obstet Gynecol* 1991;165:1857–64.

Calcitonin

Background

CAL-3-F5 was raised against the synthetic peptide corresponding to the C-terminal portion of human calcitonin (amino acids 24–32). In the human calcitonin precursor, calcitonin is flanked by two molecules: PDN (peptide-aspartic acid-asparagine), a 21–amino acid C-terminal flanking peptide, and a larger N-terminal peptide. Calcitonin gene-related peptide (CGRP) alpha is also encoded by the calcitonin gene and is produced as a result of differential RNA processing. The differential production of CGRP and calcitonin from the calcitonin gene is regulated in a tissue-specific manner, with CGRP being produced in nervous tissue and calcitonin in thyroid C-cells. However, CGRP and calcitonin are found in normal, hyperplastic, and neoplastic C-cells.

Applications

Antibodies to calcitonin are useful to identify normal, hyperplastic, and neoplastic C-cells (medullary thyroid carcinoma [MTC]). Given the morphologic (solid, trabecular, papillary, follicular, or insular patterns) and cellular heterogeneity of MTC (spindle, polyhedral, angular, round, clear, oncocytic, and anaplastic), calcitonin is crucial to making the correct diagnosis. All MTCs, classical and variants, demonstrate immunoreaction with antibodies to calcitonin.

Interpretation

Normal parafollicular C-cells are suitable as positive control tissue. Antibodies to calcitonin are also useful to identify C-cell hyperplasia in benign and malignant thyroid glands.

Selected references

Allison J, Hall L, MacIntyre I, et al. The construction and partial characterisation of plasmids containing complementary DNA sequences to human calcitonin precursor polyprotein. *Biochem J* 1981;199:725–31.

Saad MF, Ordonez NG, Guido JJ, et al. The prognostic value of calcitonin immunostaining in medullary carcinoma of the thyroid. *J Clin Endocrinol Metab* 1984;59:850–6.

NOTES

Calponin

Background

Calponin is a 34 kDa smooth muscle-specific protein implicated in the regulation of smooth contraction as a result of its ability to inhibit actin-activated MgATPase of smooth muscle myosin. Calponin is a calmodulin-negative, F-actin-negative, and tropomyosin-negative binding protein. Calponin has been demonstrated in all periacinar and periductal myoepithelial cells in salivary glands and normal breast ducts, and it also stains smooth muscle.

Applications

1. Calponin immunoexpression in pleomorphic adenomas and myoepithelial carcinomas.
2. In mesenchymal tumors, calponin immunoexpression has been demonstrated in smooth muscle tumors. However, caution is advised, as calponin also reacted with myofibroblasts, both reactive and in myofibroblastic lesions.
3. Myofibrosarcoma, angiomatoid fibrous histiocytoma, neurothekeoma (including cellular and mixed variants), atypical fibroxanthoma, glomus tumor, nodular fasciitis, solitary fibrous tumors, and synovial sarcoma.

Selected references

Miettinen MM, Sarloma-Rikala M, Kovatich AJ, et al. Calponin and h-Caldesmon in soft tissue tumors: Consistent h-Caldesmon immunoreactivity in gastrointestinal stromal tumors indicates traits of smooth muscle differentiation. *Mod Pathol* 1999;12:756–62.

Savera AT, Gown AM, Zarbo RJ. Immunolocalization of three novel smooth muscle-specific proteins in salivary gland pleomorphic adenoma: Assessment of the morphogenetic role of myoepithelium. *Mod Pathol* 1997;10:1093–100.

NOTES

Calreticulin

Background

Calreticulin (CALR) is a multifunctional protein of 417 amino acids (48,142 Da) and consists of three domains: a 180-aa N-terminal globular region, a 111-aa P-, or proline-rich, domain, and a 109-aa C-terminus. It acts as a major Ca(2^+)-binding (storage) protein in the lumen of the endoplasmic reticulum and sarcoplasmic reticulum. It is also a molecular chaperone and is involved in protein folding events. It is also found in the nucleus, suggesting that it may have a role in transcription regulation. CALR can play a role as modulator of the regulation of gene transcription by nuclear hormone receptors. It interacts with the DNA-binding domain of NR3C1 and mediates its nuclear export. The amino terminus of CALR interacts with the DNA-binding domain of the glucocorticoid receptor and prevents the receptor from binding to its specific glucocorticoid response element. All CALR mutations lead to a frameshift mutation generating a new 36–amino acid C-terminus, which can be identifiable by immunohistochemistry. Therefore, if there is an absence of a CALR mutation, there is no staining with the CALR marker.

Applications

1. CALR mutations are associated with primary myelofibrosis and essential thrombocythemia. In these conditions, staining specificity is 100%, sensitivity 82–91%, positive predictive value 100%, and negative predictive value 90–95%.
2. CALR may be useful together with other markers in the diagnosis of the upper urothelial carcinomas.
3. It is also overexpressed in adrenocortical carcinomas, ductal breast carcinomas, and lung cancer.

Interpretation

It is expressed in the endoplasmic reticulum lumen, cytoplasm and cytosol, and cell surface. It may be secreted into the extracellular space and extracellular matrix. It is also present in the cell surface (T cells) and associated with the lytic granules in the cytolytic T lymphocytes.

Selected references

Andrici J, Farzin M, Clarkson A, et al. Mutation specific immunohistochemistry is highly specific for the presence of calreticulin mutations in myeloproliferative neoplasms. *Pathology* 2016;48:319–24.

Kabbage M, Trimeche M, Bergaoui S, et al. Calreticulin expression in infiltrating ductal breast carcinomas: Relationships with disease progression and humoral immune responses. *Tumour Biol* 2013;34:1177–88.

Calretinin

Background

Calretinin is a calcium-binding protein of 29 kD and is a member of the large family of EF-hand proteins, to which S-100 protein also belongs. EF-hand proteins are characterized by a peculiar amino acid sequence, which folds up into a helix–loop–helix that acts as a calcium-binding site. Calretinin is abundantly expressed in central and peripheral neural tissues, particularly in the retina and in neurons of the sensory pathways. Although the function of calretinin is unknown, a possible role as a calcium buffer has been postulated. Consistent calretinin immunoreactivity has been found in a variety of normal tissues, including mesothelial cell lining of all serosal membranes, eccrine glands of skin, convoluted tubules of kidney, Leydig and Sertoli cells of the testis, epithelium of rete testis, mast cells, endometrium and ovarian stromal cells, and adrenal cortical cells. Calretinin is expressed abundantly in neurons and ganglion cells of the central and peripheral nervous system.

Applications

1. Calretinin represents one of the more sensitive and specific markers for mesothelial differentiation. Applicable to both histologic and cytologic material, it is recommended for inclusion in a panel of antibodies when investigating the differential diagnosis between epithelioid mesothelioma and adenocarcinoma. The E-cadherin/calretinin combination has been shown to demonstrate both a high specificity and sensitivity in distinguishing between mesothelioma and metastatic adenocarcinoma, with E-cadherin highlighting the latter. A note of caution is that calretinin stains both normal/hyperplastic and neoplastic mesothelial cells.
2. It is particularly useful for distinguishing central neurocytoma from oligodendroglioma, being negative in the latter. It has a wider potential application in distinguishing between brain tumors with glial and neuronal differentiation and those without.
3. Calretinin is a sensitive marker of ovarian sex cord–stromal tumors and is of value in this diagnostic setting as part of a larger panel. In ovarian sex cord–stromal tumors, strong calretinin immunostaining was seen in all hilus cell tumors and Leydig cell component of Sertoli–Leydig cell tumors. It was negative in fibrothecomas and granulosa cell tumor.
4. Calretinin has been shown to be an important diagnostic marker for both solid and cystic ameloblastomas, which are positive.
5. It is also positive in adrenal cortical neoplasms, medullary-type colon cancers, adenomatoid tumor, schwannoma (neurofibromas are weak/negative), granular cell tumor, neuroblastoma, focally in biphasic synovial sarcomas, and cardiac myxoma.

Interpretation

Calretinin immunoexpression occurs in both the nucleus and the cytoplasm. Adipocytes are an often useful "built-in" positive control. Purkinje cells of mature cerebellum may be used as controls. Specificity with the calretinin antibody AB 149 is high but sensitivity is low; in contrast, anti-calretinin antibody 7696 has both high specificity and high sensitivity.

Selected references

Barberis MCP, Faleri M, Veronese S, et al. Calretinin: A selective marker of normal and neoplastic mesothelial cells in serous effusions. *Acta Cytol* 1997;41:1757–61.

Cao QJ, Jones JG, Li M . Expression of calretinin in human ovary, testis, and ovarian sex cord-stromal tumors. *Int J Gynecol Pathol* 2001;20:346–52.

Dei Tos AP, Doglioni C. Calretinin: A novel tool for diagnostic immunohistochemistry. *Adv Anat Pathol* 1998;5:61–6.

Candida albicans

Candida albicans

Background

The diagnosis of oral candidiasis requires the sampling of the mucosal surface for the culture and identification of *Candida* spp. In chronic hyperplastic candidiasis, the fungal hyphae of *Candida* spp invade the superficial layers of the epithelium, making diagnosis difficult on candidal culture alone. Hence, biopsy of such lesions for microscopic examination is essential for diagnosis. Staining with periodic acid-Schiff (PAS) or methenamine-silver stains detects hyphal structures consistent with *Candida* spp in formalin-fixed tissue sections. However, these stains do not permit identification of individual *Candida* species. Further, the variable sensitivity of *Candida* spp to antifungal agents makes identification of the infecting species important.

The mouse monoclonal antibody IB12 was raised against the high-molecular-weight mannoproteins of *Candida albicans* (BioGenex). This antibody is species specific and suitable for use with formalin-fixed, paraffin-embedded material.

Interpretation

Identification of the infecting species is not only important for therapeutic purposes but may help clarify the association of chronic hyperplastic candidiasis with the development of squamous cell carcinoma.

Selected references

Monteagudo C, Marcilla A, Mormeneo S, et al. Specific immunohistochemical identification of *Candida albicans* in paraffin-embedded tissue with a new monoclonal antibody (1B12). *Am J Clin Pathol* 1995;103:130–5.

Williams DW, Jones HS, Allison RT, et al. Immunocytochemical detection of *Candida albicans* in formalin fixed, paraffin embedded material. *J Clin Pathol* 1998;51:857–9.

Carbonic anhydrase IX

Background

Carbonic anhydrase IX (CAIX), one of the four transmembrane members of the carbonic anhydrase family, regulates intracellular and extracellular pH by transmembrane transportation of CO_2. It is thought to play a major role in the survival of rapidly proliferating tumors by efficiently controlling the intracellular and extracellular pH in an attempt to adapt to progressively hypoxic conditions.

Applications

1. CAIX is highly expressed in clear cell renal cell carcinoma (CCRCC) and used to guide patient treatment because high CAIX expression is associated with a better prognosis.

   Clear cell (CC), papillary (PRCC), clear cell papillary, unclassified RCC, and Xp11.2 translocation RCC all reveal some degree of CAIX expression, which is consistently high in CC and CCPRCC variants (no luminal staining; just basolateral staining, resulting in a cup-like staining pattern). The expression of CAIX in papillary and Xp11.2 translocation RCC is focal or patchy. Chromophobe RCC and oncocytomas are mostly negative. A panel with CK7, CAIX, and racemase with or without CD10 and RCC can be used to distinguish CCRCC, PRCC, and CCPRCC.
   - CCRCC is strongly diffusely positive for CAIX but negative for CK7 and racemase
   - PRCC may be focally positive for CAIX but strongly diffusely positive for CK7 and racemase
   - CCPRCC is positive for CK7 and CAIX but negative for racemase.
2. In a workup of renal pelvic tumors where the differential diagnosis includes poorly differentiated RCC and urothelial carcinoma, it should be remembered that CAIX expression is high in both CCRCC and urothelial carcinoma, and therefore this marker should not be used in this context.
3. Metastatic CCRCC: This may be due to CCRCC presenting for the first time as a metastasis in a patient with no known history of a renal mass or a metastasis discovered in a patient who had a remote history of renal cancer.
4. In the gynecological tract it is expressed in ovarian and cervical carcinomas.
5. Gastrointestinal (GI) tract tumors involving esophagus and colorectal region show an increased expression of CAIX.
6. Carcinomas of nasopharynx, breast, and lung and some soft tissue sarcomas can all show expression of CAIX.

Interpretation

Because CAIX is constitutively activated in CCRCC it is uniformly expressed over the entire tumor. In other tumors the upregulation of CAIX is secondary to true tumor hypoxia; hence, its expression is primarily seen in the perinecrotic region.

Selected references

Al-Ahmadie HA, Alden D, Qin L-X, et al. Carbonic anhydrase IX expression in clear cell renal cell carcinoma: An immunohistochemical study comparing 2 antibodies. *Am J Surg Pathol* 2008;32: 377–82.

Bing Z, Lal P, Lu S, et al. Role of carbonic anhydrase IX, α-methylacyl coenzyme a racemase, cytokeratin 7, and galectin-3 in the evaluation of renal neoplasms: A tissue microarray immunohistochemical study. *Ann Diagn Pathol* 2013;17:58–62.

Bui MH, Visapaa H, Seligson D, et al. Prognostic value of carbonic anhydrase IX and KI67 as predictors of survival for renal clear cell carcinoma. *J Urol* 2004;171:2461–6.

Genega E, Ghebremichael M, Najarian R, et al. Carbonic anhydrase IX in renal neoplasms. Correlation with tumor type and grade. *Am J Clin Pathol* 2010;134:873–9.

Stillebroer AB, Mulders PFA, Boerman OC, et al. Carbonic anhydrase IX in renal cell carcinoma: Implications for prognosis, diagnosis and therapy. *Eur Urol* 2010;58:75–83.

NOTES

48

Carcinoembryonic antigen (CEA)

Background

CEA (also called CEACAM5) consists of a heterogeneous family of related oncofetal glycoproteins (approximately 200 kD molecular weight), which is secreted into the glycocalyx surface of gastrointestinal cells. CEA is a complex glycoprotein; hence, even after purification some degree of molecular heterogeneity exists. Therefore, antibodies to CEA, particularly polyclonal, commonly react against nonspecific cross-reactive antigens (NCA) located in normal colon and granulocytes. It is recommended that positive results obtained with a polyclonal anti-CEA antibody without preabsorption with NCA be interpreted as being nonspecific. Even monoclonal antibodies to CEA may cross-react with other molecules of the CEA family, including NCA.

Applications

1. CEA is found in several adenocarcinomas, such as colon, lung, breast, stomach, and pancreas. Its absence in mesothelioma helps in the discrimination of mesotheliomas from morphologically similar adenocarcinomas involving any organ. Occasional hyaluronate-rich epithelial mesotheliomas may produce false positivity with CEA, although this staining can be abolished by prior hyaluronidase digestion.
2. Polyclonal CEA is also useful for the demonstration of bile canaliculi in hepatocytes and the cells of hepatocellular carcinoma in both cytologic preparations and tissue sections. Although the presence of bile canaliculi is specific for hepatocytes, its sensitivity is low.

Interpretation

The fact that no single antibody is sufficiently specific and sensitive for the distinction of mesothelioma from adenocarcinoma necessitates the use of a panel of antibodies.

Selected references

Robb JA. Mesothelioma versus adenocarcinoma: False positive CEA and Leu-M1 staining due to hyaluronic acid (Letter). *Hum Pathol* 1989;20:400.

Catenins α, β, γ

Background

Catenins, the α-subunit (102 kD), β-subunit (88 kD), and γ-subunit (82 kD), are a group of proteins that interact with the intercellular domain of E-cadherin, resulting in complexes of E-cadherin/β-catenin/α-catenin or E-cadherin/γ-catenin/α-catenin, and are involved in the wnt pathway. α-Catenin shows sequence homology to vinculin and interacts with the actin cytoskeleton, either directly or indirectly via α-actinin; β-catenin is the vertebrate homologue of the Drosophila segment polarity gene armadillo; and γ-catenin is identical to plakoglobin and is also found in desmosomes. The regions of both α- and β-catenin, located on 5q21–22 and 3p21, have been shown to be involved in the development of certain tumors, and reduced expressions of both α- and β-catenin have been described in breast carcinoma. Besides adhesion functions, β-catenin binds to APC (adenomatous polyposis coli) protein, a putative tumor suppressor. β-Catenin has been shown to have a function in signal transduction when bound with members of the Tcf-LEF family of DNA-binding proteins. Somatic mutations of β-catenin and APC genes result in nuclear translocation of β-catenin in both sporadic and familial adenomatous polyposis (FAP).

Applications

1. Loss of expression of the catenin proteins and their localization are potentially important markers to predict the motility and invasiveness of epithelial neoplasms.
2. Abnormality of the wnt pathway in a tumor leads to nuclear accumulation of β-catenin, such as in sporadic basal cell carcinoma, anaplastic thyroid cancer, endometrial cancer, and pancreatic solid-pseudopapillary neoplasm.
3. Nuclear staining in fibromatosis in absence of wnt pathway/FAP abnormality.
4. Miscellaneous tumors showing nuclear staining: neuroblastoma, rhabdomyosarcoma, solitary fibrous tumor, and some PEComas.

Selected references

Birchmeier W, Behrens J. Cadherin expression in carcinomas: Role in the formation of cell junctions and the prevention of invasiveness. *Biochim Biophys Acta* 1994;1198:11–26.

Hinck L, Nathke IS, Papkoff J, et al. Dynamics of cadherin/catenin complex formation: Novel protein interactions and pathways of complex assembly. *J Cell Biol* 1994;125:1327–40.

Cathepsin B, D, and K

Background

The cathepsins are ubiquitous lysosomal proteases and are classified both functionally and according to their active site. Cathepsin B, cathepsin D, and to a lesser extent other cathepsins have been described as prognostic markers in cancer.

Cathepsin B, which catalyzes the degradation of laminin, may also play a role in the rupture of the basal membrane and may be of relevance in colorectal and pancreatic cancer.

Cathepsin D is the most widely studied of the cathepsins. It is an estrogen-regulated protease. A precursor form of 52 kD is processed in lysosomes into the mature 14 kD and 34 kD forms. This enzyme is thought to have proteolytic activity, which may facilitate the spread of neoplastic cells through different mechanisms and at different levels of the metastatic cascade. Cathepsin D is thought to promote tumor cell proliferation by acting as an autocrine mitogen through the activation of latent forms of growth factors or by interacting with growth factor receptors. The enzyme has also been shown, in vitro, to be able to degrade extracellular matrix and to activate latent precursor forms of other proteinases involved in the invasive steps of cancer metastasis.

Cathepsin K is a lysosomal cysteine protease that is responsible for bone resorption and remodeling.

Applications

1. In breast cancer, cathepsin D expression is significantly associated with poor outcomes overall, with significant associations with high tumor grade, increased tendency to local recurrence, regional recurrence, poorer disease-free survival, and poorer overall patient survival. Cathepsin D expression has been studied in a variety of other tumors with variable results.
2. Cathepsin D has been advocated as a marker of immature ganglion cells in suspected cases of Hirschsprung's disease, with intense granular cytoplasmic reactivity forming a collarette around the nucleus.
3. Cathepsin K is expressed in Xp11 (especially those bearing a PRCC-TFE3 fusion) and t(6;11) translocation renal cell cancers.
4. Cathepsin K is expressed in the majority of PEComas.

Interpretation

The staining is cytoplasmic and sometimes granular.

Selected references

Leto G, Gebbia N, Rausa L, et al. Cathepsin D in the malignant progression of neoplastic diseases (review). *Anticancer Res* 1992;12:235–40.

Schwartz MK. Tissue cathepsins as tumor markers. *Clin Chim Acta* 1995;237:67–78.

CD1A

Background

Human CD1 proteins are a family of five nonpolymorphic proteins that are homologous to both class I and II major histocompatibility complex proteins. CD1 proteins, like major histocompatibility complex proteins, are antigen-presenting proteins to T cells. However, CD1 proteins mostly present lipids, whereas major histocompatibility proteins mostly present peptides. The four isoforms of the CD1 proteins, CD1A, -B, -C, and -D, are membranous proteins and present lipids, whereas CD1E is a cytoplasmic protein and is involved in lipid transfer. Only CD1A is of interest for diagnostic purposes. CD1A is expressed by cortical thymocytes and Langerhans cells in the skin as well as a subset of dermal dendritic cells and similar antigen-presenting cells in the lymph node. CD1A is not expressed in early thymocytes or by mature resting or activated T lymphocytes.

Applications

CD1A staining is used as part of a panel of antibodies for the diagnosis of T-lymphoblastic lymphoma/leukemia. All types of mature T-cell neoplasms do not express CD1A.

CD1A staining is further used as a panel for the diagnosis of histiocytic neoplasms. CD1A is typically expressed in Langerhans cell histiocytosis and Langerhans cell sarcoma.

Interpretation

CD1A is expressed on the cell membrane.

Selected references

Chancellor A, Gadola SD, Mansour S. The versatility of the CD1 lipid antigen presentation pathway. *Immunology* 2018;154:196–203.

Krenacs L, Tiszalvicz LT, Krenacs T, et al. Immunohistochemical detection of CD1A antigen in formalin-fixed and paraffin-embedded tissue sections with monoclonal antibody 010. *J Pathol* 1993; 171: 99–104.

Porcelli SA, Modlin RL. CD 1 and the expanding universe of T cell antigens. *J Immunol* 1995;55:709–10.

CD2

Background

CD2 is a cell membrane glycoprotein expressed by T cells and NK cells. CD2 interacts with CD58 (LFA-3) on antigen-presenting cells and other cells. It is involved in the formation and organization of the immunological synapse formed between T cells and antigen-presenting cells prior to activation of the T-cell receptor by antigen delivered by the antigen-presenting cells. It is also involved in signal transduction and is considered a costimulatory molecule. CD2 is one of the earliest T-cell lineage–restricted antigens to appear during T-cell differentiation. CD2 is expressed after CD7 but before CD1 on immature T cells.

Applications

CD2 is considered a pan-T-cell antigen and is therefore useful for the identification of virtually all normal T lymphocytes and T-cell neoplasms. As with other pan-T-cell antigens, CD2 may be absent in some T-cell lymphomas and if so, may serve as an indication of T-cell neoplasia. CD2 is not expressed by B neoplasms. However, between 5% and 10% of classical Hodgkin lymphomas may aberrantly express T-cell antigens, among which CD4 and CD2 are the most common.

CD2 is also expressed by NK neoplasms and may aid in the correct diagnosis of these lesions.

CD2 is not expressed in mast cells but it may be aberrantly expressed in mastocytosis. Aberrant CD25 staining, however, is more frequently observed and is used as a minor criterion for the diagnosis of mastocytosis.

Selected references

Binder C, Cvetkovski F, Sellberg F, et al. CD2 immunobiology. *Front Immunol* 2020;11:1090.

Gonzalez L, Anderson I, Deane D, et al. Detection of immune system cells in paraffin wax-embedded ovine tissues. *J Comp Pathol* 2001; 125: 41–7.

CD3

Background

CD3 is a multisubunit complex comprising three dimers: CD3ε/δ, CD3ε/γ, and CD3ζ/ζ. It serves as the signaling complex for the T-cell receptor, to which it is noncovalently bound. Stimulation of the T-cell receptor by antigen and subsequent signaling through the CD3 complex results in T-cell activation, proliferation, and survival. Whereas the CD3γ, CD3ε, and CD3δ proteins have an extracellular immunoglobulin domain and have a short intracytoplasmic domain (with one ITAM motif), the CD3ζ has only a short extracellular domain and a longer intracytoplasmic domain (with three ITAM motifs). Anti-CD3 antibodies used in diagnosis may target different CD3 proteins and either extracellular or intracellular domains. During T-cell ontogeny, CD3 is present in the cytoplasm prior to its detection on the cell surface of thymocytes. Apart from CD7, CD3 is one of the earliest T-cell markers expressed by T cells. CD3 is not expressed by NK cells, though it is expressed by CD1-restricted NK/T cells.

Applications

CD3 is the most specific T-cell antibody. It is therefore a useful marker to distinguish both precursor T-cell and mature T-cell lymphoproliferative diseases from other hematolymphoid neoplasms. Although CD3 is not expressed by NK cells, it may be expressed, especially cytoplasmic

CD3ε, by NK-cell and NK/T-cell neoplasms. Exceptionally, cytoplasmic CD3 may also be expressed by Reed–Sternberg cells in classic Hodgkin lymphoma. Further, CD3 is also expressed by mixed-phenotype acute T/myeloid leukemia. CD3 expression other than CD3ε is part of the diagnostic requirements for the latter entity.

CD3 expression may also be lost in mature T-cell neoplasms of any type, but most often in anaplastic large-cell lymphoma.

Interpretation

As explained earlier, depending on the particular CD3 component targeted by the antibody, either surface expression or cytoplasmic expression, or both, may be observed. Most commonly, anti-CDε/δ antibodies are used, resulting in both a cytoplasmic and a membranous staining pattern, or depending on the entity (e.g., NK/T-cell lymphoma), only a cytoplasmic staining pattern may be seen.

Selected references

Birnbaum ME, Berry R, Hsiao Y-S, et al. Molecular architecture of the ab T cell receptor-CD3 complex. *Proc Natl Acad Sci* 2014;111:17,576–81.
Chetty R, Gatter K. CD3 structure, function, and role of immunostaining in clinical practice. *J Pathol* 1994:173; 303–7.

CD4

Background

After the discovery that lymphocytes could be divided into B cells and T cells, discrete subsets of T cells, which function as helper, suppressor, and cytotoxic cells, were recognized. The CD4 molecule is a nonpolymorphic glycoprotein belonging to the Ig gene superfamily that is expressed on the surface membrane of a functionally distinct subpopulation of T cells, mutually exclusive of the CD8 molecule. The CD4 molecule is a 55 kD glycoprotein with five external domains, each homologous to an Ig light chain variable region, a transmembrane domain, and a highly conserved intracellular domain. The CD4 gene has been mapped to the short arm of chromosome 12.

The CD4 molecule acts as a coreceptor with the TCR complex, appears to bind to the nonpolymorphic region of the MHC class II molecule, and may serve to increase the avidity of cell-to-cell interactions. The CD4 molecule also serves as a receptor for the human immunodeficiency virus on T cells, on monocytes/macrophages, and in some neural cells.

The CD4 antigen, like CD8, appears at the common thymocyte stage of T-cell differentiation and is expressed in about 80–90% of normal thymocytes. CD4 thus marks helper/inducer T cells and is expressed in 55–65% of mature peripheral T cells. It should be noted that the phenotype–functional association of CD4 to helper and CD8 to suppressor/cytotoxic function is not universal.

Subpopulations of suppressor or cytotoxic T cells can be identified among CD4-positive T cells. Although it is also expressed on monocytes/macrophages, Langerhans cells, and other dendritic cells, B cells do not express CD4.

Applications

The CD4 antibody is useful for the identification of T-helper/inducer cells and plays an important role in the immunophenotyping of reactive lymphocytes and in lymphoproliferative disorders. The majority of peripheral T-cell lymphomas are derived from the helper T-cell subset, so that most post-thymic T-cell neoplasms are CD4+CD8–. Tγ lymphoproliferative disease is an exception where the proliferative cells are CD4–CD8+. As with other T-cell antigens, CD4 may be aberrantly deleted in neoplastic T cells, so that the evaluation of such tumors requires the application of a panel of markers in order to identify tumors with such anomalous antigenic expression. CD4 immunostaining is seen in thymocytes (80–90%), mature T cells (65%, T-helper and CD4/CD8 thymocytes), macrophages, Langerhans cells, dendritic cells, granulocytes, and acute myeloid leukemia cells.

Selected references

Brady RL, Barclay AN. The structure of CD4. *Curr Top Microbiol Immunol* 1996;205:1–18.

CD5

Background

The CD5 molecule is a transmembrane glycoprotein of 67 kD with the typical tripartite structure of a signal peptide. The human CD5 has a sequence similar to that of the Ly-1 antigen in mouse, and both are distantly related members of the immunoglobulin superfamily of genes. CD5 is expressed on both T and some B lymphocytes. It is weakly positive in the most immature T-cell precursors, which are CD34 positive, with the intensity of expression increasing with maturation. CD5 expression is first seen in intrathymic T-cell progenitors (CD5+/CD34+), which differentiate into CD3+/CD4+/CD8+ T cells. This antigen is expressed in the majority of T cells, with as few as 11% of CD4+ lymphocytes being CD5 negative. Two-thirds of these CD5-negative cells are αβ T-cell receptor-positive cells and one-third are γδ T cells. Anti-CD5 antibodies have been shown to prolong the proliferative response of anti-CD3 activated T lymphocytes by enhancing signal transduction by the T-cell receptor antigen, a process associated with increased interleukin (IL)-2 production and increased IL-2 receptor expression by the T cells. The CD5 antigen may also act as a signal-transducing molecule in a manner independent of CD3. It has also been suggested that the B-cell surface protein CD72 (Lyb-2) is the ligand or counterstructure for CD5, and occupancy of CD72 by anti-CD72 antibodies, and possibly CD5-positive T cells, enhances IL-4-dependent CD23 expression on resting B lymphocytes.

When CD5 is expressed on B lymphocytes, it is usually weakly staining compared with the strong expression of mature T lymphocytes. This weak expression makes precise identification of the CD5-positive and CD5-negative B-cell populations difficult. CD5-positive B cells (B-1 cells) are first seen in the peritoneal and pleural cavities of the fetus at gestation week 15. The cells become prominent in the fetal spleen, with 60% or more of splenic B cells expressing the antigen. At birth, about 68% of cord blood B cells and approximately half of the peripheral blood B lymphocytes are CD5 positive, and this level drops dramatically in the peripheral blood, to near adult levels, within the first year of life. In adults, 15–25% of peripheral blood B lymphocytes are positive for CD5.

There is some suggestion that CD5-positive B lymphocytes represent a distinct subpopulation. Although both CD5-positive and CD5-negative B cells produce immunoglobulin, upon activation CD5-positive cells selectively produce primarily IgM antibodies, while CD5-negative B cells make primarily IgG antibodies, an observation made in cord blood. CD-positive B cells have also been reported to be associated with usually low-affinity, polyreactive antibody production, often called auto-antibodies. About 50% of auto-antibody-associated cross-reactive idiotype-bearing B lymphocytes are CD5 positive. It is possible that some of these differences may be due to lineage differences or simply secondary to some type of B-cell activation, which requires further investigation.

Applications

CD5 is a fairly specific and sensitive marker of T-cell lineage. Almost 85% of T-cell acute lymphoblastic leukemias (ALLs) are CD5 positive, and lack of CD5 expression in T-ALL in patients with a white cell count of less than 50,000/ml is reported to be associated with a worse prognosis than corresponding patients with CD5-positive T cells. CD5 expression has been reported in 3–10% of cases of acute myeloid leukemia. As CD5 is a pan-T-cell marker, it is not surprising that the majority of T-cell malignancies (76%) are CD5 positive. In peripheral T-cell lymphomas, including cutaneous T-cell lymphomas, the loss of CD5 expression can be employed to support a diagnosis of malignancy. In cutaneous T-cell lymphoma, CD5 is not as frequently lost as CD7.

With B-cell neoplasms, CD5 expression has been considered an almost defining characteristic of many entities. Chronic lymphocytic leukemia (CLL) is the most common CD5-positive B-cell malignancy. It is assumed that the small population of CD5-positive B cells found in normal healthy adults and prominent in cord blood is the nonneoplastic counterpart of this type of CLL. B-cell CLL is also associated with poly-specific antibodies or auto-antibodies and frequently expresses cross-reactive idiotypes. Over 90% of cases of typical CLL are CD5 positive. CD5 expression may be lost when the large-cell lymphoma of Richter's syndrome supervenes in CD5-positive CLL.

Unlike small lymphocytic lymphoma (chronic lymphocytic leukemia) and mantle cell lymphoma, with rare exceptions, monocytoid B-cell lymphoma and low-grade B-cell lymphoma of mucosa-associated lymphoid tissue are usually CD5 negative, a feature that can be employed to distinguish the small B-cell lymphoid neoplasms. CD5-positive B cells have been reported to be increased in some patients with monoclonal gammopathy of undetermined significance and in cases of multiple myeloma. De novo expression of CD 5 in diffuse large B-cell lymphoma was shown to be an indicator of poor prognosis associated with a centroblastic phenotype, interfollicular growth pattern, and intravascular or sinusoidal infiltration.

CD5-positive neoplastic cells have been found in cases of thymic carcinomas and some cases of atypical thymomas but not in typical thymomas. Carcinomas of the lung, breast, esophagus, stomach, colon, and uterine cervix have been reported to be all CD5 negative.

Positive staining for CD5 is seen in almost all T cells and most T-cell malignancies, B cells of the mantle zone of the spleen and lymph node and the corresponding mantle cell lymphomas, B cells in peritoneal and pleural cavities, B-cell small cell lymphomas, and hairy cell leukemia.

Selected references

Arber DA, Weiss LM. CD5: A review. *Appl Immunohistochem* 1995;3: 1–22.

CD7

Background

CD7 antigen is a cell surface glycoprotein of 40 kD expressed on the surface of immature and mature T cells and natural killer (NK) cells. It is a member of the immunoglobulin gene superfamily and is the first T-cell lineage-associated antigen to appear in T-cell ontogeny, being expressed in prethymic T-cell precursors (preceding CD2 expression) and in myeloid precursors in fetal liver and bone marrow, and persisting in circulating T cells. While its precise function is not known, there is a recent suggestion that the molecule functions as an Fc receptor for IgM.

Applications

CD7 is the most consistently expressed T-cell antigen in lymphoblastic lymphomas and leukemias. It is specific for T-cell lineage and is therefore a useful marker in the identification of such neoplastic proliferations. In mature post-thymic T-cell neoplasms, it is the most common pan-T antigen to be aberrantly absent, and its absence in a T-cell population is a useful pointer to a neoplastic conversion.

CD7 is immunoexpressed on 85% of mature peripheral T cells, the majority of post-thymic T cells, NK cells, some myeloid cells, T-cell acute lymphoblastic leukemia/lymphoma, acute myelogenous leukemia (especially M4/5), and chronic myelogenous leukemia. Interestingly, CD7 is conspicuously absent in adult T-cell leukemia/lymphoma and is not expressed in Sezary cells.

Selected references

Lazarovits AI, Osman N, Le Feuvre CE, et al. CD7 is associated with CD3 and CD45 in human T cells. *J Immunol* 1994:153;3956–66.

Saati TA, Alibaud L, Lamant L, et al. A new monoclonal anti-CD7 antibody reactive in paraffin sections. *Appl Immunohistochem Mol Morphol* 2001;9:289–96.

CD8

Background

Like CD4, the CD8 molecule is composed of nonpolymorphic glycoproteins, belonging to the Ig superfamily, which are expressed on the surface membrane of mutually exclusive, functionally distinct T-cell populations. The CD8 molecule is a 34 kD glycoprotein that forms disulfide-linked homodimers and homomultimers on the cell surface of peripheral T cells, the CD8 gene being linked to the κ locus on chromosome 2. The CD8 molecule comprises an external domain and highly conserved transmembrane and intracellular domains, the external domain showing striking homology with other members of the Ig gene superfamily. The CD8 molecule functions as a TCR coreceptor on suppressor/cytotoxic T cells and recognizes foreign antigens as peptides presented by MHC class I molecules. In the thymus, the CD8 molecule forms complexes with the CD1 glycoprotein, an MHC class I-like molecule. CD8 appears to bind to the nonpolymorphic regions of MHC class I molecules and may thus serve to enhance the avidity of cell-to-cell interactions. Both CD4 and CD8 antigens appear during the common thymocyte stage of T-cell differentiation and CD8 is expressed by about 80% of normal thymocytes. Thereafter, CD4 and CD8 are retained by those maturing thymocytes destined to become helper/inducer and suppressor/cytotoxic T cells, respectively, CD8 being expressed by about 25–35% of peripheral T cells, specifically of the suppressor/cytotoxic subset. In addition, about 30% of NK cells express low levels of CD8. This phenotypic–functional association is not universal and subpopulations of suppressor/cytotoxic T cells can be identified among CD4-positive cells.

Applications

As with the CD4 marker, CD8 has an important role in the immunophenotypic analysis of reactive and neoplastic populations of T cells, being used to identify a mature T-cell subset with suppressor/cytotoxic function. Like the CD4 marker, CD8 may also be aberrantly deleted from neoplastic T cells. The CD8 antigen is expressed on T-cell lymphoblastic lymphomas.

A hypopigmented form of mycosis fungoides has been shown to frequently express CD8+ phenotype.

Also, 25–35% of mature peripheral T cells stain for CD8, these mostly being cytotoxic T cells. CD8 positivity is also seen in NK cells, including 30% that are CD3 negative and 70–80% of cortical thymocytes.

Comments

The development of clones C8/144B and 1A5, which are immunoreactive in fixed, paraffin-embedded sections, has allowed the study of CD8+ T cells in a variety of diseases, including the inflammatory dermatoses, cutaneous T-cell lymphomas, gastrointestinal diseases and colorectal carcinoma, and neuronal destruction.

Selected references

Eichmann K, Boyce NW, Schmidt UR, et al. Distinct functions of CD8 (CD4) are utilised at different stages of T lymphocyte differentiation. *Immunol Rev* 1989;109:39–75.

Martz E, Davignon D, Kurzinger K, et al. The molecular basis for cytotoxic T lymphocyte function: Analysis with blocking monoclonal antibodies. *Adv Exp Med Biol* 1982;146:447–65.

Parnes JR. Molecular biology and function of CD4 and CD8. *Adv Immunol* 1989;44:265–311.

CD9

Background

The CD9 antigen is a cell surface glycoprotein (p24) of MW 24 kDa belonging to the tetra-membrane-spanning protein family (tetraspanins) coded by chromosome 12. The antigen is present on pre-B cells, monocytes, and platelets and has protein kinase activity. The majority of mature peripheral blood or lymphoid tissue B cells or other normal circulating hematopoietic cells other than platelets do not express it. It is present on activated T cells, mast cells, and some dendritic reticulum cells. CD9 also regulates motility in a variety of cell lines and appears to be an important regulator of Schwann cell behavior in the peripheral nervous system.

Applications

The expression of CD9 in malignant cells is complex and not strictly lineage, activation, or differentiation associated. It is found in >75% of precursor B-cell acute lymphoblastic leukemia/lymphoma (ALL/LBL), about 50% of B-cell chronic lymphocytic leukemia (CLL) and some better-differentiated B-cell neoplasms such as prolymphocytic leukemia and multiple myeloma, as well as some T-cell lymphomas and acute myeloid leukemias. Other B-cell lymphomas, including centrocytic lymphoma, follicle center cell lymphoma, and Burkitt's lymphoma, may also express this antigen,

and there is also variable expression on neuroblastomas and some epithelial tumors. CD9 immunoexpression has been claimed to indicate a favorable prognosis in breast carcinoma, although a recent study showed no benefit. Anti-CD9 antibodies were found to specifically inhibit the transendothelial migration of melanoma cells, and the protein immunostaining was suggested to be useful in the differential diagnosis of papillary renal cell carcinoma and collecting duct carcinomas and also between chromophobe and conventional renal cell carcinomas, being consistently positive in papillary and chromophobe carcinomas.

Selected references

Carbone A, Poletti A, Manconi R, et al. Heterogenous in situ immunotyping of follicular dendritic reticulum cells in malignant lymphomas of B cell origin. *Cancer* 1987;60:2919–26.

Lardelli P, Bookman MA, Sundeen J, et al. Lymphocytic lymphoma of intermediate differentiation: Morphologic and immunophenotypic spectrum and clinical correlations. *Am J Surg Pathol* 1990;14:752–63.

San Miguel JF, Caballero MD, Gonzalez M, et al. Immunological phenotype of neoplasms involving the B cell in the last step of differentiation. *Br J Haematol* 1986;62:75–83.

CD10

Background

CD10 is also called membrane metalloendopeptidase (MME). CD10 is a type II transmembrane glycoprotein with enzymatic activity that requires zinc as a cofactor. It inactivates short peptide hormones such as enkephalins, substance P, neurotensin, oxytocin, glucagon, and bradykinin in the extracellular space. The protein is expressed on the membrane of a wide variety of tissues, including immature B cells, germinal center B cells, endometrial stromal cells, proximal tubules and glomeruli of the kidney, myoepithelial cells for the breast, epithelial cells of the prostate, liver canaliculi, and epithelial cells of the stomach and colon.

Applications

It is expressed in approximately 75% of precursor B-cell acute lymphoblastic leukemia and a small subset of T-cell acute lymphoblastic leukemia and is used as part of the diagnostic panel. CD10 is also expressed in follicular lymphoma. This is part of its immunophenotype, and in many instances it can also be used to distinguish it from follicular hyperplasia by virtue of the detection of interfollicular CD10+ cells being present in lymphoma but not in follicular hyperplasia. CD10 expression is also evaluated to diagnose Burkitt lymphoma, where it is typically strongly expressed. In the diagnosis of diffuse large B-cell lymphoma NOS, CD10 is used as part of a panel of three markers (including also BCL6 and MUM1) to evaluate the cell of origin using the Hans algorithm. Cell of origin is of prognostic significance in diffuse large B-cell lymphoma NOS. Finally, CD10 is part of a set of markers that defines the T-follicular helper cell origin. These markers include BCL6, CXCL13, CXCR5, CD278, and CD279. The demonstration of the T-follicular helper cell immunophenotype is important for the typing of T-cell lymphoma, as it is present in angioimmunoblastic T-cell lymphoma, follicular T-cell lymphoma, and nodal peripheral T-cell lymphoma with T-follicular helper phenotype. Very rarely, aberrant CD10 expression is also seen in hairy cell leukemia, mantle cell lymphoma, marginal zone lymphoma, and chronic lymphocytic leukemia.

Apart from hematolymphoid diseases, CD10 expression is used, among other things, in the diagnosis of endometrial stromal nodules and endometrial stromal sarcoma to distinguish these lesions from uterine cellular leiomyoma and leiomyosarcoma, adult granulosa cell tumor, and undifferentiated endometrial carcinoma.

CD10 has also been shown to be expressed in melanoma, renal cell carcinoma, and mesenchymal cells of the skin, including tumors such as dermatofibroma, dermatofibrosarcoma protuberans, neurofibromas, and as many as 47% of malignant melanoma cases. The demonstration of CD10 expression in stromal cells of breast carcinoma has been correlated with prognosis.

CD10 expression has also been employed to stain canaliculi to aid the diagnosis of hepatocellular carcinoma.

Interpretation

CD10 marks cell membranes and to a lesser degree the cytoplasm of cells. Rarely, Golgi staining is seen. Of note, evaluation of CD10 on lymphoma, most often diffuse large B-cell lymphoma NOS, may in some instances be difficult to interpret because of low levels of expression.

Selected references

Chu P, Arber D. Paraffin section detection of CD10 in 505 non-hematopoietic neoplasms: Frequent expression in renal cell carcinoma and endometrial stromal sarcoma. *Am J Clin Pathol* 2000;113:374–82.

Maguer-Sata V, Besançon R, Bachelard-Cascales E. Concise review: Neutral endopeptidase (CD10): A multifaceted environment actor in stem cells, physiological mechanisms and cancer. *Stem Cells* 2011;29:389–96.

CD11

Background

Each of the CDU subtypes represents a different a chain, which forms one of the β2 family of integrin adhesion receptors when linked noncovalently to β2 (CD18) to form a heterodimer. CD11a, leukocyte function–associated protein (LFA-1), with a MW 180 kD, is present on B cells, T cells, NK cells, monocytes, granulocytes, megakaryocytes, and activated platelets. CD11b (Mac-1), the C3bi receptor, has a MW of 165 kD and is present on granulocytes, monocytes, and some histiocytes. CD11c, which has a MW of 150 kD, is present on monocytes, tissue macrophages, granulocytes, some suppressor/cytotoxic T cells, and a subset of B cells. It is usually positive on true histiocytic malignancies and some B-cell lymphomas, including hairy cell leukemia and monocytoid B-cell lymphoma.

CD11/CD18 integrins have a function in intercellular communication between lymphocytes and between lymphocytes and endothelial cells. The interaction between leukocytes and endothelial cells involves CD11/CD18 integrins, which bind to intercellular adhesion molecules ICAM-1 (CD-45) and ICAM-2.

Applications

Currently, the diagnostic applications for this marker are very limited and available antibodies are reactive only in frozen sections. Differential expression of CD11a (LFA-1) has been described in small cell lymphocytic lymphoma and chronic lymphocytic leukemia (CLL) and has been used to account for the difference in peripheral blood involvement in these entities, but the findings require confirmation. In the immunophenotypic separation of monocytoid B-cell lymphoma from other small cell lymphomas such as plasmacytoid small cell lymphoma, CLL, and mantle cell lymphoma, CD11c has been suggested to be a useful discriminant, being more frequently expressed in monocytoid lymphoma.

CD11a is found on all leukocytes. CD11b is found on granulocytes, macrophages, NK cells, follicular dendritic cells, myeloid cells, and some B and T lymphocytes. Hairy cell leukemia expresses this antigen. CD11c stains 50% of activated CD4/8+ T cells, granulocytes, lymphocytes, macrophages, and NK cells. In B-CLL, expression is associated with good prognosis, and it is expressed in virtually all cases of hairy cell leukemia.

Selected references

Chadburn A, Inghirami G, Knowles DM. Hairy cell leukemia-associated antigen Leu M5 (CD11c) is preferentially expressed by benign activated and neoplastic CD8 cells. *Am J Pathol* 1990;136:29–37.

CD15

Background

CD15 is a common glycan, also referred to as the Lewis x or Lex blood group antigen. The glycan is found as part of several glycolipids, such as glycoproteins. The CD15 antigen exists in a sialylated (sCD15) or unsialylated form. The unsialylated form is mostly of interest for tissue-based diagnosis.

Applications

CD15 is used for the diagnosis of classic Hodgkin lymphoma and for the diagnosis of myelosarcoma. CD15 expression, together with expression of CD30, weak expression of PAX5, and absence of expression of more than one B-cell surface marker, such as CD19, CD20, and CD79a, is characteristic for the immunophenotype of classic Reed–Sternberg cells and Hodgkin cell variants. CD15 expression is also important for the diagnosis of diffuse B-cell lymphoma, unclassifiable, with features intermediate between diffuse large B-cell lymphoma and Hodgkin lymphoma, as it confirms its partial Hodgkin cell immunophenotype.

Typically, CD15 is typically not expressed in nodular lymphocyte-predominant Hodgkin lymphoma, where LP Hodgkin cells display a B-cell immunophenotype.

CD15 expression can also be used as a marker for myeloid cell differentiation in cases of suspected myelosarcoma.

However, it needs to be used with more specific markers such as myeloperoxidase, as CD15 may also be expressed in acute lymphoblastic leukemia.

Interpretation

In Reed–Sternberg cells and Hodgkin cells, expression may be membranous, cytoplasmic, or both. Cytoplasmic expression is intense in the Golgi region. CD15 expression in classic Hodgkin lymphoma may stain only a subpopulation of Hodgkin cells. CD15 expression in myelosarcoma is mostly cytoplasmic.

CD15 expression is also found on normal neutrophilic granulocytes (membranous), a subpopulation of histiocytes and epithelioid histiocytes (cytoplasmic), and glandular epithelium. Its use for diagnosis of neoplastic hematologic disease must be interpreted in the context of other markers as outlined earlier, as it can be expressed in anaplastic large-cell lymphoma, T-cell lymphoma, lymphoblastic leukemia/lymphoma, and histiocytic sarcoma.

Selected references

Aber DA, Weiss LM. CD15: A review. *Appl Immunohistochem* 1993;1:17–30.

CD16

Background

CD16, also known as Fc fragment of IgG receptor III (FcγRIII), includes CD16a (FCGR3A) and CD16b (FCGR3B). They are members of the immunoglobulin superfamily and are low-affinity receptors for gamma immunoglobulin (IgG). CD16a is a transmembrane protein expressed on NK (natural killer) cells, monocytes, and macrophages and mediates antibody-dependent cellular toxicity (ADCC). CD16b, anchored by a glycosyl phosphatidylinositol (GPI) linker to the cell membrane, is present on neutrophils and subsets of basophils, which plays a role in pathogen clearance by neutrophils through activation of phagocytosis, degranulation, and oxidative burst.

CD16 is also variably expressed by granulocytes, T large granular lymphocytes, and gamma/delta T cells.

Applications

CD16 is a marker mainly used in flow cytometric analysis and is rarely used for immunohistochemical staining.

However, it may be used for demonstrating, together with other markers, an NK-cell immunophenotype for diagnosis of rare NK-cell disorders such as NK-cell enteropathy and tissue infiltration with aggressive NK-cell leukemia. CD16 is less frequently expressed in extranodal NK/T-cell lymphoma. Diminished CD16 expression by granulocytes in chronic myelomonocytic leukemia may help establishing the diagnosis.

Interpretation

Positive staining is cell membrane and cytoplasmic in location.

Selected references

Bruhns P. Properties of mouse and human IgG receptors and their contribution to disease models. *Blood* 2012;119(24):5640–9.

Cherian S and Wood B. ed. *Flow cytometry in evaluation of hematopoietic neoplasms*. CAP, Northfield, Illinois, 2012.

Feng R, Bhatt VR, Fu K, Pirruccello S, et al. Application of immunophenotypic analysis in distinguishing chronic myelomonocytic leukemia from reactive monocytosis. *Cytometry B Clin Cytom* 2018;94(6):901–9.

Qubaja M, Marmey B, Tourneau AL, et al. The detection of CD14 and CD16 in paraffin-embedded bone marrow biopsies is useful for the diagnosis of chronic myelomonocytic leukemia. *Virchows Arch* 2009;454(4):411–19.

Zhang Y, Boesen CC, Radaev S, et al. Crystal structure of the extracellular domain of a human Fc gamma RIII. *Immunity* 2000;13(3):387–95.

CD19

Background

CD19 is a transmembrane glycoprotein with two extracellular immunoglobulin-like domains and a large cytoplasmic tail. It is a coreceptor for the B-cell receptor complex and diminishes the threshold for antigen stimulation. In addition, it is an adaptor that recruits several signaling proteins, eventually leading to B-cell activation. CD19 is B-cell specific and expressed from B-cell lineage commitment of stem cells all the way to the early plasma cell stage, and disappears from the most mature plasma cells. Since CD19 is not expressed in pluripotent stem cells, it is targeted by a variety of immunotherapeutic agents, most notably in chimeric antigen receptor (CAR)-T-cell therapy.

Applications

CD19 staining is used as a pan-B-cell marker for the diagnosis of B-cell lymphoproliferative disease. A subset of plasma cell neoplasms also express CD19. Additionally, CD19 is useful to demonstrate the B-cell phenotype in the case of B-cell lymphoma, unclassifiable, with features intermediate between diffuse large B-cell lymphoma and classic Hodgkin lymphoma. Indeed, classic Hodgkin lymphoma, although of B-cell origin, is typically CD19 negative.

Interpretation

CD19 stains the cell membrane.

Selected references

Otero DC, Anzelon AN, Rickert RC. CD19 function in early and late B cell development: I. Maintenance of follicular and marginal zone B cells requires CD19-dependent survival signals. *J Immunol* 2003;170:73–83.

Otero DC, Rickert RC. CD19 function in early and late B cell development: II. CD19 facilitates the pro-B/pre-B transition. *J Immunol* 2003;171:5921–30.

CD20

Background

CD20 is a transmembrane, nonglycosylated phosphoprotein that plays a role in the regulation of cellular calcium influx, important for B-cell development, differentiation, and activation. As such, it appears in early pre-B cells and throughout their maturation into late pre-B cells. The CD20 antigen appears on the cell surface after light chain gene rearrangement and before the expression of intact surface Ig, remaining throughout the course of B-cell development. It is no longer expressed when the cells mature into plasma cells. For these reasons, CD20 is considered a pan-B-cell antigen. CD20 is not expressed on other cells.

Applications

CD20 is a commonly used immunohistochemical marker for B-cell neoplasms. It marks virtually all mature B-cell lymphomas, with the exception of most proliferative diseases showing pronounced plasma cell differentiation, such as plasma cell neoplasms and plasmablastic lymphoma. Other lymphomas with plasmablastic features, such as primary effusion lymphoma, ALK-positive large B-cell lymphoma, HHV8-positive diffuse large B-cell lymphoma, and the rare HHV-8 positive germinotropic lymphoproliferative disease, variably express CD20. However, a subset of multiple myeloma, most notably the subset with CCND1 gene translocation, may also express CD20.

CD20 is only variably expressed in B-lymphoblastic leukemia/lymphoma.

Reed–Sternberg cells in classic Hodgkin lymphoma, although of B-cell origin, only express CD20 in a subset of cases with variable levels of expression in the neoplastic cells. By contrast, LP Hodgkin cells in nodular lymphocyte-predominant Hodgkin lymphoma almost invariably express CD20.

CD20 staining is also useful in the follow-up of B-cell lymphoma, especially when treated with anti-CD20 antibody. Recurrent lymphoma may be CD20 negative, indicating resistance to further treatment with anti-CD20.

Aberrant expression of CD20 may be seen in myeloid disorders and peripheral T-cell lymphoma but is rare. Especially, monomorphic epitheliotropic intestinal T-cell lymphoma may show CD20 expression in up to 20% of cases.

Comments

Antibodies to CD20 are mostly reactive in formalin-fixed paraffin-embedded tissues. The staining pattern is membranous.

Selected references

Pavlasova G, Mraz M. The regulation and function of CD20: An "enigma" of B-cell biology and targeted therapy. *Haematologica* 2020;105:1494–506.

Bellizzi AM, Montgomery EA, Hornick JL. American Registry of Pathology Expert Opinions: Evaluation of poorly differentiated malignant neoplasms on limited samples – gastrointestinal mucosal biopsies. *Ann Diagn Pathol* 2020;44:151419.

CD21

Background

CD21 is a surface glycoprotein, also named human complement receptor type 2 (CR2). It is a receptor for various endogenous ligands, not least for complement C3 fragments iC3b, C3dg, and C3d, but also for CD23 and interferon-alpha. By virtue of binding C3d, which is covalently bound to targets, CD21 activation reduces the threshold for B-cell activation. CD21 also binds to pathogens such as Epstein–Barr virus, HIV, or prions, either directly or indirectly through C3d.

CD21 is expressed by all mature B cells and by follicular dendritic cells (FDCs), thymocytes, and a subset of peripheral T cells.

Applications

Antibodies to the CD21 antigen are useful to demonstrate FDC meshwork in lymphoid proliferations where the germinal centers may be ill-defined and difficult to delineate morphologically, e.g., HIV lymphadenopathy. In the early stages of progressive generalized lymphadenopathy (PGL, stage I), the large geographic reactive germinal centers may occupy large areas of the lymph node, giving an appearance of effacement of the architecture. Similarly, in the late stage of PGL (stage III), the atrophic germinal centers are not easily definable.

The demonstration of the nodular dense FDC meshwork in the stroma of follicular lymphomas is used for diagnosis, especially for high-grade follicular lymphomas that warrant a differential diagnosis with diffuse large B-cell lymphomas, which do not show a dense FDC network. Similarly, the nodular architecture of nodular lymphocyte-predominant Hodgkin lymphoma may be highlighted. Residual germinal centers that have been colonized in low-grade B-cell MALT lymphomas may also be demonstrated with antibody to CD21, which reveals an expanded and usually a looser FDC meshwork than is seen in follicular lymphoma.

The demonstration of irregular FDC meshworks, incorporating high endothelial venules, in the T-cell area is also characteristic of angioimmunoblastic T-cell lymphoma and sets it apart from peripheral T-cell lymphomas, including those with T-follicular helper cell immunophenotype.

The diagnosis of angiofollicular lymph node hyperplasia or Castleman disease (hyaline vascular type) may also benefit from highlighting the follicles with anti-CD21.

Dysplastic FDCs have been demonstrated in association with Castleman disease of the hyaline vascular type and are thought to be the precursor to FDC tumors. Likewise, CD21, together with CD23 and CD35, is used as a marker for the diagnosis of FDC sarcoma.

Interpretation

CD21 expression is membranous. It will stain the long extensions of FDCs and may result in misinterpretation of staining of neighboring cells.

Selected references

Bagdi E, Krenacs L, Krenacs T, et al. Follicular dendritic cells in reactive and neoplastic lymphoid tissues: A reevaluation of staining patterns of CD21, CD23, and CD35 antibodies in paraffin sections after wet heat-induced epitope retrieval. *Appl Immunohistochem Mol Morphol* 2001;9:117–24.

Hannan JP. The structure-function relationships of complement receptor type 2 (CR2; CD21). *Curr Protein Pept Sci* 2016;17(5):463–87.

CD23

Background

CD23 is a transmembrane glycoprotein. It is the low-affinity receptor for IgE and is involved in the regulation of IgE responses. In addition, it is the receptor for many ligands, including CD21, MHC class II, and integrins. CD23 can also be cleaved from the surface, yielding various soluble CD23 molecules with cytokine-like activity. CD23 is predominantly expressed in B lymphocytes and follicular dendritic cells but also to a lesser degree on other hematolymphoid cells.

Following cross-linkage of antigen and surface immunoglobulin on B cells, CD23 becomes expressed and serves as an autocrine stimulus driving B-cell proliferation. Surface CD23 has a half-life of only one to two hours and is shed in the form of soluble CD23 displaying autocrine activity. Two isoforms of CD23, CD23a and CD23b, exist, activating different signaling pathways.

CD23a is expressed on the surface IgM- and IgD-positive cells and not on circulating B cells or B cells that have undergone isotype switch and express IgG, IgA, or IgE.

CD23b is expressed weakly on a range of cell types, including monocytes, eosinophils, platelets, some T cells, and natural killer (NK) cells. Interleukin (IL)-4-treated monocytes show stronger staining. CD23 is strongly expressed on Epstein–Barr virus (EBV)-transformed lymphoblastoid B-cell lines.

Applications

Immunohistochemical analysis has been most useful as an additional marker to CD21 (and CD35) to stain follicular dendritic cells in benign and neoplastic lymphoproliferative disease (*see applications for* CD21) and helps to better type these diseases.

The use of CD23 as a B-cell marker to type B-cell lymphoma is more limited, especially with the advent of novel markers. CD23 is usually expressed by chronic lymphocytic leukemia and is usually performed as part of the panel, together with CD5, to type this lymphoproliferative disease. However, novel markers for use with flow cytometry have proven more specific, such as loss of CD79b and bright expression of CD200.

CD23 may also be useful as a marker for primary mediastinal large B-cell lymphoma.

CD23 is only variably expressed by other lymphoma types, such as marginal zone lymphoma, follicular lymphoma, diffuse large B-cell lymphoma, and classic Hodgkin lymphoma. It is thus of limited use for typing these lymphomas. Nonetheless, certain subtypes of follicular lymphoma, such as the diffuse variant, are typically CD23 expressing and may aid in this diagnosis.

Interpretation

CD23 is a membranous marker. Difficulties with interpretation of expression on B cells may arise in the presence of stromal follicular dendritic cells, which display long interstitial cytoplasmic extensions.

Selected references

Acharya M, Borland G, Edkins AL, et al. CD23/FcεRII: Molecular multi-tasking. *Clin Exp Immunol* 2010;162(1):12–23.

CD24

Background

Antibodies to CD24 react with a 42 kD single-chain cell surface sialoglycoprotein, which is expressed throughout B-cell differentiation but, like other pan-B-cell antigens, is lost following activation and before the secretory (plasma cell) stage. CD24 is not entirely restricted to B cells and is expressed on granulocytes, interdigitating cells, and renal epithelial cells as well as some benign and malignant epithelial tumors. CD24 can function as a ligand for β-selectin, may have a role in the lung colonization of human tumors, and, through glycolipid-enriched membrane fractions, may mediate intracellular signaling and apoptosis in human B lymphocytes. CD24 has adhesion molecule functions and promotes invasion of glioma cells in vivo. In breast carcinoma, the binding of tumor cells to platelets and the rolling of these cells on endothelial β-selectin facilitates metastasis.

Applications

CD24 is expressed on the majority of precursor B-cell acute lymphoblastic leukemia/lymphomas (ALL/LBLs) and by virtually all mature, TdT-negative, SIg-positive, and SIg-negative B-cell non-Hodgkin's lymphomas. It is not found in multiple myeloma or on either benign or neoplastic T cells. Anti-CD24 has been used for purging bone marrow of B-ALL cells in autologous bone marrow transplantation.

CD24 is abundantly expressed on breast cancer cell lines and tumor tissues and has been suggested as a possible marker for breast carcinoma, with cytoplasmic expression in carcinoma cells compared with apical expression in benign cells.

CD24 is positive on all B cells, granulocytes, kidney cells, epithelial cells, both benign and malignant, most pre-B-ALL/LBL, and virtually all B-cell lymphomas. It is not expressed on plasma cells, myeloma, T cells, monocytes, red blood cells, and platelets.

Selected references

Abramson CS, Kersey JH, LeBien TW. A monoclonal antibody (BA-1) reactive with cells of human B lymphocyte lineage. *J Immunol* 1981;126:83 8.

CD25

Background

CD25 is the α-chain of the interleukin-2 receptor (IL2 R-α). It is a transmembrane protein that forms a complex with the beta- (CD122) and gamma- (CD132) subunits to form a high-affinity receptor for IL-2. CD25 is expressed on a variety of normal hematopoietic cell types, including activated lymphocytes, monocytes, and a subset of myeloid precursors. Of note, CD25 is typically expressed by regulatory T cells. CD25 is reportedly also a marker of bile canaliculus.

Applications

CD25 immunostaining is mostly used for typing certain hematolymphoid neoplasias.

CD25 immunostaining is used in the workup of adult T-cell leukemia/lymphoma (ATLL), where, together with FOXP3 expression, it enables the regulatory T-cell immunophenotype these lymphomas usually display to be established. Although CD25 expression is distinctive for ATLL, it is not unique to it. CD25 marks activated T cells; hence, a variety of other T-cell lymphoma types may variably express it. However, the most notable expression is seen in anaplastic large-cell lymphoma, although the marker is not used for this diagnosis.

CD25 is also important in the diagnostic workup of certain B-cell neoplasms. CD25 is used for the diagnosis of hairy cell leukemia, although immunophenotyping is usually performed by flow cytometry of a blood or bone marrow sample and includes a panel of markers. The typical immunophenotype includes expression of CD25, CD103, and CD123 with strong coexpression of CD19, CD20, CD22, and CD11c. If diagnosis is performed by immunohistochemistry, the panel includes CD25 and annexin A1 in addition to pan-B-cell markers.

Absence of CD25 expression is particularly important to exclude a diagnosis of hairy cell leukemia-variant, which may resemble hairy cell leukemia but is resistant to conventional hairy cell leukemia therapies.

CD25 is also expressed in other B-cell neoplasms, including lymphoplasmacytic lymphomas, follicular lymphoma, chronic lymphocytic leukemia/small lymphocytic lymphoma, diffuse large B-cell lymphomas, and classic Hodgkin lymphoma. While expression of CD25 in these entities is not diagnostic, the demonstration of CD25 positivity may have prognostic and therapeutic implications in some B-cell neoplasms.

CD25 expression has diagnostic implications in systemic mastocytosis. While normal mast cells do not express CD25, it may aberrantly be expressed in mastocytosis. Aberrant expression of CD25 is included in the diagnostic criteria for the disease.

CD25 immunohistochemistry is not widely used in the workup of nonhematopoietic neoplasms.

Selected references

Bayer AL, Pugliese A, Malek TR. The IL-2/IL-2 R system: From basic science to therapeutic applications to enhance immune regulation. *Immunol Res* 2013;57(1–3):197–209. doi:10.1007/s12026-013-8452-5

O'Malley DP, Chizhevsky V, Grimm KE, et al. Utility of BCL2, PD1, and CD25 immunohistochemical expression in the diagnosis of T cell lymphomas. *Appl Immunohistochem Mol Morphol* 2014;22:99–104.

NOTES

CD30

Background

CD30 is a transmembrane glycoprotein and member of the tumor necrosis factor receptor superfamily. Through binding with its ligand, CD153 (CD30L), expressed by antigen-presenting cells, CD30 expressed by T cells provides additional costimulatory signals. This promotes proliferation and differentiation of naïve T cells into effector and memory T cells. CD30 is also expressed by activated B cells as well as to some degree in histiocytes. Exocrine pancreatic cells, a subset of cortical neurons, and Purkinje cells may also express CD30. The function of CD30 cells in those cell types is as yet unclear.

In reactive lymph nodes, CD30-expressing scattered large B and T cells are localized around lymphoid follicles and at the margin of germinal centers.

Applications

CD30 immunohistochemistry is widely used for diagnosis of hematolymphoid neoplasia, including Hodgkin lymphoma, anaplastic large-cell lymphoma, lymphomatoid papulosis, and to a lesser extent for peripheral T-cell lymphoma as well as subsets of B-cell lymphoma. Nonetheless, evaluation of CD30 expression in the latter entities may be important for determining eligibility for anti-CD30 antibody treatment.

Hodgkin and Reed–Sternberg cells in classic Hodgkin are typically strongly positive for CD30. By contrast, LP Hodgkin cells in nodular lymphocyte-predominant Hodgkin lymphoma are negative or only variably positive. Anaplastic large-cell lymphoma is homogeneously and strongly positive for CD30. Likewise, the large atypical cells in lymphomatoid papulosis are strongly CD30 positive.

Strong and homogeneous CD30 expression is also a characteristic feature of anaplastic large-cell lymphoma and should be stained for whenever this diagnosis is suspected. The small-cell variant of anaplastic large-cell lymphoma is the only variant that may only variably express CD30, with CD30 only strongly expressed by the largest cells.

CD30 expression is typically weak and variably expressed in primary mediastinal large B-cell lymphoma, a staining pattern that is helpful for making this diagnosis in the proper context of a large-cell lymphoma presentation in the anterior mediastinum.

Peripheral T-cell lymphoma, extranodal NK/T-cell lymphoma, and large B-cell lymphoma may be variably positive. CD30 is less useful for these diagnoses. Of note, EBV-positive large B-cell lymphoma is usually, but variably, CD30 positive. CD30 expression in diffuse large B-cell lymphoma, NOS has been reported to be associated with improved prognosis. CD30 may also be expressed in mycosis fungoides, where it may indicate large-cell transformation.

CD30 positivity has been reported in embryonal carcinomas and in the embryonal elements of mixed germ cell tumors and, less commonly, has been observed in pancreatic and salivary gland carcinomas. CD30 expression in metastatic embryonal carcinoma may be lost following chemotherapy. The combination of CD30 and CD117 staining has been used for the distinction of embryonal carcinoma from seminoma, these tumors staining CD30+/CD117– and CD30–/CD117+, respectively.

CD30 positivity has less commonly been observed in mesenchymal tumors, including leiomyoma, leiomyosarcoma, rhabdomyosarcoma, synovial sarcoma, giant cell tumor of tendon sheath, malignant fibrous histiocytoma, osteogenic sarcoma, Ewing's sarcoma, malignant schwannoma, ganglioneuromas, and aggressive fibromatosis. Occasional lipoblasts in liposarcoma may show positivity.

Interpretation

In Hodgkin lymphoma, anaplastic large-cell lymphoma, and lymphomatoid papulosis, the CD30 staining pattern is membranous, often with a strong paranuclear Golgi region staining and weaker cytoplasmic staining. In other lymphomas, less distinct CD30 expression is seen with some membrane as well as cytoplasmic expression.

Semiquantitative evaluation of staining has been advocated prior to treatment of lymphoma with anti-CD30 antibody therapy. Guidelines do not really exist, but estimating the percentage of tumor cells staining with CD30 is recommended, with 10% being the cut-off for anti-CD30 treatment mostly used in the clinical trial setting. Alternatively, an H-score may be provided (using the formula $[1 \times (\% \text{ cells } 1+) + 2 \times (\% \text{ cells } 2+) + 3 \times (\% \text{ cells } 3+)]$).

Selected references

Hang KL, Arber DA, Weiss LM. CD30: A review. *Appl Immunohistochem* 1993;1:244–55.

So T, Ishii N. The TNF-TNFR family of co-signal molecules. *Adv Exp Med Biol* 2019;1189:53–84.

Xu ML, Gabali A, Hsi ED, et al. Practical approaches on CD30 detection and reporting in lymphoma diagnosis. *Am J Surg Pathol* 2020;44(2):e1–e14.

CD31

Background

CD31 is a 130 kD glycoprotein, also designated platelet endothelial cell adhesion molecule-1 (PECAM-1), that is normally expressed on endothelial cells and circulating and tissue-phase hematopoietic cells, including platelets, monocytes/macrophages, granulocytes, and B cells. This antigen is also expressed in sinusoidal endothelial cells in the liver, lymph node, and spleen The same endothelial cells display variable staining with *Ulex europeaus* agglutinin-I (UEA-1) and for von Willebrand factor (Factor VIII-related protein), indicating that the sinusoidal endothelium differs from other vascular endothelium. CD 31 does not label connective tissue, basement membrane, squamous epithelium, or adnexal structures of the skin. The exact function of CD 31 has not been fully elucidated, but CD 31 appears to mediate platelet adhesion to endothelial cells and may promote vascular adhesion of leukocytes.

Applications

1. The main application of CD31 is as a marker of both benign and malignant endothelial cells. CD31 is an apparently more sensitive marker than CD34, von Willebrand factor, or UEA-1 as a marker of malignant vascular endothelium. Despite the earlier suggestion that CD31 is specific for vascular endothelium with no expression by lymphangiomas, we clearly showed that there was distinct staining for CD31 in all 19 cases of lymphangioma studied, albeit of lesser intensity than that observed in vascular endothelium. Indeed, the endothelium of blood and lymphatic vessels share many common antigens, such as CD 34, von Willebrand factor, and UEA-1, and none provides absolute distinction between the two types of vessels. In the light of these findings, claims that Kaposi's sarcoma shows vascular endothelial differentiation or derivation will need to be reassessed. CD31 is thus employed as a marker of endothelial cells in the evaluation of tumor angiogenesis.

2. While CD31 is only occasionally found on Ewing's sarcoma/peripheral neuroendocrine tumors, it was consistently found in small lymphocytic lymphoma and lymphoblastic lymphoma and less often in mantle cell and follicular center cell lymphomas. Rhabdomyosarcomas and desmoplastic small round-cell tumors did not express the antigen.

Selected references

Albelda SM, Muller WA, Buck CA, et al. Molecular and cellular properties of PECAM-1 (endoCAM/CD31): A novel vascular cell-cell adhesion molecule. *J Cell Biol* 1991;114:1059–61.

DeYoung BR, Wick MR, Fitzgibbon JF, et al. CD 31: An immunospecific marker for endothelial differentiation in human neoplasms. *Appl Immunohistochem* 1993;1:97–100.

Stokinger H, Gadd SJ, Eher R, et al. Molecular characterization and functional analysis of the leukocyte surface protein CD31. *J Immunol* 1990;145:3889–97.

Suthipintawong C, Leong AS-Y, Vinyuvat S. A comparative study of immunomarkers for lymphangiomas and hemangiomas. *Appl Immunohistochem* 1995;3:239–44.

Teo NB, Shoker BS, Jarvis C, et al. Vascular density and phenotype around ductal carcinoma in situ (DCIS) of the breast. *Br J Cancer* 2002;86:905–11.

CD33

Background

CD33 is a sialic-acid-binding immunoglobulin-like lectin (SIGLEC), which is part of a large family with differential expression on leukocyte subsets. It consists of extracellular, transmembrane, and intracellular domains and is involved in binding of carbohydrates and other lectins containing sialic acid. CD33 is post-translationally modified by N-linked glycosylation. CD33 plays a role in the regulation of diverse immunological and inflammatory activity of the cells. It is a pan-myeloid antigen, universally expressed on myeloid progenitors, monocytes/macrophages, and granulocytes. However, lower expression is found on mature eosinophils and neutrophils. CD33 may also be expressed, very weakly, on plasma cells. CD33 is not expressed in nonhematopoietic cells.

Applications

CD33 is widely used for typing of leukemia by flow cytometry. Its expression is part of the myeloid immunophenotype. Since typing of leukemia is mostly performed by flow cytometry, its use for immunohistochemistry is more limited. It is useful in the diagnosis of myelosarcoma to differentiate it from other neoplasia with blastoid morphology. One should be aware that B-lymphoblastic leukemia/lymphoma may also aberrantly express CD33, especially those cases with BCR-ABL1 gene translocation. Although not used for this diagnosis, CD33 may be expressed in plasma cell neoplasms and very rarely in ALK-positive anaplastic large-cell lymphoma.

CD33 assessment is not only important for assigning lineage to cells of interest but also represents a potential therapeutic target.

Interpretation

CD33 stains the plasma membrane and, variably, the cytoplasm.

Selected references

Bovio I, Allan RW. The expression of myeloid antigens CD13 and/or CD33 is a marker of ALK+ anaplastic large cell lymphomas. *Am J Clin Pathol* 2008; 130: 628–34.

Crocker PR, McMillan SJ, Richards HE. CD33-related siglecs as potential modulators of inflammatory responses. *Ann NY Acad Sci* 2012;1253:102–111.

Hoyer JD, Grogg KL, Hanson CA, et al. CD33 detection by immunohistochemistry in paraffin-embedded tissues: A new antibody shows excellent specificity and sensitivity for cells of myelomonocytic lineage. *Am J Clin Pathol* 2008; 129: 316–23.

CD34

Background

The CD34 antigen is a heavily glycosylated transmembrane protein, the function of which is as yet incompletely known. Some evidence suggests that CD34 might play a role in cell adhesion, cell differentiation, and proliferation. It acts as a ligand for lectins, among others CD62L (S-selectin). In this way, CD34+ hematopoietic precursors might bind to lectin-expressing cells of the bone marrow stroma.

CD34 is a marker of resident progenitor cells of many tissues, including hematopoietic tissue, fatty tissue, fibrous tissue, skeletal muscle, epidermis, and endothelium. However, it is also a marker of mature endothelial cells, although it may be absent from large veins and arteries and from sinuses in the placenta and spleen.

Applications

CD34 immunohistology is mainly used for the diagnosis of acute leukemias, myelodysplastic syndromes, and vascular neoplasms and for the diagnosis of some other soft tissue tumors.

CD34 is expressed in 40% of acute myeloid leukemia but also in acute B- and T-lymphoblastic leukemia. Although these diagnoses are usually made by bone marrow smear interpretation and flow cytometry, CD34 immunostaining on the trephine biopsy may help to quantify the number of blasts in the marrow, as aspirates may be hemodilute. Quantification of blasts is required for acute myeloid leukemia, requiring 20% blasts to be present, but also for myelodysplastic syndromes to define cases with excess of blasts, which have a worse prognosis. Two cut-off values are being used, excess of blasts 1, with 5–9% blasts, and excess of blasts 2, with 10–19% of blasts. CD34 immunostaining is also used with a panel of other markers for diagnosis of myelosarcoma.

The expression of CD34 is a good marker for vascular tumors. The endothelial cells of both vascular and lymphatic vessels express the antigen. The expression of CD34 is also helpful for diagnosis of other soft tissue tumors as part of a panel of markers to diagnose these tumors.

Solitary fibrous tumor, dermatofibrosarcoma protuberans, epithelioid sarcoma, spindle cell and pleomorphic lipoma, cellular digital fibroma, gastrointestinal stroma tumor (GIST), and superficial CD34 positive fibroblastic tumors, as the name implies for the last, typically express CD34.

Epithelioid smooth muscle tumors stain less frequently, but the marker may serve as a useful discriminator from epithelial tumors, which are generally negative for CD34. The antigen is displayed by nerve sheath tumors, although in some series both neurofibromas and schwannomas failed to stain. In the latter, staining may be mainly in the Antoni B areas. While the staining in malignant nerve sheath tumors is largely negative, some series report a high frequency of reactivity, suggesting that CD34 may be a useful inclusion in the diagnostic panel for such tumors, in which S100 and CD57 are negative. CD34 expression was also described in some cases of angiomyofibroblastomas, giant cell fibroblastomas, and Bednar tumor.

Interpretation

CD34 is expressed on the cell membrane but also in the cytoplasm.

Selected references

Sidney LE, Branch MJ, Dunphy SE, et al. Concise review: Evidence for CD34 as a common marker for diverse progenitors. *Stem Cells* 2014;32:1380–9.

Hughes MR, Hernaez DC, Cait J, et al. A sticky wicket: Defining molecular functions for CD34 in hematopoietic cells. *Exp Hematol* 2020;86:1–14.

CD35

Background

CD35 is complement receptor type 1 (CR1). It is a type I membrane-bound glycoprotein belonging to the family of complement regulators. The receptor binds complement fragment C3b, the activated form of complement protein C3. The receptor has lower-affinity binding with complement proteins C4b, C1q, and a degraded form of C3b. CD3b is an opsonin released during the inflammatory response and will trigger cells expressing CD35 to phagocytosis of the pathogen or cells coated with it.

CD35 is expressed on erythrocytes, granulocytes, monocytes, and a subset of mantle cells as well as some T cells, follicular dendritic cells, and glomerular podocytes.

Applications

The use of CD35 in diagnostic immunohistochemistry is mostly as a marker for follicular dendritic cells and sarcomas derived from follicular dendritic cells. The demonstration of expanded follicular dendritic cell networks is an important part of the diagnosis of B-cell lymphoma subsets as well as T-cell lymphoma subsets. However, CD21 is the more widely used marker for this purpose. With regard to B-cell lymphoma, well-defined nodular meshworks of follicular dendritic cells are characteristic of follicular lymphoma, whereas mantle cell lymphoma and marginal zone lymphoma show more loosely arranged networks. The demonstration of well-defined nodular follicular dendritic cell networks is of particular importance to distinguish follicular lymphoma grade 3B from diffuse large B-cell lymphoma. Follicular T-cell lymphoma derived from T-follicular helper cells also shows well-defined, often irregularly expanded, networks of follicular helper cells, whereas angio-immunoblastic T-cell lymphoma, equally derived from T-follicular helper cells, shows highly irregular and loose follicular dendritic cell networks, often with high endothelial venules entrapped. Nodular lymphocyte-predominant Hodgkin lymphoma shows typically expanded well-defined nodular follicular dendritic cell networks in the stroma, although rare variants of this disease may show a more diffuse architecture with absence of follicular dendritic cell networks.

CD35 has great utility in the typing of follicular dendritic cell tumors, together with CD21 and CD23.

Aberrant expression of CD35 is seen on mast cells in mastocytosis but is not used for this diagnosis in tissue sections.

Interpretation

CD35 stains the membrane of cells, including the long membranous extensions of the follicular dendritic cells.

Selected references

Badgi E, Krenacs L, Krenacs T, et al. Follicular dendritic cells in reactive and neoplastic lymphoid tissues: A reevaluation of staining patterns of CD21, CD23, and CD35 antibodies in paraffin sections after wet heat-induced epitope retrieval. *Appl Immunohistochem* 2001;9:117–24.

Liu D, Niu Z-X. The structure, genetic polymorphisms, expression and biological functions of complement receptor type 1 (CR1/CD35). *Immunopharmacol Immunotoxicol* 2009;31:524–35.

CD38

Background

CD38 is a transmembrane glycoprotein expressed in a wide variety of cells. CD38 is the ligand of CD31, expressed by endothelial cells, but also binds laterally to professional signaling complexes, such as the CD3/TCR complex in T cells, the CD19/CD21/BCR complex in B cells, and the CD16/CD61 complex in natural killer (NK) cells. These receptor complexes with CD38 are located in lipid rafts of the cell membrane and play a critical role in transducing activating signals. Cells expressing CD38 have an important immunomodulatory function. CD38 is expressed early upon differentiation of CD34+ stem cells but disappears from resting mature B-, T-, and NK cells, monocytes, and granulocytes to be re-expressed upon activation. It is also highly expressed on plasma cells. In solid tissues, CD38 is expressed in the brain (pyramidal neurons, astrocytes), eye, prostate (basal and secretory epithelial cells), gut, pancreas, muscle, bone, and kidney. Apart from signal transduction, CD38 also has a role in the control of intracellular $Ca2^+$ and functions as an ecto-enzyme; the latter involves a hydrolase enzymatic activity converting NAD^+ to cyclin ADP-ribose. These functions are important for cell activation. In the pancreas, insulin secretion is one of the functions mediated by CD38. The molecule is the target of an autoimmune response, and serum auto-antibodies to CD38 have been detected in diabetic patients. Anti-CD38 auto-antibodies have been suggested to be a new diagnostic marker of β-cell autoimmunity in diabetes.

Applications

Despite its wide expression, CD38 immunostaining is mainly of value for identifying plasma cells and typing of plasma cell neoplasia as an alternative or additional marker to CD138. Importantly, the successful use of anti-CD38 immunotherapy in plasma cell neoplasia and increasingly in autoimmune disorders has increased the interest in CD38 as a marker. Although its expression is mostly analyzed by flow cytometry in those conditions, tissue immunohistochemistry is of use when flow cytometry is not available.

Interpretation

CD38 stains the plasma membrane and, variably, the cytoplasm.

Selected references

Morandi F, Airoldi I, Marimpietri D, et al. CD38, a receptor with multifunctional activities: From modulatory functions on regulatory cell subsets and extracellular vesicles, to a target for therapeutic strategies. *Cells* 2019;8:1527.

CD40

Background

CD40 is a 48 kD integral membrane protein expressed by
B lymphocytes, follicular dendritic cells, interdigitating
reticulum cells, monocytes, epithelial cells, endothelial cells,
and tumor cells, including carcinomas, B-cell lymphomas/
leukemia, and Reed–Sternberg cells of Hodgkin's disease.
CD40 has been clustered as a member of the nerve growth
factor (NGF)/tumor necrosis factor (TNF) receptor
superfamily. Its corresponding counterstructure, the CD40
ligand (CD40L), is mainly expressed by activated CD4+
T cells and also some activated CD8+ T cells, basophils,
eosinophils, mast cells, and stromal cells. CD40L shares
significant amino acid homology with TNF, particularly in
its extracellular domain, and is therefore viewed as a member
of the TNF ligand superfamily. The flurry of publications
relating to CD40 suggests that this receptor may have a pivotal
role in the function of B lymphocytes and their survival.
Binding of CD40L+ T cells to CD40+ B cells is thought to
play a major role in T-cell-dependent B-cell activation, B-cell
proliferation, Ig isotype switching, memory B-cell formation,
and rescue of B cells from apoptotic death in germinal
centers. Mutations of the CD40L gene have been associated
with the X-linked hyper-IgM immunodeficiency syndrome,
indicating the critical role of the CD40/CD40L interaction
in the T-cell–B-cell interplay. Accordingly, expression of
CD40 has been found in most of the B-cell neoplasms, Reed–
Sternberg cells of Hodgkin's disease, and some carcinomas.
In contrast, functional CD40/CD40L interactions appear
to be critical for cellular activation signals during immune
responses and neoplastic tumor cell growth. Lack of this
important interaction results in greatly reduced activation of
CD4+ T cells, while successful interaction of these molecules
results in full activation of T-cell effector functions, such as
help for B-cell differentiation and class switch, activation of
monocytes and macrophages to produce lymphokines and
to kill intracellular pathogens, and activation of autoreactive

T cells to mount an autoimmune response. CD40 may also
play a similar role in the transduction of regulatory signals
for cell functions such as proliferation and differentiation
in nonlymphoid cells and has a role in the binding of tumor
cells to endothelium, cell migration, and enhancement of
cell motility, so that it is of interest in tumor metastasis and
prognostication.

Applications

The intense research interest in CD40 and its ligand has yet
to be translated into diagnostic applications. Current uses
of CD40 have mostly been for the immunodetection and
identification of tumor cells in all subtypes of Hodgkin's
disease. As many as 100% of Hodgkin's disease cells have
displayed positivity for CD40, irrespective of their antigenic
phenotype. In contrast, CD40 was immunodetected in only
one-third of anaplastic large-cell lymphomas, whereas almost
83% of B-cell non-Hodgkin's lymphomas were positive.
In vitro engagement of CD40 by its soluble ligand CD40L
enhanced both clonogenic capacity and colony cell survival
of Hodgkin's disease cell lines. Recombinant CD40L induced
interleukin (IL)-8 secretion and enhanced IL-6, TNF, and
lymphotoxin-alpha release from cultured Reed–Sternberg
cells. These cytokines play a significant role in the clinical
presentation and pathology of Hodgkin's disease, a tumor
of cytokine-producing cells. CD40L has pleiotropic biologic
activities on Reed–Sternberg cells, and the CD40–CD40L
interaction might be a critical element in the deregulated
cytokine network and cell contact–dependent activation
cascade typical of Hodgkin's disease.

Comments

CD40 shows distinctive immunolocalization to the cell
membrane and as a paranuclear dot similar to that of CD30
and CD15.

CD40 is expressed on B cells, macrophages, dendritic cells, endothelial cells, fibroblasts, keratinocytes, carcinomas, most B-cell lymphomas, and some B-cell acute lymphoblastic leukemia (B-ALL) and is not expressed on plasma cells.

Selected references

Carbone A, Gloghini A, Gruss HJ, et al. CD40 ligand is constitutively expressed in a subset of T cell lymphomas and on the microenvironmental reactive T cells of follicular lymphomas and Hodgkin's disease. *Am J Pathol* 1995;147:912–22.

CD43

Background

MT1 and the identical antibody DFT-1 recognize a sialoantigen present on normal T cells, myeloid cells, and macrophages. Megakaryocytes are variably positive. Both antibodies belong to the CD43 cluster. There is evidence that the antibody MT1, originally thought to belong to CD45, binds to an entirely unrelated molecule. Both MT1 and DFT-1 recognize surface antigens (190, 110, and 100 kD).

Applications

In a review of several published series, CD43 (MT1) was shown to immunoreact with 30% low-grade B-cell lymphomas, approximately 90% T-cell lymphomas, 69% B-cell and 97% T-cell lymphoblastic lymphomas, and 44% anaplastic large-cell lymphomas. However, it should be noted that CD43 also highlights myeloid cells and macrophages and may be employed as a marker of granulocytic tumors. Although normal small B lymphocytes are CD43 negative, most low-grade B-cell lymphomas are CD43 positive. However, hairy cell leukemia, MALT lymphoma, and follicle center cell lymphomas are notable exceptions. Therefore, CD43 is not useful to distinguish between T- and B-cell lymphocytic lymphoma. Furthermore, although CD43 is a reliable marker of mantle cell lymphoma (MCL), it cannot immunophenotypically distinguish MCL from T- or B-cell lymphoblastic lymphomas. CD43 marks plasmacytoma/myeloma and is more often positive than negative in peripheral T-cell lymphomas.

Comments

CD43 is positive on most T cells, activated B cells, natural killer (NK) cells, granulocytes, monocytes, megakaryocytes, and 90% of T-cell lymphomas, and coexpressed with CD20 in small lymphocyte lymphoma, but not in benign cells, granulocytic sarcomas, acute myeloid leukemia, most acute lymphocytic leukemia, plasmacytomas, and mast cell disease.

Selected references

Flavell DJ, Flavell SU, Jones DB, et al. Two new monoclonal antibodies recognising T-cells (DF-T1) and B-cells (DF-B1) in formalin fixed paraffin embedded tissue sections. *J Pathol* 1988;155:343A.

Poppema S, Hollema H, Visser L, et al. Monoclonal antibodies (MT1, MT2, MB1, MB2, MB3) reactive with leukocyte subsets in paraffin-embedded tissue sections. *Am J Pathol* 1987;127:418–29.

CD44

Background

The CD44 receptor is also known as phagocytic glycoprotein (Pgp-1), extracellular matrix receptor III (ECM-III), B-cell p80 antigen, lymphocyte homing receptor (Hermes antigen), and hyaluronate cellular adhesion molecule (H-CAM). CD44 shows considerable homology with the cartilage link proteins involved in adhesion between hyaluronate and other proteoglycans in the extracellular matrix, including collagen, fibronectin, and ankyrin. Besides this function, CD44 has since been found to have a role in recognition between lymphocytes and endothelial cells and in lymphocyte homing to the reticuloendothelial tissues. This latter function has led to interest in its possible role in the regulation of tumor cell dissemination.

The CD 44 family of glycoproteins exists in a number of variant isoforms, the most common being the standard 85–95 kD or hematopoietic variant (CD44s) that is found in mesodermal cells such as hematopoietic, fibroblastic, and glial cells, and in some carcinoma cell lines. The receptor is coded in five distinct domains located on the short arm of chromosome 11. The heterogeneity in the CD44 molecule results from post-translational modification of the protein and/or alternative splicing of up to 10 exons resulting in variant isoforms of higher molecular mass (140–160 kD), which may be expressed individually or in various combinations, with potentially diverse functions. Higher-molecular-weight isoforms have been described in epithelial cells (CD44v) and are thought to function in intercellular adhesion and stomal binding. While the other functions and distributions of the CD44 family have not yet been completely elucidated, they are also known to participate in embryonic development and angiogenesis as well as other molecular processes associated with specific adhesions, signal transduction, and cell migration. The recent demonstration of a concordance of the cell proliferation nuclear antigen

Ki-67 and CD44 expression in adenomatous polyps, colonic carcinomas, and adjacent mucosa raises the possibility of involvement of CD44 in stimulating cell growth.

While many human tumors express CD44, a positive correlation between increased CD44v expression and tumor progression and/or dedifferentiation has been demonstrated in only some. Such tumors include non-Hodgkin's lymphoma, hepatocellular carcinoma, breast carcinoma, renal cell carcinoma, colonic carcinoma, and some soft tissue tumors. More recent additions to the list include metastatic melanoma, prostatic carcinoma, and gastric cancer. Conversely, CD44v expression is downgraded in other tumors, including neuroblastoma and squamous cell and basal cell carcinomas of the skin.

Applications

The suggestion that there is a positive association between CD44 isoform expression and progression in human tumors has important implications for diagnosis and prognosis. Unfortunately, the situation is not yet clear-cut. Confusion over the complicated exon boundaries together with the different nomenclature employed by researchers has added to problems of identifying the true metastasis-associated isoform. Furthermore, stromal cells may contribute to the isoform pattern detected. For example, activated lymphocytes may express the so-called metastasis-associated variant of CD44, emphasizing the importance of immunohistological assessment as a method that allows morphologic discrimination.

Selected references

East JE, Hart IR. CD 44 and its role in tumor progression and metastasis. *Eur J Cancer* 1993;29A: 1921–2.

CD45 (leukocyte common antigen)

Background

The CD45 cluster of antibodies recognizes a family of proteins known as the leukocyte common antigen (LCA), exclusively expressed on the surface of almost all hematolymphoid cells and their progenitors. The CD45 antibody is one of the most specific antibodies currently available for diagnostic use. Virtually all hematolymphoid cells, including T and B lymphocytes, granulocytes and monocytes, and macrophages, with the exception of maturing erythrocytes and megakaryocytes, express CD45. This family of proteins, to date, has not been conclusively shown on any nonhematolymphoid cells.

The CD45 proteins are coded for by a single gene located on chromosome lq31–32. The gene is composed of 33 exons that code for the cDNA sequence as well as both 5′ and 3′ nontranslated regions. Differential usage of three exons termed A, B, and C is known to generate eight different mRNAs and at least five proteins in the CD45 protein family. The complete CD45 protein consists of a large cytoplasmic domain of 707 amino acids, a transmembrane region of 22 amino acids, and an external domain of 391–552 amino acids depending on the pattern of exon splicing. By electron microscopy, the CD45 proteins consist of a globular structure of 12 nm, representing the cytoplasmic domain, and a rod-like structure of 18 nm, representing the external domain.

There is high conservation of the cytoplasmic domain among mammals and it shows homology with placental tyrosine phosphatases. Consistently with this homology, the CD45 protein has intrinsic tyrosine phosphatase activity and belongs to a family of protein tyrosine phosphatases that includes 16 other members, at least 7 of which are transmembrane proteins.

The precise function of the CD45 proteins is not known, but they appear to play an important role in early lymphocyte activation. Protein tyrosine phosphatase can counter the actions of protein tyrosine kinases, enzymes known to be induced in early T-cell activation that may represent the primary signaling event initiated by the T-cell receptor. CD45 expression is inversely related to spontaneous tyrosine phosphorylation of multiple proteins, which has a fundamental role in regulating T-cell calcium levels. CD45 is required for both T-cell antigen receptor and CD2-mediated activation of T-lymphocyte protein tyrosine kinase, and CD45 is physically linked to both CD2 and the T-cell receptor on the surface of memory T lymphocytes. The difference in structure among the external domains of the different CD45 proteins probably determines the specific target stimuli for the different cell types expressing CD45. Similarly, CD45 may also be important for B-cell function. Antibodies to CD45 inhibit an early phase in the activation of resting B cells and are able to inhibit c-myc induction in B cells.

As a result of post-translocational change of the mRNA of the A, B, and C exons, several isoforms are produced. By strict definition, CD45 antibodies are monoclonal antibodies, which react with all isoforms of CD45 proteins, and there are several subclusters of antibodies that detect different species of CD45 proteins. These have molecular weights of 220 kD representing the ABC isoform, 205 kD probably representing distinct AB and BC isoforms, 190 kD representing the B isoform, and 180 kD representing the O isoform. The restricted CD45 antibody refers to those that recognize subsets of CD45 proteins but not the entire class, and these CD45R antibodies can be further subdivided into CD45RA, CD45RB, and CD45RO depending on the isoform recognized by the antibody. To date, there are no monoclonal antibodies that specifically recognize the C isoform. CD45RA antibodies generally precipitate the 200 and 205 kD (ABC and AB isoforms), CD45RB the 220, 205, and 190 kD (ABC, AB, BC, and B isoform), and CD45RO the 180 kD protein (O isoform).

Many of the CD45 antibodies are sensitive to neuraminidase, which is consistent with the suggestion that these antibodies recognize epitopes that are associated with carbohydrates and, possibly, terminal sialic acids. PD 7 is a CD 45RB antibody and labels all known CD45 proteins with the exception of the ones lacking exons A, B, and C, whereas 2B11 reacts against AB protein but not others. The combination of PD 7 with 2B11 as a CD45–CD45RB cocktail (Dako) allows a reliable method of detecting LCA in hematolymphoid cells. CD45 proteins are major components of the membranes of lymphocytes and form about 10% of the lymphocyte surface, accounting for much of the carbohydrate present on the membrane. The staining with CD45 antibodies is membranous, although there may be some staining of the Golgi. Histiocytes exhibit minimal cell membrane staining and phagocytic cells show immuno-localization of the antigen to secondary lysosomes.

Applications

It is an essential component of the panel to distinguish anaplastic large-cell tumors, which include the entities malignant lymphoma, melanoma, and carcinoma. The reactivity of anti-LCA antibodies is 93–99% for a cross-spectrum of different subtypes of B- and T-cell lymphomas.

In classic Hodgkin's disease, excluding the nodular L and H lymphocyte predominant subtype, membrane staining for LCA is rare, although cytoplasmic staining may be seen. Cytoplasmic staining may be spurious, as similar cytoplasmic staining can be found in nonhematolymphoid neoplasms. By contrast, the majority of nodular L and H lymphocyte predominant Hodgkin's disease shows positivity for PD 7 and/or 2B11, and this subtype is now thought to be distinctly different from classic Hodgkin's disease.

Anaplastic large-cell lymphoma may show positivity for LCA in only 50–87% of cases, although this figure may be higher in frozen section material. Furthermore, anaplastic large-cell lymphoma may also show staining for epithelial membrane antigen, making its immunohistochemical differentiation from anaplastic carcinoma difficult. These tumors express CD30 and, in 60% of cases, are of activated T-cell phenotype, showing staining for CD45RO and/or CD43 in paraffin sections.

Among other hematolymphoid neoplasms, plasmacytomas show a variable degree of positivity for LCA, ranging from 0 to 20% of cases. Hairy cell leukemia has been found to be uniformly positive for PD 7–2B11, and CD45 expression has been found in all cases of acute leukemias of T-cell lineage and in over 80% of cases of B-cell lineage. Failure of expression of CD45 in acute childhood lymphoblastic leukemia appears to be associated with other favorable prognostic features, such as lower leukocyte counts and serum lactic dehydrogenase levels, and is associated with chromosomal hyperdiploidy. Mast cell disease appears to be positive for PD 1–2B11, and polycythemia vera and extramedullary hematopoiesis were reported to be negative, although only a few cases were studied. In keeping with the low expression in histiocytes, true histiocytic tumors were found to be negative for PD 7–2B11, whereas cases of Langerhans' histiocytosis were reported to be positive. The rare cases of interdigitating reticulum cell sarcoma that have been studied have been reported to be positive for PD 7, similarly to nonneoplastic interdigitating reticulum cells. Cases of CD45-negative, keratin-positive large-cell lymphomas have been reported, but these are exceptionally rare.

While larger series have reported a total absence of staining for LCA in nonhematolymphoid neoplasms, there have been rare case reports of staining examples of primitive sarcoma, probably rhabdomyosarcoma.

CD45RA (4KB5, MB1, KiB3, and MT2)

The CD45RA group of antibodies recognize the 220 kD and 205 kD variants of CD45 encoded by exon A. These isoforms are expressed on the surface of most B cells as well as post-thymic, naive T cells and some medullary thymocytes. MT2 is thought to recognize a carbohydrate moiety and is negative in normal germinal centers, unlike antibodies MB1 and KiB3, which appear to bind to the peptide backbone of CD45RA, staining mantle zone and follicular center cells. In the paracortical areas of lymph nodes, there are approximately equal numbers of CD45RO-positive and CD45RA-positive cells. In paraffin-embedded sections, MB1 and 4KB5 stain over 80% of cases of B-cell lymphomas, while MT2 stains only 57% of such cases. Small lymphocytic lymphoma has the highest rate of positivity while small noncleaved cell lymphoma has the lowest. Fifty-seven percent of cases of follicular center lymphoma are positive for MT2, and this pattern of staining has been exploited for diagnostic purposes, as only weak or absent scattered positivity for MT2 is seen in reactive germinal center cells. Neoplastic follicles are labeled by MT2, whereas reactive follicles are not. This difference in staining patterns with MT2 has been postulated to be due to differences in the sialylation of the CD45 protein present on these B cells. T-cell lymphoma has a much lower incidence of positivity with CD45RA antibodies and is seen in about 10% of cases.

CD45RA+ mycosis fungoides is a rare form of the disease with T-helper phenotype (CD3+, CD4+, CD8−, CD45RO+), often with loss of lineage markers.

CD45RO (UCHL1, A6, OPD4)

CD45RO antibodies recognize the 180 kD (O isoform) variant of CD45. UCHL1 antibody reacts with approximately 90% of cortical thymocytes, 50% of medullary thymocytes, and approximately 50–70% of CD2-negative and CD3-positive peripheral blood and lymph node T cells. It rarely, if ever, reacts with benign B cells. While most mature T cells are CD45RO positive, some normal T-cell subsets are constitutively CD45RO negative and CD45RA positive, and the CD45RO-positive cells slowly increase in number to reach the adult level of about 50% by the age of 10–20 years. CD45RO-negative cells include naive CD4-positive T cells, which predominate in neonates, and some CD8-positive or CD4-negative CD8-negative subsets found in intestinal intraepithelial T cells and enteropathy-associated T-cell lymphoma.

In the differentiation of low-grade B-cell from T-cell lymphomas, the approximated test analysis figures for UCHL1 are as follows: sensitivity 95%, specificity 95%, accuracy 95%. In contrast, in high-grade lymphomas, the same parameters are 80%, 85%, and 83%, respectively. Stem cells giving rise to both erythroid and myeloid cells as well as primitive erythroid colony-forming cells express the 180 kD isoform of the CD45 protein recognized by CD45RO, but more mature erythroid forms lack CD45 expression. Most granulopoietic colony-forming cells are CD45RO negative, while mature monocytes or macrophages and myeloid cells are generally CD45RO positive. These latter cells do not stain with the antibody OPD4; the difference in reactivity is possibly due to a difference in the carbohydrate structure of the epitope presented on these cells.

Enumeration of CD45RO+ inflammatory cells together with CD8, neutrophil elastase, CD68, and mast cell tryptase has been employed in an attempt to distinguish ulcerative colitis and Crohn's disease, but the results require confirmation.

The OPD4 antibody is not, as originally claimed, specific for CD4-positive T cells. It reacts very similarly to clone UCHL1, differing only in having a low sensitivity for T-cell lymphoma, and is not reactive with monocytic cells.

CD45 is positive on all hematopoietic cells, and strong expression is seen on lymphocytes. The antigen may not be found on nonhematopoietic cells, lymphoplasmacytic lymphoma, lymphoblastic lymphoma, anaplastic lymphoma, and multiple myeloma. CD45RA is expressed on naïve and activated T cells and medullary thymocytes. CD45RO is expressed on memory and activated T cells, thymocytes, some B cells, and weakly on granulocytes and macrophages. The antigen is expressed on about 75% of T-cell lymphomas, with variable expression of T-cell lymphoblastic lymphoma.

Selected references

Poppema S, Lai R, Visser L. Monoclonal antibody OPD4 is reactive with CD45RO but differs from UCHL1 by the absence of monocyte activity. *Am J Pathol* 1991;139:725–9.

Weiss LM, Arber DA, Chang KL. CD45: A review. *Appl Immunohistochem* 1993;1:166–81.

CD54 (ICAM-1)

Background

Cell–cell adhesion is critical in the generation of effective immune responses and is dependent upon the generation of a variety of cell surface receptors. Intercellular adhesion molecule-1 (ICAM-1; CD54) is an inducible cell surface glycoprotein expressed at a low level on a subpopulation of hematopoietic cells, vascular endothelium, fibroblasts, and certain epithelial cells. However, its expression is dramatically increased at sites of inflammation, providing an important means of regulating cell–cell interactions and hence inflammatory responses. ICAM-1 is induced by proinflammatory cytokines such as interleukin-1, tumor necrosis factor-alpha, or interferon-gamma.

The CD54 antigen (ICAM-1) is a 90 kD integral membrane glycoprotein with seven potential N-linked glycosylation sites.

Applications

The CD54 antigen is expressed on monocytes and endothelial cells. It is also a lymphokine-inducible molecule and has been shown to be a ligand for LFA-1-mediated adhesion. Expression of the antigen can be induced or upregulated on many cell types, including B and T lymphocytes, thymocytes, fibroblasts, keratinocytes, and epithelial cells. In its function of mediating immune and inflammatory responses, CD54 antigen mediates adhesion of T cells with antigen-presenting cells and is involved in T-cell to T-cell and T-cell to B-cell interactions.

CD54 may be strongly positive on mantle cell lymphomas of the spleen.

Increased expression of ICAM-1 has been associated with many types of atherosclerotic lesions. In rejecting kidneys the antibody strongly highlights all infiltrating cells as well as glomerulus epithelium, endothelium on capillaries, vessels, and mesangium.

Comments

CD54 is expressed on both B and T cells, monocytes, endothelial cells, and a variety of epithelial cells and thus has low specificity.

Selected references

Ohh M, Takei F. New insights into the regulation of ICAM-1 gene expression. *Leuk Lymphoma* 1996;20:223–8.

CD56 (neural cell adhesion molecule)

Background

CD56, the neural cell adhesion molecule (NCAM), was discovered in a search for cell-surface molecules that contribute to cell–cell interactions during neural development. Human peripheral cells capable of non-MHC-restricted cytotoxicity express the CD56 antigen. NCAM has at least three isoforms, generated by differential splicing of the RNA transcript from a single gene located on chromosome 11. The core polypeptide of the CD56 appears to be the 140\kD isoform of NCAM, which is variably glycosylated and sialylated to produce mature species with molecular weights ranging from 175 to 220 kD. The CD56 antigen itself appears not to participate directly in the cytolytic activity of natural killer (NK) cells. Subsequent immunohistochemical studies have shown that NCAM is widely expressed in neural and neuroendocrine tissues. CD56 also marks thyroid follicular epithelium, proximal renal tubules, hepatocytes, gastric parietal cells, and pancreatic islet cells.

Applications

Merkel cell carcinoma, neuroblastoma, ganglioglioma, oligodendroglioma, glioblastoma multiforme, pheochromocytoma, retinoblastoma, laryngeal and pulmonary squamous cell carcinoma, pulmonary and intestinal carcinoid, pulmonary small cell undifferentiated carcinoma, pancreatic islet cell tumor, hepatocellular carcinoma, renal cell carcinoma, and follicular and papillary thyroid carcinoma mark positively with CD56 antibodies.

The current major application of CD56 on paraffin sections is in the diagnosis of NK and NK-like T-cell lymphoma, i.e., CD56 is a marker for NK cells. CD56-positive lymphomas are heterogeneous, encompassing several entities: nasal/nasopharyngeal NK/T-cell lymphoma, nasal type (extranasal) NK/T-cell lymphoma, aggressive NK-cell leukemia/ lymphoma, and the newly described blastoid NK-cell lymphoma. The nasal form represents the prototype of this group and is referred to as angiocentric lymphoma.

Two other types of T-cell lymphoma show a particularly high frequency of CD56 expression: hepatosplenic δγT-cell lymphoma (63% CD56+) and S-100 protein-positive T-cell lymphoma.

Microvillous lymphomas are a group of B-cell lymphomas that frequently express CD56. These rare, poorly defined transformed cell lymphomas are characterized by a cohesive sinus growth pattern and ultrastructural cytoplasmic processes. They have been compared to transformed follicle center cells and follicular dendritic cells and show clonal heavy chain immunoglobulin rearrangement. They mark with CD74, CDw75, and CD20 but not DBA.44, CD21, or CD35. About half of such tumors express CD56, suggesting a role for adhesion molecules in the distribution of these lymphomas.

An unusual cutaneous blastic tumor coexpresses CD56 and terminal deoxynucleatidyl transferase (TdT) and has been termed blastic natural killer cell lymphoma. These tumors are likely to be of primitive/undifferentiated hematopoietic origin and may progressively develop bone marrow involvement by blast cells with myeloid immunophenotype that are negative for CD56 and TdT.

Another rare malignancy with CD56+CD4+ immunophenotype was recently shown to correspond to the so-called type 2 dendritic cell or plasmacytoid dendritic cell. Such tumors typically present with cutaneous nodules associated with lymphadenopathy or splenic enlargement or both and massive bone marrow infiltration. The disease is rapidly fatal, but there is a purely cutaneous form that is indolent.

Comments

Clearly, CD56 antibodies are essential for the diagnosis of NK/T-cell lymphomas, which show a predilection for the upper aerodigestive tract, skin, testes, skeletal muscle, gastrointestinal tract, and other extranodal sites and pursue an aggressive clinical course. Furthermore, this antibody may be used to detect residual disease in CD56-positive NK-T-cell lymphoma in which the neoplastic lymphoid cells are small and show minimal atypia, especially in small biopsies.

CD56 is expressed on NK cells, activated T cells, cerebellum, and brain, at neuromuscular junctions, and in normal and neoplastic neuroendocrine tissues, myeloma, and myeloid leukemia.

Selected references

Chan JKC. CD56-positive putative natural killer (NK) cell lymphomas: Nasal, nasal-type, blastoid, and leukemic forms. *Adv Anat Pathol* 1997;4:163–72.

CD57

Background

CD57 antibodies detect a 38 kD protein encoded by a gene on chromosome 11. The protein is present on some peripheral lymphocytes but not in monocytes, granulocytes, platelets, or erythrocytes. CD57+ lymphocytes increase with age and represent 10–20% of lymphocytes in most adults. They mostly include a subset of CD8+ T lymphocytes as well as natural killer (NK) cells. A subpopulation of peripheral lymphocytes that reacts with this marker includes large granular lymphocytes. This antibody also reacts with both CD3+ and CD3– non-B lymphocytes. The CD3– lymphocytes demonstrate NK-cell activity and have large cytoplasmic granules that are not seen in the CD3+ cells. CD3+/CD57+ T cells are primarily suppressor lymphocytes with CD8 expression, though CD4+/CD8–/CD57+ T cells have been described and CD8+/CD57+/HLA-DR+ T cells have also been identified. CD3+/CD8+/CD57+ lymphocytes are positive for CD45RA but not CD45RO. While this phenotype is characteristic of naïve T lymphocytes, the CD57+ cells differ from other naïve T cells by failing to lose the CD45RA antigen when stimulated with allo-antigens. These cells also differ from other T lymphocytes by their increased ability to acquire the HLA-DR antigen in the absence of antigen-specific cytotoxic activity against allogeneic target cells.

The frequency of CD57+ lymphocytes in solid tissues varies according to site. CD57+ lymphocytes are increased in term placental tissue but not in decidua of early pregnancy. CD57+ lymphocytes are decreased in bronchoalveolar lavage specimens compared with peripheral blood in the same patient, and they represent fewer than 2% of all nasal mucosal lymphocytes. CD57+ lymphocytes are rare in both the endometrium and uterine cervix. They are also rare in the thymus and in the bone marrow; they constitute no more than 1% of all nucleated cells.

CD57+ lymphocytes have a different distribution from that of CD8+ cells in the tonsils and lymph nodes, with the CD57+ cells located primarily within the germinal centers. These germinal center cells are CD3+ T cells, which also express the CD4 antigen. Similarly to the CD57+/CD4+ T cells in cytomegalovirus (CMV) carriers, the CD4+ germinal center cells do not display the usual helper activity of classic CD4+ lymphocytes.

CD57+ cells in the spleen are seen mostly in the germinal centers of the white pulp or as a rim of cells around the central white pulp.

The HNK-1/Leu 7 antibody also reacts with cells other than lymphocytes. CD57 antibodies react with an antigen present in the central and peripheral nervous system myelin and with oligodendroglia and Schwann cells. Some neural adhesion molecules also contain a carbohydrate epitope that is recognized by CD57 antibodies. The reactivity is due to part of the myelin-associated glycoprotein having a similar molecular mass (110 kD) to the CD57 lymphocyte antigen.

Besides neural-associated cells, CD57 antibodies immunoreact with prostatic epithelium, pancreatic islets, adrenal medulla, renal loops of Henle and proximal tubules, chromaffin cells of the gut, gastric chief cells, epithelial cells of the outer thymic cortex, and some cells in the fetal bronchus. CD57 is also detected in the prostatic seminal fluid.

Applications

CD57+ lymphocytes are increased in patients following bone marrow transplantation. This increase often persists for years after the procedure. The majority of these cells are CD57–/CD8+ T lymphocytes, which form up to two-thirds of the peripheral blood T lymphocytes, with a small expansion in CD57+/CD4+ cells.

The relationship between this increase in CD57+ cells and graft versus host disease is controversial, some workers finding a correlation between the increase in CD57+ cells and the onset of disease while others have not. Some investigators have noted the expansion of the CD57+ population with reactivation of CMV after transplantation, similar to the increase in CD57+ cells seen in healthy carriers of CMV.

CD57+ cells are also elevated in the peripheral blood in some solid organ transplant patients. Up to 20% of renal allograft, 66% of cardiac allograft, and 44% of liver allograft recipients had greater than 20% peripheral blood CD57+/CD3+ lymphocytes, the majority of these cells also being CD8+. As with bone marrow transplantation, the elevation of CD57+ is correlated with a rise in CMV titers and may show poorer graft survival.

CD57+ cells are also elevated in human immunodeficiency virus infections. CD57+/CD8+ lymphocytes are increased through the clinical progression of the infection while CD57+/NK and CD57− NK cells remain normal.

Peripheral blood CD57+ cells may be increased in patients with adult-onset cyclic neutropenia, whereas no elevation was seen in childhood onset cases. The adult-onset variant of cyclic neutropenia was found to be steroid responsive.

Circulating CD57− lymphocytes are elevated in patients with Crohn's disease, with many of these cells being CD8+, corresponding to the increase in suppressor cell function found in such patients. Elevations in peripheral blood CD57+ cells may also be seen in rheumatoid arthritis.

Large granular lymphocytosis (LGL) is by far the most common CD57-positive lymphoproliferative disorder. LGL is usually CD2+ and may be divided into T-cell and NK-cell types based on CD3 expression. CD3+ cases are generally associated with clonal T-cell gene rearrangement. The T-cell cases are usually CD57 and CD8 positive, and may be further typed according to the presence (Type 1) or absence (Type 2) of the NK-associated antigen CD16. Immunostaining of the spleen may be useful in the evaluation of resected spleens in LGL patients. CD 57+ lymphocytes are found in the splenic red pulp, while the expanded white pulp nodules are usually not involved.

Elevations of peripheral blood CD57+ lymphocytes may be associated with nonneoplastic states, such as in CMV carriers, possibly in chronic hepatitis, in ankylosing spondylitis, and more frequently in rheumatoid arthritis and Felty's syndrome. Synovial fluid CD 57+ cells may also be elevated in rheumatoid arthritis. Clonal T-cell receptor gene rearrangement has been demonstrated in some cases of rheumatoid arthritis, especially those with Felty's syndrome.

NK/T-cell lymphomas frequently affect the nasal and extranodal sites and show similarities to LGL. The lymphoma cells display large cytoplasmic granules with either a T-cell or an NK-cell phenotype. They are also mostly positive for the Epstein–Barr virus and display an angiocentric pattern of infiltration with necrosis and an aggressive clinical course. Unlike LGL, NK/T-cell lymphomas are CD57 positive in fewer than 10% of cases, with most cases being CD56+, so that CD57 antibodies alone are unreliable NK-cell markers of such lymphomas.

CD57 expression is seen in just over 20% of T-lymphoblastic lymphomas, but the expression of CD57 does not correlate with NK activity in these cases, and the significance of expression of this antigen is unknown. Fewer than 2% of other types of T-cell lymphoma are CD57+ and the antigen does not appear to be expressed in B-cell lymphomas, monocytic leukemia, or Langerhans' histiocytosis. Increases in presumably nonneoplastic CD 57+ cells may be seen in the neoplastic follicles of follicular lymphomas, especially of the small cleaved cell type and in cases of nodular L & H Hodgkin's disease, where the + cells often rosette around CD20-positive L & H cells, providing a useful pointer to the diagnosis. The CD57+ cells in the latter condition are also CD4+ and can be seen in about 25–30% of cases of nodular lymphocyte-predominant Hodgkin's disease. Interestingly, a recently described variant of classic Hodgkin's disease that produces follicles with small, eccentric germinal centers and expanded mantle zones that contained classic Reed–Sternberg cells showed similar CD57+ resetting of the latter cells, mimicking nodular L & H Hodgkin's disease. Similar distribution and increases in CD57+ cells were not found in nodular sclerosing Hodgkin's disease, T-cell rich B-cell lymphoma, or follicular lymphoma.

CD57 expression may be observed in a variety of solid tumors, the most common of which are lung tumors. Almost half of small cell lung carcinomas and about 85% of carcinoid tumors are CD57+. In non-small cell lung carcinoma, the identification of neuroendocrine-associated antigens such as CD57 has been shown to be predictive of response to chemotherapy. The expression of CD57 antigen in small cell carcinoma and carcinoid is generally widespread in the tumor but only focal in non-small cell lung carcinomas. Sampling errors should be taken into consideration in the assessment, and because of the low sensitivity and specificity of CD57 antibodies, other neuroendocrine-associated markers such as chromogranin, synaptophysin, and neuron specific enolase should be employed.

Other nonhematopoietic neoplasms that express CD57 include the majority of thyroid carcinomas, especially papillary carcinoma, while it is present in only 30% of benign thyroid proliferations. CD57 may be used to separate medullary carcinomas from other thyroid carcinomas, although there have been some reported examples of positivity in medullary carcinomas. Strong CD57-staining of the majority of the tumor cells is indicative of papillary or follicular carcinoma and uncommon in benign thyroid proliferations and medullary carcinoma.

The CD57 antigen is expressed in prostatic epithelium, but the marker does not discriminate between benign and neoplastic cells. Metanephric adenomas were strongly and diffusely positive for CD57 and WT1, with focal staining for

CK7 but no staining for CD56 and desmin. While Wilm's tumor was also strongly positive for WT1 in the blastema and epithelial components, there was no staining for CD57 in these components, and some cases were diffusely positive for CD56.

Epithelial cells of thymomas are usually CD57 positive, while only some thymic carcinomas express the antigen. Over half of malignant mesotheliomas are reported to express CD57, although they generally do not react with other neuroendocrine markers. Among the soft tissue tumors, the majority of neural tumors, especially neuromas, schwannomas, and neurofibromas, react with CD57 antibodies. Most malignant peripheral nerve sheath tumors are CD57 positive but the antigen may also be expressed by other sarcomas, such as synovial sarcoma and leiomyosarcoma. Therefore, the marker on its own is not a useful diagnostic discriminant and should be used in an appropriate panel of antibodies in order to separate the various spindled and pleomorphic soft tissue tumors. Similarly, because CD57 may be expressed by a variety of small round-cell tumors, including neuroblastomas, it is not a useful diagnostic discriminant for this group of poorly differentiated tumors.

In the central nervous system, CD57 expression may be seen in normal oligodendroglia and other nervous system cells as well as in their corresponding tumors. Oligodendrogliomas perhaps show the most extensive degree of CD57 positivity compared with astrocytomas and glioblastomas, which demonstrate fewer positive cells. Among skin tumors, the expression of CD57 closely paralleled that of S100 protein although the two were not identical. Neither was useful in the distinction of eccrine from apocrine tumors. Melanocytic proliferations and melanomas may show variable positivity for CD57, whereas reports of the expression of this antigen in Merkel cell carcinoma are conflicting, the antigen being absent in some series and positive in half the tumors in another study. CD57 positivity is also seen in other tumors, including a large proportion of granular cell tumors, paragangliomas, and pheochromocytomas. Embryonal carcinomas and dysgerminomas are also reported to be positive for CD57 in most cases.

Selected references

Arber DA, Weiss LM. CD57: A review. *Appl Immunohistochem* 1995;3:137–52.

CD68

Background

The best macrophage reagents produced to date are those recognizing the CD68 antigen. This 110 kD antigen belongs to a family of acidic, highly glycosylated lysosomal glycoproteins that include the lamp-1 and lamp-2 molecules. CD68 is the human homologue of the murine macrosialin antigen and is present in the cytoplasmic granules of monocytes, macrophages, neutrophils, basophils, and large lymphocytes. This antigen is also expressed to some degree in the cytoplasm of some nonhemopoietic tissue. However, the function of the molecule is to date unknown.

The monoclonal antibody KP1 (IgG1, Kappa) was raised against lysosomal granules prepared from lung macrophages and recognizes the 110 kD CD68 antigen. This antibody labels monocytes and macrophages in a wide range of tissues, e.g., lung macrophages, germinal center macrophages, and Kupffer cells. Osteoclasts and myeloid precursors in bone marrow are also strongly labeled. In frozen sections, KP1 stains endothelium and hepatocytes weakly. Strong labeling of blood monocytes (granular/cytoplasmic), neutrophils, and basophils is also demonstrated with KP1. KP1 antigen is expressed as an intracytoplasmic molecule associated with lysosomal granules.

The murine PG-M1 monoclonal antibody (IgG3, Kappa) was raised against spleen cells of Gaucher's disease. Reactivity with cells transfected with a human cDNA encoding for the CD68 antigen confirms PG-M1 as a member of the CD68 cluster. In normal tissue, PG-M1 is comparable to KP-1; however, in bone marrow paraffin sections, PG-M1 strongly stains macrophages but not granulocytes and myeloid precursors. PG-M1 also shows immunopositivity with mast cells and synovial cells.

Applications

Malignant histiocytosis and true histiocytic lymphoma express the CD68 macrophage marker. These tumors should be CD68 positive but unlabeled with antibodies to CD30,

T- and B-cell antigens, and cytokeratins. Acute myeloid leukemias (AML) are identified by the presence of CD68 antigen. Whilst KP1 recognizes M1–M5 types, PG-M1 immunoreaction is confined to M4 (myelomonocytic) and M5 (monocytic) types of AML. The CD68 antibodies are also able to distinguish between monocyte/macrophage and lymphoid leukemias (Appendix 2.4). Whilst this is useful in identifying granulocytic sarcoma, some B-cell neoplasms (notably small lymphocytic lymphoma and hairy cell leukemia) show weak cytoplasmic staining in the form of a few scattered granules. Mast cell proliferations and "plasmacytoid monocytes" are usually stained by both the KP1 and PG-M1 antibodies. The CD68 antigen is also expressed to varying degrees in Langerhans' and interdigitating reticulum cell sarcomas as well as Langerhans' cell histiocytosis. Other accessory cell tumors, such as follicular dendritic cell sarcomas, may be positive for CD68.

Macrophages may be present as either rare scattered cells or large cellular infiltrates in some T- and B-cell lymphomas, leading to erroneous diagnoses of histiocytic malignancies. Dual immunocytochemical labeling with CD68 antigen and T/B-cell antigen is useful in delineating the two populations. The identification of macrophages is also crucial in the diagnosis of granulomatous diseases, storage diseases, and certain types of lymphadenitis, e.g., Kikuchi's lymphadenitis. In the latter condition, macrophages phagocytosing apoptotic bodies and cells, known as "plasmacytoid monocytes" and "crescentic histiocytes," are easily recognized with antibodies against CD68, avoiding a misdiagnosis of a high-grade lymphoma.

Comments

Caution is advised in the immunophenotypic interpretation of histiocytes, since the distinction between "uptake" and "synthetic" patterns should be borne in mind. KP1 would appear to be superior to PG-M1, particularly with respect to the wider recognition of AML. The latter antibody also carries the distinct disadvantage of being demonstrated in about 10% of melanomas. Tissue rich in macrophages is suitable as a positive control.

CD68 is expressed on macrophages/monocytes, basophils, neutrophils, mast cells, dendritic cells, myeloid and CD34+ progenitor cells, B and T cells, 50% of acute myeloid leukemias, some B-cell lymphomas, hairy cell leukemia, Langerhans cell histiocytosis, mastocytosis, and some melanomas.

Selected references

Pulford KAF, Rigney EM, Micklem KJ, et al. KP1: A new monoclonal antibody that detects a monocyte/macrophage associated antigen in routinely processed tissue sections. *J Clin Pathol* 1989;42:414–21.

Pulford KAF, Sipos A, Cordell JL, et al. Distribution of the CD68 macrophage/myeloid associated antigen. *Immunology* 1990;2:973–80.

CD71

Background

CD71, also known as a transferrin receptor, represents a major cellular receptor for iron. CD71 is highly expressed in all proliferating cells because of their metabolic need for iron. Among specific cell lineages, CD71 is most highly expressed among the erythroid precursors, whose great need for iron is necessitated by heme synthesis and differentiation rather than proliferation. In iron-replete nonerythroid cells, CD71 is downregulated to prevent excessive iron intake, which can be toxic to the cell.

Applications

In the immunohistochemistry lab, where other markers of cellular proliferation are more standard than CD71 (e.g., Ki-67), CD71 is of greatest utility in identifying erythroid precursors in bone marrow specimens. Because of the high expression of CD71 on the surface erythroid precursors (it stains in a membranous pattern), it represents the best marker of this cell population in our experience. While CD71 would be expressed at lower levels among nonerythroid proliferating cells in the marrow, the disparity in expression levels between nonerythroid and erythroid cells leads to minimal background staining of nonerythroid tissues. Importantly, because of the very high level of CD71 expression in erythroid precursors, the antibody works well on virtually all decalcified bone marrow biopsies in addition to outstanding performance in nondecalcified bone marrow clots and particle preparations.

Because CD71 expression is turned on at high levels as soon as a myeloid progenitor commits to the erythroid lineage and is significantly downregulated when erythroid precursors

extrude their nuclei and become mature erythrocytes, CD71 identifies the full spectrum of nucleated erythroid precursors in the marrow, from proerythroblasts up through orthochromatic erythroblasts. Because it marks the entirety of nucleate erythroid differentiation, CD71 represents the single best marker to assess the proportion of erythroid cells among the bone marrow hematopoietic cells for the purpose of determining a myeloid to erythroid ratio. For the latter ratio, we favor using CD15 as the myeloid marker by immunohistochemistry, since it identifies all maturing granulocytes at high level and most maturing monocytes at moderate level at least.

When combined with antibodies to E-cadherin (a proerythroblast marker) and glycophorin-A (a marker of post-proerythroblast cells), this combination of antibodies can yield valuable insight about the extent to which the erythroid maturation is "left shifted" to immaturity.

While CD71 is not uncommonly used as a proliferation marker in flow cytometric evaluation of neoplastic hematolymphoid populations, other antigens such as Ki-67 are more robust for this purpose in formalin-fixed paraffin-embedded tissue.

Selected references

Dong, H., Wilkes, S., Yang, H. CD71 is selectively and ubiquitously expressed at high levels in erythroid precursors of all maturation stages: A comparative immunochemical study with glycophorin A and hemoglobin A. *Am J Surg Path* 2011;35:723–32.

Marsee, D., Pinkus, G. S., Yu, H. CD71 (transferrin receptor): An effective marker for erythroid precursors in bone marrow biopsy specimens. *Am J Clin Path* 2010;134:429–35.

CD74

Background

The CD74 antigen represents a membrane-bound subunit of the MHC Class II associated invariant chain that is encoded by the gene located on chromosome 5 region q31-q33. The monoclonal antibody LN2 recognizes nuclear and cytoplasmic antigens of molecular weights 35 kD and 31 kD, respectively, in routinely processed tissues. MB-3, another mononuclear antibody, is thought to be identical to LN2. LN2 reacts with about 50% and 75% of activated and resting L20-positive B cells in the peripheral blood and tonsils, respectively. LN2 is positive in fewer than 3% of CD 3-positive T cells. Very weak staining may be seen on circulating monocytes, and granulocytes are negative.

In lymph nodes, LN2 positivity is seen primarily in germinal center and mantle cells. Staining is strongest in small germinal center cells and in mantle cells. Plasma cells are not labeled. The vast majority of cells in the interfollicular areas are negative except for interdigitating dendritic reticular cells, which are often strongly positive. Besides distinct staining of the nuclear membrane, there may be diffuse or paranuclear cytoplasmic staining, the pattern of staining being similar in both fixed and frozen tissue sections.

Thymocytes are negative for LN2 but thymic dendritic cells may often be positive. Other cells that may be positive for LN2 include sinusoidal histiocytes, epithelioid histiocytes, splenic red pulp histiocytes, and Langhans' type giant cells. In addition, some epithelial cells and corresponding carcinomas may be positive but the staining of LN2 in these cells is often diffuse in the cytoplasm and the distinctive nuclear membrane staining is not observed.

Applications

CD74 is expressed on B cells, activated T cells, macrophages, endothelial cells, and a variety of epithelial cells and corresponding tumors.

The LN2 antibody stains about 90% and 20% of low-grade B- and T-cell lymphomas, respectively. In high-grade lymphomas, the corresponding figures are 85% and 75%, respectively, so that its value as a discriminator is lower in large-cell lymphomas. The pattern of labeling is also different. In small lymphocytic lymphoma, LN2 shows either nuclear membrane or dot-like cytoplasmic positivity, whereas in small cleaved cells nuclear membrane staining is the predominant pattern. In the mixed cell lymphomas and large-cell lymphomas, LN2 stains the nuclear membranes of the small cleaved cells, but only some of the larger cells exhibit cytoplasmic staining, the minority displaying bright cytoplasmic globules.

Reed–Sternberg cells also stain with LN2, exhibiting cytoplasmic, cytoplasmic membrane, and nuclear membrane staining in about two-thirds of cases. The antigen is expressed in about 60% of precursor B-cell acute lymphoblastic leukemia/lymphomas (ALLs/LBLs), about 50% of acute myeloid leukemias (AMLs) (excluding FAB M6 AML), most cases of chronic myeloid leukemia (CML), granulocytic sarcomas, and true histiocytic sarcomas.

LN2 has also been observed to label some epithelial tumors, including adenocarcinoma of the uterus, squamous cell carcinoma of the lung and transitional cell carcinoma of the bladder, and renal cell carcinoma.

Selected references

Schroder B. The multifaceted roles of the invariant chain CD74: More than just a chaperone. *Biochem Biophys Acta Mol Cell Res* 2016;1863:1269–81.

NOTES

CD79a

Background

Membrane-bound immunoglobulin (mIg) on human B lymphocytes is noncovalently associated with a disulfide-linked heterodimer, which consists of two phosphoproteins of 47 kD and 37 kD, encoded by the mb-1 and B29 genes, respectively. Association of IgM with the mb-1 protein is necessary for membrane expression of the B-cell antigen receptor complex. When antigen is bound to this B-cell complex, a signal transduction is transmitted to the interior of the cell, accompanied by phosphorylation of several components following induction of tyrosine kinase activity. The mb-1/B29 dimer seems to be analogous to the association of the T-cell receptor with the CD3 components.

Studies have shown that mb-1 is present throughout B-cell differentiation and is B-cell specific. Its high degree of specificity is probably a reflection of its crucial role in signal transduction after antigen binding to the B-cell antigen receptor complex.

Applications

CD79a is a marker of precursor B cells, expressed early in B-cell differentiation, and often positive when other mature B-cell markers are negative. It is expressed on megakaryocytes. CD79a has been shown on pre-T-acute lymphoblastic leukemia and rarely in peripheral T-cell lymphomas, normal T cells being negative for the antigen. As CD79a is only weakly positive in some B-cell lymphomas, it is preferable to use CD20 as the first-line marker of mature B-cell lymphomas.

The mb-1 (CD79a) chain appears before the pre-B-cell stage and is still present at the plasma cell stage. JCB117 reacts with human B cells in paraffin-embedded tissue sections, including decalcified bone marrow trephines. When applied to 454 paraffin-embedded tissue biopsies, it reacted with the majority (97%) of B-cell neoplasms. This covered the full range of B-cell maturation including 10/20 cases of myeloma/plasmacytoma. This antibody also labeled precursor B-cell acute lymphoblastic leukemia, making it the most reliable B-cell marker detectable on paraffin-embedded specimens. T-cell and nonlymphoid neoplasms were negative, indicating that JCB117 may be of value in identification of B-cell neoplasms.

The mb-1 protein has also been detected in nodular lymphocyte-predominant Hodgkin's disease using monoclonal antibody JCB117; however, only 20% of non-lymphocyte predominance cases expressed mb-1. A rare phenotypic characterization has been demonstrated in mediastinal large B-cell lymphomas, with the majority being mb-1+/Ig.

Selected references

Chu PG, Arber DA. CD79: A review. *Appl Immunohistochem Mol Morphol* 2001;9:97–106.

Mason DY, Cordell JL, Brown MH, et al. CD79a: A novel marker for B cell neoplasms in routinely processed tissue samples. *Blood* 1995;86:1453–9.

CD99 (p30/32MIC2)

Background

The p30/32MIC2 antigen, also referred to as CD99 or the MIC2 gene product, is a cell-surface glycoprotein of relative molecular mass of 30,000–32,000 that appears to be involved in cell adhesion processes. It is recognized by a number of monoclonal antibodies, including RFB-1, 12E7, HBA71, and 013, although there is some demonstrable difference in sensitivity and perhaps specificity.

CD99 was first described as a polypeptide expressed in T-cell acute lymphoblastic leukemia and T-ALL derived cell lines as well as in a subset of cortical thymocytes. CD99 was also found on a group of hematopoietic precursor cells in the human bone marrow, including terminal deoxynucleotidyl transferase-positive cells and myelo-monocyte progenitors, the expression decreasing with maturation of cells in the latter series. The MIC2 gene has been mapped to the terminal region of the short arm of the X chromosome (Xp22.32-pter) and the euchromatin region of the Y chromosome (Yq11-pter). The gene is expressed in both sexes and escapes X inactivation, making it the first described pseudo-autosomal gene in humans.

The main application of this antigen has been for the differentiation of the group of small round-cell tumors in childhood, as the marker is strongly expressed in Ewing's sarcoma and the closely related peripheral/primitive neuroectodermal tumors (PNETs). Both show strong membrane and cytoplasmic staining with clones 12E7, HBA71, and 013. Subsequent studies have also demonstrated positive staining in acute lymphoblastic lymphoma and related leukemias, and in rhabdomyosarcoma, although to a much lesser degree.

Immunoreactivity for this marker has been shown in a wide spectrum of normal tissues and ependymal cells, pancreatic islet cells, urothelium, some squamous cells, columnar epithelial cells, fibroblasts, endothelial cells, and granulosa/Sertoli cells. Among the spindle cell neoplastic tissues that show variable positivity for CD99 are synovial

sarcomas, hemangiopericytomas, meningiomas, solitary fibrous tumors, and only very rarely mesotheliomas. Epithelial tumors expressing CD99 include neuroendocrine tumors such as islet cell tumors, carcinoid tumors, and pulmonary oat cell carcinomas but apparently not Merkel cell carcinomas of the skin. Granulocytic sarcomas have been shown to stain for CD99.

Applications

CD99 antibodies have proven usefulness for the separation of Ewing's sarcoma (ES) and PNETs from the other small round-cell tumors in childhood. In addition, this marker can be employed as a diagnostic discriminator for the identification of thymic cortical T cells associated with thymic neoplasms and in the differential diagnosis of spindle cell tumors. The latter include synovial sarcoma, hemangiopericytoma, meningioma, and solitary fibrous tumors, all of which show variable extents of positivity.

The demonstration of CD99 in mesenchymal chondrosarcoma emphasizes the need for caution if this marker is to be employed as a diagnostic discriminator for small round-cell tumors. Furthermore, the immunoexpression of CD99, while most common in ES/PNET (100%), may also be seen in rhabdomyosarcoma, non-Hodgkin's lymphoma, and synovial sarcoma and needs to be used in combination with antibodies to FLI-1 and Tdt to increase the diagnostic yield.

CD99 expression in retinoblastoma is much less common compared with PNET. Ependymomas express CD99 strongly in a membranous pattern with intracytoplasmic or intercellular dots.

B-cell lymphoblastic lymphomas have also been shown to immunoexpress CD99.

Benign spindle stromal tumors of the breast, which encompass spindle cell lipoma-like tumor, solitary fibrous tumor, and myofibroblastoma, share the common immunophenotype of vimentin+/CD34+/bcl-2+/CD99+ and may have a common histogenesis.

CD99 has also been described on a number of other tumors, including superficial acral fibromyxoma, proximal epithelioid sarcoma, spindle cell epithelioma of the vagina, neuroepithelial tumors of the kidney, and tumors of sex cord–stromal differentiation.

Selected references

Stevenson AJ, Chatten J, Bertoni F, et al. CD99 (p30/32MIC2) neuroectodermal/Ewing's sarcoma antigen as an immunohistochemical marker: Review of more than 600 tumors and the literature experience. *Appl Immunohistochem* 1994;2:231–40.

Vartanian RK, Sudilovsky D, Weidner N. Immunostaining of monoclonal antibody 013 (anti MIC2 gene product) (CD99) in lymphomas: Impact of heat-induced epitope retrieval. *Appl Immunohistochem* 1996;4:43–55.

Weidner N, Tjoe J. Immunohistochemical profile of monoclonal antibody 013: Antibody that recognizes glycoprotein p30/32MIC2 and is useful in diagnosing Ewing's sarcoma and peripheral neuroepithelioma. *Am J Surg Pathol* 1994;18:486–94.

CD103

Background

The antibody to CD103, also known as anti-human mucosal lymphocyte 1 antigen (HML-1) and integrin alphaE chain, recognizes a T-cell-associated trimeric protein of 150, 125, and 105 kD, which is expressed on 95% of intraepithelial lymphocytes and only on 1–2% of peripheral blood lymphocytes. CD103 (alpha E integrin) antigen is part of the family of beta 7 integrins on human mucosal lymphocytes, which play a specific role in mucosal localization or adhesion. CD103 is a receptor for the epithelial cell-specific ligand E-cadherin and is expressed by a major subset of CD3+,CD8+,CD4– lymphocytes present in the intestinal mucosa. About 40% of isolated intestinal lamina propria lymphocytes (LPL) expressed HML-1, the majority being CD8+. Virtually all LPL expressed CD45RO, whereas only about 50% were CD29+, a percentage similar to that in peripheral blood lymphocytes. HML-1+ cells were almost exclusively CD45RA– and the in vitro expression of HML-1 was inducible on T cells by mitogen. CD103+CD8+ T lymphocytes have also been demonstrated in the bladder urothelium and its corresponding tumors, the epidermis in inflammatory skin disorders, pancreas in chronic pancreatitis, and graft epithelium during renal allograft rejection.

Applications

Antibodies to CD103 are used for the diagnosis of intestinal T-cell lymphoma. CD103 has been found to be a useful marker of B-cell hairy cell leukemia, which shows strong reactivity for CD22, CD25, CD103, and DBA.44 as well as immunoglobulin light chain restriction. The abnormal coexpression of CD103, CD25, and intense CD11c and CD20 on monomorphic, slightly large B lymphocytes has been shown to be highly characteristic of hairy cell leukemia. The antigen may be occasionally expressed by some B-cell lymphomas. The antigen has also been demonstrated in T-lymphoblastic lymphoma.

HTLV-1 associated T-cell leukemia.

Selected references

Ebert MP, Ademmer K, Muller-Ostermeyer F, et al. CD8+CD103+ T cells analogous to intestinal intraepithelial lymphocytes infiltrate the pancreas in chronic pancreatitis. *Am J Gastroenterol* 1998;93:2141–7.

Pauls K, Schon M, Kubitza RC, et al. Role of integrin alphaE (CD 103) beta 7 for tissue-specific epidermal localization of CD8+ T lymphocytes. *J Invest Dermatol* 2001;117:569–75.

CD117 (KIT)

Background

KIT is a transmembrane type III tyrosine kinase receptor for stem cell factor (SCF), a growth factor. KIT is essential for cell survival and proliferation and has a role in the proper development of hematopoietic cells, mast cells, melanocytes, and germ cells. KIT is also expressed on basal cells of the skin, breast epithelial cells, and cells of Cajal. Activation of KIT leads to subsequent activation of various transcription factors according to the cell type on which it is expressed. Congenital inactivating mutations of the KIT gene lead to a rare disorder affecting skin and hair pigmentation. Somatic activating mutations of KIT are oncogenic and have been detected in gastrointestinal stroma tumor (GIST), testicular germ cell tumor, acute myeloid leukemia, and mastocytosis. Imatinib mesylate is a tyrosine kinase inhibitor.

Applications

Expression of CD117 is of diagnostic importance in a variety of neoplastic diseases, listed in Table 1.

Table 1

Tumor	Expression Rate (%)	Notes
GIST	100	Diagnostic marker in addition to proper antibody panel
Seminoma and intratubular germ cell neoplasia	90	Diagnostic marker, in addition to proper antibody panel
Mastocytosis	100	Diagnostic marker in addition to proper antibody panel
Acute myeloid leukemia	70	Marker of myeloid origin in addition to proper antibody panel
Plasma cell neoplasms	30	Marker of neoplastic plasma cells, to be used with proper antibody panel
Merkel cell carcinoma	95	Diagnostic marker in addition to proper antibody panel
Thymic carcinoma	90	Diagnostic marker in addition to proper antibody panel; thymoma does not express CD117

CD117 is also variably expressed in a range of other tumors. One should be aware of this in order to avoid misdiagnosis of the entities in Table 1. Variable CD117 expression is seen in small cell carcinoma of the lung, large-cell neuroendocrine carcinomas of the lung, lung adenocarcinoma, squamous carcinoma of the lung, breast carcinoma, ovarian carcinoma, colon carcinoma, chromophobe renal carcinoma, and neuroblastoma. It is exceptionally seen in T-cell lymphoma, including T-cell acute lymphoblastic leukemia, and is very rarely seen in B-cell lymphoma.

Interpretation

CD117 is a membranous marker.

Selected references

Gibson PC, Cooper K. GD117 (KIT): A diverse protein with selective applications in surgical pathology. *Adv Anat Pathol* 2002;9:65–9.

Miettinen M, Lasota J. KIT (CD117): A review on expression in normal and neoplastic tissues, and mutations and their clinicopathologic correlation. *Appl Immunohistochem Mol Morphol* 2005;13:205–20.

CD123

Background

The CD123 antigen is the alpha chain of the interleukin-3 receptor (IL3 R-alpha). It is a transmembrane protein that forms a complex with the beta subunit (CD122) to form the complete, high-affinity IL3 receptor. Among normal hematopoietic cells, CD123 is most highly expressed on basophils and plasmacytoid dendritic cells and may be expressed at lower level on hematopoietic progenitor cells. Among nonhematopoietic cells that one may see in hematolymphoid tissues, CD123 tends to be highly expressed on high endothelium and may be expressed on stromal progenitor cells. Note that the common beta chain with which CD123 interacts to form the high-affinity receptor is CDw131; while an IL3-specific beta subunit has been described in the mouse, no such subunit appears present in humans.

Applications

In nonneoplastic lymphoid tissue, such as lymph node or tonsil, CD123 will uniformly identify high endothelium in a characteristic membranous pattern. Smaller numbers of nonendothelial cells identified in the nodal parenchyma will be largely plasmacytoid dendritic cells. In normal bone marrow, the scattered strongly CD123 positive cells are likely to be plasmacytoid dendritic cells, while lower-level positive hematolymphoid cells are likely to be basophils.

Again, CD123 will identify a subset of vascular endothelial cells. CD123 is expressed in the following hematolymphoid malignancies:

1) Blastic plasmacytoid dendritic cell neoplasm (BPDCN), in which CD123 is one of the important lineage-defining antigens for this entity, along with CD4, TCL1, and aberrantly expressed CD56
2) Neoplastic myeloid progenitors in a variety of myeloid neoplasms, including acute myeloid leukemia (AML) bearing the FLT3 internal tandem duplication1
3) The abnormal basophils in chronic myelogenous leukemia (CML)
4) The neoplastic B cells in hairy cell leukemia,2 but not in potential HCL mimics such as HCL-variant and splenic marginal zone lymphoma with villous lymphocytes.

Selected references

Del Giudice I, Matutes E, Morilla R, et al. The diagnostic value of CD123 in B-cell disorders with hairy or villous lymphocytes. *Haematologica* 2004;89(3):303–8.

Kussick, SJ, Stirewalt DL, Yi HS, et al. A distinctive nuclear morphology in acute myeloid leukemia is strongly associated with loss of HLA-DR expression and FLT3 internal tandem duplication. *Leukemia* 2004;18(10):1591–8.

CD138

Background

CD138 is a transmembrane heparan sulfate proteoglycan and member of the syndecan family of proteoglycans. CD138 binds to many different growth factors, cytokines, chemokines, and integrins by its heparan sulfate chains. CD138 also binds to extracellular matrix proteins such as collagen and fibronectin. It mediates cell adhesion, cell signaling, and cytoskeletal reorganization. CD138 also binds to extracellular matrix proteins such as collagen and fibronectin.

Applications

CD138 is mainly expressed in plasma cells and many mature epithelia. Its routine use is in highlighting plasma cells as part of an inflammatory infiltrate that may aid in the diagnosis of certain diseases with an important plasma cell stromal component, such as Castleman disease or IGG4-related disease; further, and more importantly, it is used in the diagnosis of plasma cell neoplasms (MGUS, smoldering myeloma, multiple myeloma, and plasmacytoma), small B-cell lymphoma with plasma cell differentiation (marginal zone lymphoma, lymphoplasmacytic lymphoma, and more rarely follicular lymphoma or chronic lymphocytic lymphoma/leukemia), or large B-cell lymphoma with plasma cell

differentiation (plasmablastic lymphoma, primary effusion lymphoma, and ALK-positive large B-cell lymphoma). It is also often used in the follow-up of plasma cell neoplasm to quantify plasma cells in the bone marrow trephine. Because of its presence in neoplasms of epithelial origin, CD138 cannot be used as proof of plasma cell origin in cases with a broad differential diagnosis. If proof of a plasma cell origin is needed, expression of cytoplasmic immunoglobulins should additionally be performed as well as other markers such as IRF4 (MUM1) or CD38.

Interpretation

CD138 is expressed on the cell membrane.

Selected references

Kambham N, Kong C, Longacre TA, et al. Utility of syndecan-1 (CD138) expression in the diagnosis of undifferentiated malignant neoplasms: A tissue microarray study of 1,754 cases. *Appl Immunohistochem Mol Morphol* 2005;13: 304–10.

O'Connell FP, Pinkus JL, Pinkus GS. CD138 (syndecan-1), a plasma cell marker: Immunohistochemical profile in hematopoietic and nonhematopoietic neoplasms. *Am J Clin Pathol* 2004;121:254–63.

CD163

Background

CD163 is a membrane protein that functions as a scavenger receptor and is part of a family of scavenger receptors including CD6 and Scart1. It is a receptor for hemoglobin–haptoglobin complexes formed during erythrocyte hemolysis. In addition, it is a receptor for the TNF-alpha-like weak inducer of apoptosis protein and for certain bacteria, including *Streptococcus mutans*, *Escherichia coli*, and *Staphylococcus aureus*, as well as certain viruses. While CD163 functions as a scavenger for the hemoglobin–haptoglobin complex, the binding of bacteria does not induce endocytosis. It leads to the production of cytokines and thus functions as a sensor. CD163 is weakly expressed in monocytes and strongly expressed in the M2 subset of macrophages, i.e., macrophages with anti-inflammatory characteristics involved in tissue repair. These macrophages do not belong to a separate lineage but represent a versatile differentiation state. Dendritic cells, including Langerhans cells, do not express CD163. CD68, lysozyme, and CD4 are, by contrast, markers of all monocyte-derived cells.

The extracellular domain of the protein may be shed into plasma. Therefore, soluble CD163 (sCD163) can be measured in serum and is associated with a variety of inflammatory conditions, including macrophage activation/hemophagocytic syndrome, Gaucher's disease, sepsis, cirrhosis, and HIV infection.

CD163 stains the membrane and cytoplasm of macrophages. Because of the membrane staining and because macrophages may have elaborate cellular extensions, care should be taken to avoid falsely ascribing CD163 expression to neoplastic cells in tumors that usually contain variable numbers of macrophages. Careful evaluation of the presence of cytoplasmic CD163 should allow the true expression to be ascribed to neoplastic cells or only to tumor-infiltrating macrophages.

Applications

CD163 is a highly specific marker of M2 macrophages. It will therefore stain many macrophages in normal lymphoid tissue as well as inflamed tissue. CD163 is relatively underexpressed on tingible body macrophages in germinal centers. By contrast, interfollicular macrophages typically do express CD163. The abnormal histiocytes in Rosai–Dorfman disease (sinus histiocytosis with massive lymphadenopathy) express CD163 in addition to S100, and both are used in diagnosis of the disease. In the majority of cases, intracellular defects in CD163 positivity in the abnormal macrophages can help identify the phenomenon of emperipolesis, in which lymphocytes or other inflammatory cells migrate through the macrophage cytoplasm, a characteristic finding of Rosai–Dorfman disease. Both markers can highlight the typical emperipolesis of lymphoid cells and plasma cells seen in the macrophages of the disease.

CD163 staining may also be used, although mostly for research purposes, for semi-quantification of M2 macrophages in several neoplasms, in which it may be correlated with prognosis. An increase of M2 macrophages is correlated with adverse prognosis in Hodgkin lymphoma and follicular lymphoma.

CD163 is one of the macrophage markers that are routinely used to diagnose histiocytic sarcoma and to differentiate it from dendritic cell sarcomas. Langerhans cell histiocytosis does not mark with CD163.

Selected references

Klein JL, Nguyen TT, Bien-Willner GA, et al. CD163 immunohistochemistry is superior to CD68 in predicting outcome in classical Hodgkin lymphoma. *Am J Clin Pathol* 2014;141:381–7.

Kridel R, Xerri L, Gelas-Dore B, et al. The prognostic impact of CD163-positive macrophages in follicular lymphoma: A study from the BC Cancer Agency and the Lymphoma Study Association. *Clin Cancer Res* 2015;21:3428–35.

Lau SK, Chu PG, Weiss LM. CD163: A specific marker of macrophages in paraffin-embedded tissue samples. *Am J Clin Pathol* 2004;122:794–801.

Nguyen TT, Schwartz EJ, West RB, et al. Expression of CD163 (hemoglobin scavenger receptor) in normal tissues, lymphomas, carcinomas and sarcomas is largely restricted to the monocyte/macrophage lineage. *Am J Surg Pathol* 2005;29:617–24.

CDK4

Background

Cyclin-dependent kinase 4 (CDK4) regulates the cell cycle by inhibiting retinoblastoma 1. The CDK4 gene is located at chromosome 12q13. Aberrant cytogenetic karyotypes containing 12q13-15 within supernumerary ring chromosomes or giant rod chromosomes including amplified copies of the CDK4 and MDM2 genes are characteristic of most cases of atypical lipomatous tumors/well-differentiated liposarcoma (ALT/WDLPS) and dedifferentiated liposarcoma (DDLPS). Amplification of chromosome 12q13-15 has been observed in well-differentiated osteosarcoma.

Applications

1. CDK4 is overexpressed in nearly all well-differentiated and dedifferentiated liposarcomas, most often in concert with MDM2. This phenomenon reflects the common presence of ring or giant marker chromosomes that contain amplified copies of the CDK4 and MDM2 genes. Diagnostic application of CDK4 or MDM2 immunohistochemistry can be used to diagnose DDLPS, as opposed to other high-grade sarcomas, and in the distinction between benign lipocytic neoplasms and ALT/WDLPS, when the latter show very minimal atypical histologic features. CDK4 also can be used to differentiate retroperitoneal liposarcoma with myxoid differentiation from myxoid/round-cell liposarcoma.

   Analogous to liposarcoma, 12q13-15 chromosome amplification has been shown to correlate with CDK4 immunoreactivity in well-differentiated osteosarcoma. This CDK4 reactivity can be useful to distinguish low-grade osteosarcoma from morphologic stimulants. Acidic decalcifying solution was reported to minimally decrease CDK4 staining intensity. Differences in CDK4 immunoreactivity in intermediate and high-grade osteosarcoma have been reported in the literature.

2. CDK4 reactivity in other types of sarcoma: chondrosarcoma of the jaw (60%), leiomyosarcoma (40%), malignant peripheral nerve sheath tumor (10%), myxofibrosarcoma (20%), embryonal rhabdomyosarcoma (25–55%), alveolar rhabdomyosarcoma (35%), undifferentiated pleomorphic sarcoma (3%), and myxoid/round-cell liposarcoma (5%).

Selected references

Binh MB, Sastre-Garau X, Guillou L, et al. MDM2 and CDK4 immunostainings are useful adjuncts in diagnosing well-differentiated and dedifferentiated liposarcoma subtypes: A comparative analysis of 559 soft tissue neoplasms with genetic data. *Am J Surg Pathol* 2005;29:1340–7.

Coindre JM, Hostein I, Maire G, et al. Inflammatory malignant fibrous histiocytomas and dedifferentiated liposarcomas: Histological review, genomic profile, and MDM2 and CDK4 status favour a single entity. *J Pathol* 2004;203(3):822–30.

Dei Tos AP, Doglioni C, Piccinin S, et al. Coordinated expression and amplification of the MDM2, CDK4, and HMGI-C genes in atypical lipomatous tumours. *J Pathol* 2000;190:531–6.

Dujardin F, Binh MB, Bouvier C, et al. MDM2 and CDK4 immunohistochemistry is a valuable tool in the differential diagnosis of low-grade osteosarcomas and other primary fibro-osseous lesions of the bone. *Mod Pathol* 2011;24:624–37.

Thway K, Flora R, Shah C, et al. Diagnostic utility of p16, CDK4, and MDM2 as an immunohistochemical panel in distinguishing well-differentiated and dedifferentiated liposarcomas from other adipocytic tumors. *Am J Surg Pathol* 2012;36(3):462–9.

CDw75

Background

The CDw75 epitope is a sialylated carbohydrate determinant generated by the beta-galactosyl alpha 2,6 sialyltransferase and has a molecular weight of 53 kD. Sialyltransferase catalyzes the incorporation of sialic acid to the carbohydrate group of glycoconjugates. Alterations on the cell surface of the oligosaccharide portion of glycoproteins and glycolipids are thought to play a role in tumorigenesis. Sialyltransferase has been found elevated in different tumor tissues and in serum of cancer patients. Further, the amount of sialic acid correlates with the invasiveness and metastasizing potential of several human tumors. Therefore, the CDw75 epitope can be viewed as a target for identifying biologically aggressive tumors.

LN1 belongs to the CDw75 group of antibodies and recognizes a sialo antigen (45–85 kD). LN1 stains B lymphocytes in the germinal center with no reaction with T cells. It also reacts with a variety of epithelial cells, including distal renal tubules, mammary glands, bronchus, and prostate.

Applications

CDw75 antigen expression has been examined in breast lesions. Duct carcinoma showed diffuse cytoplasmic staining in 21% of in situ and 35% of invasive carcinomas, respectively. No correlation was demonstrated between immunoreactivity for CDw75 in breast carcinomas and their metastatic potential. However, CDw75 was more frequently expressed in high-grade carcinomas. A positive immunoreaction was demonstrated in benign proliferating lesions: intraductal papillomas and epitheliosis in fibrocystic disease. This high frequency of immunoreactivity among the benign breast lesions was ascribed to activation of epithelial cells.

CDw75 epitope expression has also been examined in gastric carcinomas and their metastases. Approximately half were immunopositive for CDw75 antigen in the primary tumors or metastases. In contrast to breast carcinomas, a close relationship was found between antigen in primary tumors and their respective metastases. In addition, antigen expression correlated with an infiltrative growth pattern, lymphatic invasiveness, and aneuploidy, whilst no correlation was found with gastric carcinoma morphology, lymphoid infiltrate, vascular invasion, and gastric wall penetration. Hence, CDw75 expression appears to be a good indicator of biologic aggressiveness of gastric carcinoma, a finding recently confirmed. In view of the contrasting results between breast and gastric carcinoma, further studies examining CDw75 expression in these and other cancers is awaited.

LN1 is an excellent marker for B-cell lymphomas, especially follicular-derived lymphomas. In B cells, the LN1 antibody produces a typical membrane and cytoplasmic (paranuclear "dot-like" or Golgi) staining pattern. No immunoreaction is present with small lymphocytic lymphomas and T-cell lymphomas. LN1 also reacts with L & H cells in nodular lymphocyte-predominant Hodgkin's disease. In a study of CD10, bcl-6, and CDw75 as markers of follicle center cell lymphomas, it was found that CDw75 was the most sensitive (97%), closely followed by bcl-6 (90%), with CD10 being the least sensitive (79%). A combination of all three markers produced a sensitivity of 100%.

Selected references

Dunphy CH, Polski JM, Lance Evans H, et al. Paraffin immunoreactivity of CD10, CDw75 and bcl-6 in follicle center cell lymphoma. *Leuk Lymphoma* 2001;41:585–92.

CDX2 (caudal type homeobox 2)

Background

Caudal type homeobox transcription factor 2, also known as caudal-related homeobox gene 2 (CDX2), is a homeobox gene that encodes an intestine-specific transcription factor expressed early in development. It is also involved in the regulation of proliferation and differentiation of intestinal epithelial cells and is expressed in the nuclei of epithelial cells throughout the intestine, from the duodenum to the rectum. While it is not expressed in normal gastric mucosa and the distalmost portions of the intestinal tract (anal canal), CDX2 protein is expressed in primary and metastatic colorectal carcinomas. It is also expressed in intestinal metaplasia of the esophagus and stomach, intestinal-type gastric cancer, small intestinal adenocarcinomas, and mucinous neoplasms of the lung, breast, ovary, urinary bladder, and pancreaticobiliary tract.

Applications

1. CDX2 is a useful marker of intestinal-type differentiation and is expressed in the majority of colorectal adenocarcinomas. Its primary utility lies in determination of the site of origin of metastatic adenocarcinomas of unknown primary sites in both cytology and surgical pathology specimens. Though combined expression of CDX2 and cytokeratin 20 with absent cytokeratin 7 expression is useful in the diagnosis of lower intestinal adenocarcinomas, it is not specific and may be seen in intestinal-type adenocarcinomas of the cervix and sinonasal mucosa. Additionally, loss of CDX2 and CK20 is more frequently encountered in mismatch repair-deficient colorectal adenocarcinomas, which should be taken into consideration to differentiate between primary and metastatic colorectal cancer.

2. CDX2 expression is also frequently noted in primary and metastatic well-differentiated neuroendocrine tumors of the midgut and hindgut.

Selected references

Bellizzi AM. Assigning site of origin in metastatic neuroendocrine neoplasms: A clinically significant application of diagnostic immunohistochemistry. *Adv Anat Pathol* 2013;20:285–314.

Freund JN, Domon-Dell C, Kedinger M, et al. The Cdx-1 and Cdx-2 homeobox genes in the intestine. *Biochem Cell Biol* 1998;76:957–69.

Jaffee IM, Rahmani M, Singhal MG, et al. Expression of the intestinal transcription factor CDX2 in carcinoid tumors is a marker of midgut origin. *Arch Pathol Lab Med* 2006;130:1522–6.

Li MK, Folpe AL. CDX-2, a new marker for adenocarcinoma of gastrointestinal origin. *Adv Anat Pathol* 2004;11:101–5.

Werling RW, Yaziji H, Bacchi CE, et al. CDX2, a highly sensitive and specific marker of adenocarcinomas of intestinal origin: An immunohistochemical survey of 476 primary and metastatic carcinomas. *Am J Surg Pathol* 2003;27:303–10.

NOTES

c-erbB-2 (Her-2, neu, CD340)

Background

The c-erbB-2 gene is located on human chromosome 17q21 and codes for the c-erbB-2 protein (p185). The c-erbB-2 oncogene is homologous with, but not identical to, the c-erbB-1 gene, which is located on chromosome 7 and codes for epidermal growth factor receptor (EGFR). The c-erbB-2 protein is a normal cell membrane component of all epithelial cells with extracellular, transmembrane, and intracellular tyrosine kinase activity. Apart from a growth stimulatory function, it plays an important role in the motility of tumor cells. c-erbB-2 gene alterations have been reported in diverse human neoplasms and almost exclusively involve amplification of the gene. Amplification involves the repeated duplication of a particular gene sequence, resulting in multiple gene copies within each cell. This results in overexpression of the gene product, as reflected in the levels of mRNA and gene oncoprotein. There is generally good correlation of the c-erbB-2 gene amplification with overexpression.

Applications

1. c-erbB-2 has been shown to be amplified in about 20–30% of invasive breast carcinomas. There is a strong correlation with established adverse factors including large tumor size, unfavorable histologic subtype, high histologic grade, high mitotic index and proliferative activity, positive nodal status, presence of hematogenous spread, and aneuploidy. c-erbB-2 expression has also been shown to be an independent significant prognostic factor in both node-positive as well as node-negative breast cancer, and the combination of c-erbB-2 positivity and estrogen receptor negativity made it possible to identify a subgroup of patients with the worst clinical outcome. c-erbB-2 overexpression is more common in invasive ductal and medullary carcinomas than in lobular, colloid, and papillary carcinomas. In intraductal carcinomas, it is almost exclusively seen in large-cell, high nuclear grade, estrogen receptor negative, and comedo type intraductal carcinoma. (interestingly, a larger percentage of ductal carcinoma in situ [DCIS] compared with infiltrating ductal carcinoma is positive for c-erbB-2.) In situ lobular carcinoma seldom shows overexpression of the oncoprotein. Overexpression is more common in invasive tumors associated with an intraductal component than in those without, and there is usually concordance between the invasive and intraductal components of an individual tumor. Overexpression of c-erbB-2 may also serve as a predictor of response to adjuvant treatment, predicting a poor response to chemotherapy and a lack of response to endocrine therapy on relapse, and identifying those patients who are most likely to benefit from high-dose regimens as a target for immunotherapy with the humanized anti-HER 2/neu antibody, trastuzumab, particularly for patients with metastatic carcinoma.
2. Esophagogastric junction and gastric adenocarcinomas: if positive and anti-Her2 treatment is used, survival is improved.
3. c-erbB-2 immunoexpression has been demonstrated in a number of epithelial tumors, including carcinomas of the prostate, bile duct, colon and rectum, lung, and head and neck region, amongst others.

Interpretation

Occasional reports have noted discrepancies between the demonstration of amplification of the c-erbB-2 gene and detection of protein overexpression by immunostaining. Despite this drawback, immunohistochemistry now appears to be the method of choice in most institutions for assessing c-erbB-2 overexpression. A number of factors account for variability of immunohistochemical results, and these include fixation, storage, antigen retrieval, reagent optimization, antibody specificity and its domain, controls, scoring system employed, and interobserver variability. Numerous antibodies to c-erbB-2 are available, including both polyclonal and monoclonal antibodies. In general, monoclonal antibodies are considered more specific.

Only membrane staining should be accepted as positive staining. Disparate interpretation systems have been employed; some take into consideration the proportion of positive cells, some only regard the intensity of staining, while others combine the two parameters into one score. The heterogeneity of staining in any section is due to variability of fixation and embedding and probably not to intrinsic tumor properties.

The majority of publications score immunostaining of c-erbB-2 for breast cancer in the following manner:

Score 0 = no staining
Score 1+: occasional tumor cells show membranous staining that is fragmented and not circumferential
Score 2+: scattered tumor cells or small groups of tumor cells show circumferential staining
Score 3+: strong membrane staining throughout the tumor that may be associated with some cytoplasmic staining.

The area of highest intensity of staining is assessed: the area occupying at least 10–20% of the tumor in the section. Successful antigen retrieval will result in normal expression in benign epithelial cells, as c-erbB-2 is a normal gene. However, such internal controls of benign breast epithelium must not display >1+ staining. Data from clinical trials suggest that 3+ immunoexpression reflects gene amplification and 0 and 1+ are negative. Scores of 2+ should proceed to fluorescence in situ hybridization (FISH) analysis as a small portion of these cases represent true gene amplification.

c-erbB2 staining of esophagogastric junction and gastric adenocarcinomas:

Score 0 = no membranous staining or fewer than 10% of tumor cells staining in resection specimens; biopsy: no membranous staining or rare cells staining (fewer than five cohesive cells). This is regarded as negative.
Score 1+: weak staining or staining in one part of the membrane in ≥10% of tumor cells in resection; biopsy: weak staining or staining in one part of the membrane in at least five cohesive cells. This is regarded as negative.
Score 2+: weak/moderate complete or basolateral membranous staining in ≥10% of tumor cells in resection; biopsy: weak/moderate complete or basolateral membranous staining in at least five cohesive cells. This is regarded as equivocal staining.
Score 3+: strong complete or basolateral membranous staining in ≥10% of tumor cells in resection; biopsy: strong complete or basolateral membranous staining in at least five cohesive cells.

Selected references

Bobrow LG, Happerfield LC, Millis RR. Comparison of immunohistological staining with different antibodies to the c-erbB-2 oncoprotein. *Appl Immunohistochem* 1996;4:128–34.

DePotter CR. The new-oncogene: More than a prognostic indicator? *Hum Pathol* 1994;25:1264–8.

Chlamydia

Background

Chlamydia psittaci is the causative agent of psittacosis. It infects a diverse group of animals, including birds, humans, and other mammals. It is a cause of abortion in sheep, cattle, and goats. Transmission to humans is incidental, with a history of direct contact with contaminated products of conception. In pregnancy, the human host is especially vulnerable. Gestational psittacosis typically presents as a progressive febrile illness with headaches, complicated by abnormal liver enzymes, low-grade disseminated intravascular coagulopathy, atypical pneumonia, and abnormal renal function.

Applications

1. A monoclonal antibody specific for the outer membrane proteins of *C. trachomatis* is available. Diagnosis of gestational psittacosis is dependent on histopathological findings, which consist of an intense acute intervillositis, perivillous fibrin deposition with villous necrosis, and large irregular basophilic intracytoplasmic inclusions within the syncytiotrophoblast. The application of genus-specific monoclonal anti-chlamydial antibody is useful for the rapid confirmation of the diagnosis.

2. Inclusion bodies may also be demonstrated in lung tissue and secretions in atypical pneumonias caused by *C. trachomatis*. Trachoma inclusion conjunctivitis or TRIC infection is common in the tropical zones, where it is responsible for blindness. The organism initially infects the conjunctival epithelium and can be demonstrated in smears of these cells by the presence of characteristic intracytoplasmic inclusion bodies.

3. Chlamydia infection of the cardiovascular system is associated with pericarditis, endocarditis, and myocarditis. Chlamydia particles have also been observed in damaged heart valves and may be associated with lesions of arteriosclerosis and aortic aneurysm. *C. pneumoniae* was found most often in macrophages and less often in smooth muscle cells. The organism has similarly been demonstrated in atherosclerotic plaques in a variety of other vascular sites.

Selected references

Beatty WL, Morison RP, Byrne GI. Immunoelectron microscopic quantitation of differential levels of chlamydial proteins in cell culture model of persistent *Chlamydia trachomatis* infection. *Infect Immun* 1994;62:4059–62.

Chromogranin

Background

The chromogranins are a family of soluble acidic proteins of about 68 kD. They are the major proteins in the peptide-containing dense core (neurosecretory) granules of neuroendocrine cells and sympathetic nerves. Ultrastructural examination has confirmed the localization of chromogranins to the matrix of neurosecretory granules of neuroendocrine cells. While having different molecular weights, the chromogranin subunits are neither identical nor entirely dissimilar and may differ in only two or three amino acid residues, with a minimum homology between any pair of polypeptides of about 33%. The chromogranins in neuroendocrine tissues display both quantitative and qualitative variability. They occur in the highest concentration in the following rank order: the adrenal medulla; anterior, intermediate, and posterior pituitary; pancreatic islets; small intestine; thyroid C-cells; and hypothalamus.

Intracellularly, they play a role in targeting peptide hormones and neurotransmitters to granules of the regulated pathway by virtue of their ability to aggregate in the low-pH, high-calcium environment of the trans-Golgi network. Extracellular peptides formed as a result of proteolytic processing of chromogranins regulate hormone secretion. The synthesis of chromogranins is regulated by many different factors, including steroid hormones and agents that act through a variety of signaling pathways.

Applications

1. The identification of neuroepithelial/neuroendocrine differentiation in normal and neoplastic tissues as well as the neural elements of the brain and gut.
2. Chromogranin immunostaining has been employed to demonstrate argyrophilia seen in some breast cancers.
3. Aberrant immunoreactivity for chromogranin has been described in normal and neoplastic urothelium, particularly in the umbrella cells, attributed to reactivity with chromogranin-like proteins in the transitional cells.

Interpretation

As neurosecretory granules tend to be localized beneath the plasma membranes of neuroendocrine cells, their highest density is within the cytoplasmic processes characteristic of such cells. As such staining for chromogranin highlights the cytoplasmic processes often not visible in H & E stains, these processes when cut in cross section show dot-like staining.

Selected references

Hendy GN, Bevan S, Mattei MG, et al. Chromogranin A. *Clin Invest Med* 1995;18:47–65.

Claudin-5

Background

Claudin-5 is a transmembrane tight-junction protein that has a role in endothelial and epithelial cell junction barriers. It is expressed in endothelial cells and reported to be strongest in capillaries. It is also expressed in sinusoids of lymph node, inner hair shaft epithelium, sweat gland lumens, gastrointestinal epithelium, and epithelium of other viscera, including tonsil crypts, bile ducts, prostate, thyroid gland follicles, podocytes in glomeruli, and ductal epithelium of breast. In addition to being expressed in vascular neoplasms, claudin-5 is variably expressed in a variety of adenocarcinomas (lung, stomach, colon, pancreas, ovary, prostate, and endometrium) and squamous cell carcinomas as well. Amongst nonepithelial tumors, claudin-5 is expressed in epithelial component of biphasic synovial sarcoma.

Applications

1. Claudin-5 is a useful marker in the workup of vascular neoplasms. It is expressed in 100% of hemangiomas (including variants), hemangioendothelioma, and lymphangiomas.
2. Within epithelioid hemangioendothelioma, nearly all (51/58 cases) are positive with variable degrees of positivity.
3. The majority of angiosarcomas are positive for claudin-5, but the utility as a specific marker in a high-grade malignant tumor workup is limited given the widespread expression of claudin-5 in carcinomas. However claudin-5 is typically not seen in melanoma and epithelioid sarcoma.
4. Very few other sarcomas (biphasic synovial sarcoma) are claudin-5 positive.
5. Claudin-5 is typically negative in epithelioid mesotheliomas and can be useful in a panel of immunohistochemical markers when differentiating epithelioid mesothelioma from adenocarcinoma.

Comment

Claudin-5 is expressed as cytoplasmic and/or membranous positivity.

Claudin-5 is a sensitive marker to support the diagnosis of angiosarcoma and hemangioendothelioma. But since it is expressed in a variety of carcinomas, its specificity is limited.

Unlike CD31, which can stain histiocytes and plasma cells and make interpretation challenging, claudin-5 does not mark histiocytes.

Selected references

Miettinen M, Sarlomo-Rikala M, Wang ZF. Claudin-5 as an immunohistochemical marker for angiosarcoma and hemangioendotheliomas. *Am J Surg Pathol* 2011;35(12):1848–56.

c-Myc

Background

Myc protein is the product of the early-response gene myc. The myc family of oncogenes, c-myc and N-myc, on chromosome 8, encodes three highly related regulatory cycle cycle-specific nuclear phosphoproteins. Myc protein contains a transcriptional activation domain and a basic helix-loop-helix-leucine zipper DNA-binding and dimerization domain. As a heterodimer with a structurally related protein, Max, Myc can bind DNA in a sequence-specific manner, suggesting that the Myc/Max heterodimer functions as a transcriptional activator of genes that are critical for the regulation of cell growth. When overexpressed or hyperactivated as a result of mutation in certain types of cells, myc can cause uncontrolled proliferation. There is evidence that myc may have a critical role in the normal control of cell proliferation, and cells in which myc expression is specifically prevented in vitro will not divide even in the presence of growth factors. In follicular B-cell lymphomas, collaboration between myc and the bcl-2 gene occurs. If myc alone is overexpressed, cells are driven round the cell cycle inappropriately, but this does not result in lymphoma because the progeny of such forced divisions die by apoptosis. If bcl-2 is overexpressed at the same time, the excess progeny survive and proliferate, as bcl-2 acts as an oncogene by inhibiting apoptosis.

Applications

1. Squamous cell carcinoma of the head and neck: significant negative correlation has been shown between c-myc levels and the number of metastatic nodes and clinical stage of disease, but no correlation was found with tumor size or degree of differentiation.
2. c-myc protein expression in prostatic carcinoma, pituitary adenomas, ovary, lung, and colon.
3. c-myc in breast carcinoma correlates with proliferation index, differentiation, patient age, and estrogen receptor status.

Comments

Clone 9E10 is immunoreactive in formalin-fixed, paraffin-embedded tissue sections.

Selected references

Vastrik I, Makela TP, Koskinen PJ, et al. Myc protein: Partners and antagonists. *Crit Rev Oncol* 1994;5:59–68.

Collagen type IV

Background

Basal lamina is mostly formed by a dense 40–60 nm-thick layer called the lamina densa and an electron-lucent layer adjacent to the cell membrane known as the lamina lucida. A loose layer of connective tissue known as the lamina reticularis may be present under the lamina densa. Type IV collagen localizes exclusively to the lamina densa and by immunoelectron microscopy is found in both lamina densa and lamina lucida. Laminin has the same distribution but appears to be more intensely localized to the lamina lucida. Other components of basal lamina include heparin sulfate proteoglycan, entactin, fibronectin, and type V collagen, the last probably a stromal rather than basal lamina component.

Applications

1. Diagnostic applications of collagen type IV immunostaining have mostly centered around the demonstration of basal lamina in invasive tumors, particularly epithelial tumors. Demonstration of an intact basal lamina has been used to distinguish benign glandular proliferations such as microglandular adenosis and sclerosing adenosis from well-differentiated carcinoma like tubular carcinoma of the breast.
2. Immunostaining for collagen type IV has also been applied to discriminate between C-cell hyperplasia and microscopic medullary carcinoma of the thyroid. The former showed complete investment of the C-cells by a continuous rim of basal lamina, whereas the latter was typified by deficiencies of the basal lamina.
3. Immunostaining for basal lamina has been shown to be a useful way to distinguish major variants of congenital epidermolysis bullosa.
4. Fragmentation of the basal lamina has been demonstrated with collagen type IV immunostaining in the mucosa of patients with celiac disease.
5. Decreased or discontinuous staining for basal lamina has been employed to distinguish invasive foci of adenocarcinoma from misplaced submucosal epithelial deposits in adenomatous polyps.
6. Distinctive patterns of basal distribution were recently demonstrated in various types of soft tissue tumors.

Interpretation

The application of heat-induced epitope retrieval (HIER) combined with proteolytic digestion makes it possible to produce consistent immunostaining of paraffin-embedded, routinely prepared tissue sections.

Selected references

Birembaut P, Caron Y, Adnet J-J. Usefulness of basement membrane markers in tumoral pathology. *J Pathol* 1985;145: 283–96.

CXCL13

Background

C-X-C motif chemokine 13 (CXCL13), also known as B-lymphocyte chemoattractant (BLC), is a cytokine capable of inducing chemotaxis (i.e., a chemokine) in nearby responsive cells. As its alternative name implies, CXCL13 is thought to be selectively chemotactic for B cells. Together with its ligand CXCR5, CXCL13 plays a role in determining the organization of B cells within lymphoid follicles, including during normal lymph node development, and is important for subsequent immune system responses.

Applications

1. CXCL13 is a relatively specific marker for follicular helper T cells, the CD4 positive T-cell subset that typically resides in the germinal center and helps coordinate immunologic reactions in this location. In addition to CXCL13, follicular helper T cells (TFH) characteristically express CD10, bcl-6, and PD1.
2. Has clinical applications in the diagnostic workup of T-cell non-Hodgkin lymphomas. In angioimmunoblastic T-cell lymphoma (AITL), cytoplasmic CXCL13 expression is typically only seen in a subset of the neoplastic cells. Cases with cutaneous involvement by angioimmunoblastic T-cell lymphoma also express CXCL13, although only a subset of the cells are usually positive.
3. Strong expression of CXCL13 is unusual in other T-cell lymphoproliferative disorders but has been reported in some cases of peripheral T-cell lymphoma, not otherwise specified (PTCL-NOS), that are of TFH origin but lack the characteristic clinical and histologic features of AITL.
4. CXCL13 is not well described in other cutaneous T-cell lymphomas, although there is at least one report of TFH marker expression in rare cases of mycosis fungoides/ Sezary syndrome.

5. Expansions of TFH cells can also be seen in a variety of benign immunologic reactions. Several human autoimmune diseases, including systemic lupus erythematosus, autoimmune thyroid disease, myasthenia gravis, ankylosing spondylitis, and rheumatoid arthritis, are associated with increased numbers of TFH cells, and CXCL13 could potentially serve as a biomarker for some autoimmune disorders.

Interpretation

CXCL13 is typically expressed in the cytoplasm in a granular or perinuclear dot-like pattern. Immunoreactivity with CXCL13 is highly fixation dependent and is best interpreted in well-preserved, formalin-fixed, paraffin-embedded tissues.

Selected references

Burkle A, Neidermeier M, Schmitt-Graff A, et al. Overexpression of the CXCR5 chemokine receptor, and its ligand, CXCL13 in B cell chronic lymphocytic leukemia. *Blood* 2007;110:3316–25.

Dupuis J, Boye K, Martin N, et al. Expression of CXCL13 by neoplastic cells in angioimmunoblastic T cell lymphoma (AITL): A new diagnostic marker providing evidence that AITL derives from follicular helper T cells. *Am J Surg Pathol* 2006;30:490–4.

Nam-Cha SH, Roncador G, Sanchez-Verde L, et al. PD-1, a follicular T-cell marker useful for recognizing nodular lymphocyte-predominant Hodgkin lymphoma. *Am J Surg Pathol* 2008;32:1252–7.

Ortonne N, Dupuis J, Plonquet A, et al. Characterization of CXCL13+ neoplastic T cells in cutaneous lesions of angioimmunoblastic T cell lymphoma (AITL). *Am J Surg Pathol* 2007;31:1068–76.

Cyclin D1 (bcl-1)

Background

The G1 cyclin gene, cyclin D1 (PRAD-1, CCND-1), located on chromosome 11q13, exhibits characteristics of known cellular oncogenes. Cyclin D1 is a 36 kD protein with a maximum expression of cyclin Dl occurring at a critical point in the mid- to late G1 phase of the cell cycle. It plays an integral role in normal cell growth control and with cyclin-dependent kinase (Cdk), is required for completion of the G1/S transition in the cell cycle. Further, cyclin Dl inhibits the growth suppressive function of retinoblastoma tumor-suppressor protein.

Applications

1. Many neoplasms, including mantle cell lymphoma, parathyroid adenomas, and a spectrum of carcinomas including breast, supradiaphragmatic squamous cell, ovarian, and bladder transitional cell carcinomas, demonstrate overexpression of cyclin-D1 antibody.

2. Cyclin D1 overexpression was demonstrated in metastasizing papillary microadenocarcinomas of the thyroid.
3. Overexpression of the protein predicted poor prognosis in estrogen receptor–negative breast cancer patients, recurrence in nasopharyngeal carcinoma, and reduced disease-free survival in papillary bladder carcinoma.

Interpretation

Cyclin Dl is a nuclear stain. Breast cancer tissue may be used as positive control.

Selected references

Bartkova J, Lukas J, Strauss M, et al. Cell cycle-related variation and tissue-restricted expression of human cyclin D1 protein. *J Pathol* 1994;172:237–45.

NOTES

Cytokeratins

Cytokeratins (CKs) belong to a group of proteins known as intermediate filaments that constitute the cytoskeletal structure of virtually all epithelial cells (see Tables 2 and 3). Being intermediate between microfilaments (6 nm) and microtubules (25 nm), the intermediate filaments comprise five characteristic groups based on cellular origin: CKs (epithelium), glial (astrocytes), neurofilaments (nerve cells), desmin (muscle), and vimentin (mesenchymal cells). More recently, these families of cytoskeletal proteins – the intermediate filaments – have been reclassified into six subtypes. Intermediate filament proteins are composed of a 310 amino acid–residue central region known as the rod domain, which is flanked by end domains of varying length and sequence, known as the head and tail. It is these flanking sequences that are the most immunogenic, responsible for the different properties and functions of the intermediate filament proteins. Being exposed, these molecules are also sensitive to fixation artefacts due to the formation of cross-linkages. It is also important to note that due to the 30–50% sequence homology between the amino acid sequences of intermediate filaments of different types, monoclonal antibodies may cross-react with different intermediate filament types.

CKs are present in both benign and malignant epithelial cells independently of cellular differentiation. However, CK immunohistochemistry utilizing subset-selective antibodies has extended beyond the typing of epithelial tumors, with recent descriptions of nonepithelial cells and tumors expressing CK.

The CKs are a family of proteins coded by different genes, and the expression in epithelial cells is dependent on the embryonic development and degree of cellular differentiation. These CKs were identified by the biochemical properties in two-dimensional gel electrophoresis of tissue extracts with their identification based on their isoelectric points and molecular weight. Hence, two groups of CKs emerge: type I/A (CK 9–20), with an acidic isoelectric point, and type II/B (CK 1–8), with a basic-neutral isoelectric point. Apart from a few exceptions, CKs are numbered from the highest to the lowest molecular weight in each group.

An interesting phenomenon is the existence of the keratin intermediate filaments as pairs. With some exceptions, all other CKs form polymers with their corresponding member from each type. Hence, it follows that all epithelial cells contain at least two CKs. For example, whilst hepatocytes harbor a single pair of CK 8 and 18, keratinocytes may contain as many as 10 CKs.

Monoclonal antibodies to CKs may be divided into two categories: (i) a broad group that recognizes many members of the keratin family and (ii) a selective group that reacts with isolated CKs.

Table 2 Summary of the most important keratin subtypes of some epithelial tumors

Carcinoma Type	Keratin Composition (Moll's Catalog)									
	4	5	7	8	13	14	17	18	19	20
Squamous cell carcinoma, skin		+				+			+[a]	
Squamous cell carcinoma of esophagus	+				+	+			+	
Ductal carcinoma of breast			+	+		+[a]	+[a]	+	+	
Malignant mesothelioma		+	+	+		+		+	+	
Adenocarcinoma, lung			+	+				+	+	
Adenocarcinoma, colon				+				+	+	+
Adenocarcinoma, pancreas			+	+				+	+	+[a]
Hepatocellular carcinoma				+				+	+[a]	
Carcinoid tumor/small cell carcinoma				+				+	+[b]	
Merkel cell carcinoma				+				+	+	+
Renal (cell) adenocarcinoma				+				+	+[b]	
Transitional cell carcinoma, low grade	+		+	+	+			+	+	+[a]
Transitional cell carcinoma, high grade			+	+	+[a]			+	+	
Thyroid carcinoma, papillary				+				+	+	
Thyroid carcinoma, follicular				+				+	+[a]	
Adenocarcinoma of prostate			+[a]	+				+	+	
Adenocarcinoma of ovary			+	+				+	+	+[a]

[a] Occasionally present/minor component
[b] Often but inconsistently present
Modified from Miettinen, 1993

Table 3 Specificities of selected cytokeratin antibodies

Mol Wt (kD)	35βH11	34βE12	AE1	AE3	Anti-Bovine keratin	Anti-Callus keratin	Cam 5.2	KL1	MNF116
39							+		+
40			+					+	
45							+	+	+
48			+	+					
50		+	+						
51				+					
52			+	+					
52.5									
54	+								+
56					+	+	+	+	
56.5		+	+	+					
57		+						+	+
58		+		+	+				
60					+		+		
64						+			
65		+							
65.5									
66		+						+	
67		+							
68		+							

Selected references

Battifora H. Diagnostic uses of antibodies to keratins: A review and immunohistochemical comparison of seven monoclonal and three polyclonal antibodies. In: Fenoglio-Preiser CM, Wolff M, Rilke F. eds. *Progress in surgical pathology*, Vol. VIII. Springer-Verlag, Berlin, 1988, pp. 1–15.

Heatley MK. Cytokeratins and cytokeratin staining in diagnostic histopathology (commentary). *Histopathology* 1996;28:479–83.

Miettinen M. Keratin immunohistochemistry: Update of applications and pitfalls. In: Rosen PP, Fechner RE. eds. *Pathology annual*, Part 2/Vol 28. Appleton & Lange, New York, 1993, pp. 113–43.

C

Cytokeratins

Cytokeratin 5/6 (CK 5/6)

Background

Cytokeratins 5 and 6 correspond to keratins of 58 and 56 kD, respectively. CK 5 (58 kDa) is a high-molecular-weight, basic type of cytokeratin expressed in the basal, intermediate, and superficial layers of stratified epithelia, transitional epithelium, and mesothelium. CK 6 (56 kDa) is also a high-molecular-weight, basic cytokeratin expressed by proliferating squamous epithelium, palmoplantar cell, mucosa, and epidermal appendages. Although this combination of cytokeratins is expressed by a number of different epithelia, its popularity stems from its use in the diagnosis of mesothelioma. Morphologically, the mesothelium is similar to simple epithelium, and like adenocarcinomas, mesotheliomas express simple epithelial keratins such as CK 7, CK 8, and CK 19. Similarly to squamous cell carcinoma, mesotheliomas also express the stratified epithelial keratins such as CK 14, CK 5/6, and CK 17.

Applications

1. CK 5/6 is useful in discriminating between epithelial mesotheliomas and pulmonary adenocarcinomas but does not exclude metastatic carcinomas from some sites, as the latter may be positive for CK 5/6. Furthermore, as it is often negative in sarcomatoid mesothelioma, CK 5/6 is best utilized in a panel of antibodies for this differential diagnosis. CK5/6 also stains both reactive and neoplastic mesothelium.
2. It has also been suggested for use in the differential diagnosis of squamous cell carcinoma and adenocarcinoma, being positive in basal cells and stratum spinosum cells of squamous epithelium, so that the immunoexpression of CK 5/6 in a poorly differentiated metastatic carcinoma is highly predictive of a primary tumor of squamous differentiation.
3. It has been reported that intense CK 5/6 positivity in ductal hyperplasia, and negative staining of most cases of atypical ductal hyperplasia and ductal carcinoma in situ may assist in the differential diagnosis of atypical proliferations of the breast.
4. It should be noted that this marker is of low specificity for adenocarcinomas of the salivary gland and lung, squamous cell carcinoma of the lung, anus, esophagus, cervix, upper aerodigestive tract, and skin, and carcinomas of the urinary bladder, breast, and pancreas.
5. CK 5/6 immunostaining has been employed successfully as a substitute for 34βE12 for the identification of basal cells in benign prostatic glands, allowing their distinction from neoplastic glands.

Interpretation

CK 5/6 demonstrates a diffuse cytoplasm immunopositive reaction. Skin or prostate gland may be a useful source of positive control tissue.

Selected references

Chu PG, Weiss LM. Expression of cytokeratin 5/6 in epithelial neoplasms: An immunohistochemical study of 509 cases. *Mod Pathol* 2002;15:6–10.

Chu PG, Weiss LM. Keratin expression in human tissues and neoplasms. *Histopathology* 2002;40:403–39.

Cytokeratin 7 (CK 7)

Background

CK 7 antibody reacts with the 54 kDa cytokeratin intermediate filament protein isolated from human OTN II ovarian carcinoma cells and other cell lines. Identified as CK 7 according to Moll's catalog, it is a basic cytokeratin found in most glandular and transitional epithelia.

In normal tissue CK 7 reacts with many ductal and glandular epithelia but not stratified squamous epithelia. It is also reactive with transitional epithelium of urinary tract. Hepatocytes are negative, whilst bile ducts are positive. In addition, lung and breast epithelia are positive with this antibody, whilst colon and prostate epithelial cells are negative.

Applications

1. CK is expressed in specific subtypes of ovarian, breast, and lung adenocarcinoma, whilst carcinomas of the colon are negative.
2. A CK 7+CK 20− immunophenotype is helpful in distinguishing metastatic colonic adenocarcinoma from primary ovarian carcinomas, particularly the endometrioid type (with the exception of the mucinous type). Occasional ovarian mucinous carcinomas may show the same immunophenotype as metastatic colonic carcinomas (CK 7−CK 20+).
3. CK 7 is also useful to distinguish transitional cell carcinomas (+ve) from prostate cancer (−ve). The failure of CK 7 to interact with squamous cell carcinomas presents the potential for specificity for adenocarcinoma and transitional cell carcinoma.

Comments

The combined use of CK 7 and CK 20 is extremely useful in distinguishing ovarian carcinomas (except mucinous) from colonic adenocarcinomas. Serous ovarian carcinoma tissue is recommended for positive control tissue.

Selected references

Moll R, Franke WW, Schiller DL, et al. The catalog of human cytokeratins: Patterns of expression in normal epithelia, tumors and cultured cells. *Cell* 1982;31:11–24.

Cytokeratin 19 (CK 19)

Background

Cytokeratin 19, like other cytokeratins, is an intermediate filament protein and a component of the cell cytoskeleton. Cytokeratin 19, has a low molecular weight and is normally expressed in the cytoplasm of epithelial cells of the gastrointestinal tract (GIT), including the appendix, gallbladder, pancreas, tonsil, ureter and bronchus, cervical glands in the ectocervix and endocervix, epithelial cells and Hassall's corpuscles in thymus, basal keratinocytes in tongue, endometrial glandular epithelium, ducts in parotid gland and testis, pneumocytes in lung, bile ducts in liver, glandular epithelium in breast, trophoblasts in placenta, tubules in kidney, and ductal epithelium in skin.

Applications

1. It is also expressed in several malignant neoplasms, including squamous cell carcinomas of the head and neck, cervix, and lung, urothelial carcinoma, papillary thyroid carcinomas, a minority of follicular thyroid carcinomas, infiltrating ductal carcinomas of the breast, adenocarcinomas of the GIT, including appendix and colorectum, neuroendocrine tumors and neuroendocrine carcinomas of the GIT, pancreatic adenocarcinoma, cholangiocarcinoma, prostatic adenocarcinoma, mucinous and serous cystadenocarcinoma, and clear cell carcinomas of the ovary, endometrial adenocarcinoma, and extramammary Paget's disease.
2. Cytokeratin 19 positivity is an independent marker of aggressive behavior in pancreatic neuroendocrine tumors but has been shown to be a favorable marker of tumor cells of extramammary Paget's disease.

Interpretation

On a cellular level, CK 19 is typically expressed in a cytoplasmic pattern with coexisting complete or partial membranous expression. The other staining pattern noted is paranuclear dot-like accentuation with and without cytoplasmic/membrane staining.

Selected references

Ali A, Serra S, Asa SL, et al. The predictive value of CK19 and CD99 in pancreatic endocrine tumors. *Am J Surg Pathol* 2006;30:1588–94.

Chetty R. An overview of practical issues in the diagnosis of gastroenteropancreatic neuroendocrine pathology. *Arch Pathol Lab Med* 2008;132:1285–9.

Deshpande V, Fernandez-del Castillo C, Muzikansky A, et al. Cytokeratin 19 is a powerful predictor of survival in pancreatic endocrine tumors. *Am J Surg Pathol* 2004;28:1145–53.

Jain R, Fischer S, Serra S, et al. The use of cytokeratin 19 (CK19) immunohistochemistry in lesions of the pancreas, gastrointestinal tract, and liver. *Appl Immunohistochem* 2010;18:9–15.

Nechifor-Boila A, Borda A, Sassolas G, et al. Immunohistochemical markers in the diagnosis of papillary thyroid carcinomas: The promising role of combined immunostaining using HBME-1 and CD56. *Pathol Res Pract* 2013;209:585–92.

Rosai J. Immunohistochemical markers of thyroid tumors: Significance and diagnostic applications. *Tumori* 2003;89:517–19.

Ryu HS, Lee K, Shin E, et al. Comparative analysis of immunohistochemical markers for differential diagnosis of hepatocellular carcinoma and cholangiocarcinoma. *Tumori* 2012;98:478–84.

Cytokeratin 20 (CK 20)

Background

CK 20 is a low-molecular-weight cytokeratin that reacts with the 46 kD cytokeratin intermediate filament isolated from villi of duodenal mucosa.

CK 20 is less acidic than other type 1 cytokeratins and is particularly interesting because of its restricted range of expression.

In normal tissues it is expressed only in gastrointestinal epithelium, urothelium, and Merkel cells. Other epithelial cells, including breast epithelia, do not react with CD20, nor does it recognize other intermediate filament proteins.

Applications

1. Colorectal carcinomas consistently express CK 20, while gastric adenocarcinomas and other carcinomas of the gastrointestinal tract express this cytokeratin isotype less frequently. In addition, adenocarcinomas of the biliary tree, pancreatic duct, mucinous ovarian tumors, and transitional cell carcinomas are also CK 20 positive. The application of CK 20 antibody for determining the site of origin of carcinomas is useful due to the absence of CK 20 expression in adenocarcinomas of the breast, lung, endometrium, and nonmucinous tumors of the ovary.
2. Immunostaining for CK 7 and CK 20 has been shown to be useful in the differentiation of ovarian metastases from colonic carcinoma and primary ovarian carcinoma. A CK 7–/CK 20+ immunophenotype was seen in 94% of metastatic colonic carcinomas to the ovary, 5% of primary ovarian mucinous carcinomas, and none of the primary ovarian endometrioid or serous carcinomas.
3. The almost consistent staining of Merkel cell carcinoma for CK 20 and the very low frequency of CK 20 reactivity in other small cell carcinomas (except those of salivary gland origin) can help to resolve the diagnostic dilemma between Merkel cell carcinoma and metastatic small cell carcinoma. In fact, it was recently shown that CK 20 positivity in a small cell carcinoma of uncertain origin is strongly predictive of Merkel cell carcinoma, especially when the majority of tumor cells are positive. In contrast, a negative CK 20 reaction practically rules out Merkel cell carcinoma.
4. CK 20 positivity is often encountered in transitional cell carcinomas of the bladder but is rare in squamous carcinomas of that organ or adenocarcinoma of prostate.

Selected references

Chan JKC, Suster S, Wenig BM, et al. Cytokeratin 20 immunoreactivity distinguishes Merkel cell (primary cutaneous neuroendocrine) carcinomas and salivary gland small cell carcinomas from small cell carcinomas of various sites. *Am J Surg Pathol* 1997;21:226–34.

Cytokeratins: 34βE12

Background

34βE12 identifies keratins of approximately 66 kD and 57 kD in extracts of stratum corneum. The antibody reacts with keratins 1, 5, 10, and 14 in Moll's catalog (MW 68 kD, 58 kD, 56.5 kD, 50 kD, respectively). In normal tissue the antibody labels squamous, ductal, and other complex epithelia.

Applications

1. The most useful application for 34βE12 is in the detection of basal cells of the prostatic acini. 34βE12 is negative in adenocarcinoma of the prostate. In this context 34βE12 is also useful to demonstrate the basal cells in basal cell hyperplasia (partial or atypical) and atypical adenomatous hyperplasia of the prostate, the latter being difficult to distinguish morphologically from prostatic adenocarcinoma.
2. 34βE12 expression is confined to papillary carcinoma of the thyroid, whereas follicular neoplasms and hyperplastic nodules were either negative or showed focal staining.

3. 34βE12 is also consistently positive in squamous cell carcinomas, ductal carcinoma of breast, pancreas, bile duct, and salivary gland.
4. It has also been demonstrated in transitional cell carcinomas of the bladder, nasopharyngeal carcinoma, thymomas, and epithelioid mesotheliomas.
5. It is negative in hepatocellular carcinoma, renal cell carcinoma, endometrial carcinoma, mesenchymal tumors, lymphomas, melanomas, neural tumors, and neuroendocrine tumors.

Comments

It should be noted that different incubation protocols need to be followed for the prostatic and thyroid pathology applications of 34βE12.

Selected references

Moll R, Franke WW, Schiller DL, et al. The catalog of human cytokeratins: Patterns of expression in normal epithelia, tumors and cultured cells. *Cell* 1982;31:11–24.

Cytokeratins: AE1/AE3

Background

The antibody AE1/AE3 is a mixture of two monoclonal antibodies raised against human epidermal keratins. AE1 recognizes most of the acidic (type I) keratins with molecular weights 56.5, 50, 50, 48, and 40 kD. AE3 recognizes all known basic (type II) cytokeratins. This combination shows broad reactivity and is claimed to stain almost all epithelia and their neoplasms. It is also reputed not to cross-react with other members of the intermediate filaments.

Applications

1. Strong staining of AE1/AE3 has been demonstrated in adenocarcinomas (e.g., colorectal, gastric, breast, prostate), renal cell carcinoma, hepatocellular carcinoma, transitional cell carcinoma, small cell carcinoma, neuroendocrine tumors, epithelial component of pleomorphic adenoma, and squamous cell carcinoma of the skin (including the spindle cell variant), cervix, and bronchus.
2. Thymomas, mesotheliomas (including the sarcomatoid component), and chordomas consistently stain with AE1/AE3.
3. Nonepithelial tumors that demonstrate AE1/AE3 positivity include germ cell tumors (except seminomas), synovial sarcoma and epithelioid sarcoma, and leiomyosarcomas.

Interpretation

The pan-keratin marking potential of antibody AE1/AE3 places it in an ideal position to screen for neoplasms of epithelial origin, especially poorly differentiated carcinomas of diverse origin, and to distinguish these from melanoma and lymphoma. Another useful role is the identification of micrometastases, e.g., breast secondaries in lymph nodes and bone marrow.

Selected references

Battifora H. Diagnostic uses of antibodies to keratins: A review and immunohistochemical comparison of seven monoclonal and three polyclonal antibodies. In: Fenoglio-Preiser CM, Wolff M, Rilke F. eds. *Progress in surgical pathology*, Vol. VIII. Springer-Verlag, Berlin, 1988, pp. 1–15.

Cytokeratins: CAM 5.2

Background

CAM 5.2 was derived from hybridization of mouse P3/NS1/1-Ag4-1 cells with spleen cells from BALB/c mice immunized with a human colorectal carcinoma line, HT29. It comprises mouse IgG2a heavy chain and kappa light chains from spleen parent and myeloma cell lines. The antibody CAM 5.2 detects human cytokeratin epitopes with molecular weights 52 kDa and 45 kDa, corresponding to Moll's catalog numbers 8 and 18, respectively. In normal tissue CAM 5.2 reacts with secretory epithelia but not stratified squamous epithelium.

Applications

1. Anti-cytokeratin antibody CAM 5.2 is useful for the detection of adenocarcinomas, mesotheliomas, and certain carcinomas derived from squamous epithelia, the latter including spindle cell carcinomas. It should, however, be noted that some squamous cell carcinomas do not stain with CAM 5.2, e.g., those in the cervix, vagina, and esophagus.
2. The ability of CAM 5.2 to detect epithelial neoplasms but not normal stratified squamous epithelium (e.g., skin) can be used to distinguish between Paget's disease (both mammary and extramammary) and superficial spreading melanoma.
3. CAM 5.2 is especially useful in the demonstration of subtle metastatic deposits of breast carcinoma cells in lymph nodes and bone marrow. It also successfully reacts with renal cell carcinomas, hepatocellular carcinomas, and cholangio-carcinomas.
4. CAM 5.2 also detects neuroendocrine carcinomas (including small cell carcinoma and Merkel cell carcinomas), germ cell tumors (with the exception of seminoma), synovial and epithelioid sarcomas, and epithelial cells in thymomas.
5. Nonepithelial tissues that react with anti-cytokeratin CAM 5.2 include smooth muscle, rare sarcomas of breast, meningiomas, neuroblastomas, and B-cell anaplastic large-cell lymphoma.

Selected references

Battifora H. Diagnostic uses of antibodies to keratins: A review and immunohistochemical comparison of seven monoclonal and three polyclonal antibodies. In: Fenoglio-Preiser CM, Wolff M, Rilke F. eds. *Progress in surgical pathology* (Vol VIII), Springer-Verlag, Berlin, 1988, pp. 10–15.

Cytokeratins: MAK-6

Background

MAK-6 antibody cocktail contains an optimized mixture of two murine monoclonal antibodies of IgG1 isotype. Antibody kA 4 recognizes human cytokeratin types, 14, 15, 16, and 19, while antibody UCD/PR-10.11 recognizes human cytokeratin 8 and 18.

Antibody UCD/PR 10.11 was produced using shed extracellular antigen purified from MCF-7 tissue culture media and was selected for its specificity to cytokeratin types 8 and 18. Antibody KA4 was produced against human sole epidermis and was selected for its specificity to cytokeratin types 14, 15, 16, and 19.

Applications

1. Stains all cases of squamous cell carcinomas and the majority of adenocarcinomas, neuroendocrine tumors, and undifferentiated carcinomas.

2. Some expression in synovial sarcomas and epithelioid sarcomas.

Interpretation

When it is used in conjunction with other pan-keratin markers, the majority of neoplasms showing cytokeratin expression may be identified.

Selected references

Cooper D, Schermer A, Sun T-T. Classification of human epithelia and their neoplasms using monoclonal antibodies to keratins: Strategies, applications, and limitations. *Lab Invest* 1985;52:243–56.

Cytokeratins: MNF 116

Background

MNF 116 antibody detects an epitope that is present in a wide range of keratins. These comprise a number of discrete polypeptides, whose molecular weights range from 45 to 56.5 kD. These correspond to Moll's keratin numbers 5, 6, 8, 17, and probably 19. In normal tissue, the MNF 116 antibody shows a broad pattern of reactivity with epithelial cells from simple glandular to stratified squamous epithelium. Epithelial cells are labeled irrespective of ectodermal, mesodermal, or endodermal origin. However, due to the cross-reactivity with the other members of the family of intermediate filaments, this antibody (not unlike other monoclonal anti-keratin antibodies) cross-reacts with nonepithelial cells including smooth muscle, dendritic cells in lymph nodes, syncytiotrophoblasts, some cortical neurons, and a minority of plasma cells.

Applications

1. A strong pattern of staining is observed in squamous cell carcinoma (including nasopharyngeal carcinoma), small cell carcinoma, sarcomatoid carcinoma, spindle cell carcinoma, adenocarcinoma, and mesotheliomas. In small cell carcinomas, a characteristic juxtanuclear globular pattern of staining has been found to be extremely useful in identifying these neoplasms. Both epithelioid and spindle cell components of mesotheliomas react with this antibody.
2. MNF 116 is also useful in confirming the diagnosis in a wide range of soft tissue neoplasms. Monophasic and biphasic synovial sarcomas demonstrate strong positivity (albeit focal in the spindle cells).
3. Vascular neoplasms that react with this broad-range cytokeratin antibody include epithelioid hemangioendothelioma (focal), epithelioid angiosarcoma, and sinonasal hemangiopericytoma. Epithelioid sarcoma, desmoplastic small round-cell tumors, chordomas, and extra-renal rhabdoid tumors are consistently positive.
4. Mixed tumors and myoepitheliomas also express pan-keratin.
5. Among germ cell tumors, embryonal carcinoma and yolk sac tumors are consistently positive with MNF 116.
6. Aberrant staining with MNF 116 is seen in smooth muscle tumors, plasmacytoma, and primitive neuroectodermal tumors, and rarely, myofibroblasts may demonstrate focal cytokeratin positivity.

Comments

Any epithelial tissue – glandular or squamous – is suitable for use as positive control for MNF116.

Selected references

Miettinen M. Keratin immunohistochemistry: Update of applications and pitfalls. In: Rosen PP, Fechner RE. eds. *Pathology Annual*, Part 2/Vol 28. Appleton & Lange, New York, 1993, pp. 113–43.

Moll R, Franke WW, Schiller DL, et al. The catalog of human cytokeratins: Patterns of expression in normal epithelia, tumors and cultured cells. *Cell* 1982;31:11–24.

Cytomegalovirus (CMV)

Background

The CCH2 clone recognizes a 43 kD protein, whilst the DDG9 clone recognizes a 76 kD protein, both having been demonstrated in glycine-extracted CMV antigen. These proteins are expressed in the immediate early and early stage of CMV replication in infected cells. Early viral proteins are expressed in the nucleus of infected cells within 6–24 hours of infection and prior to viral DNA replication. Several late viral proteins may be demonstrated in the nucleus and the cytoplasm of infected cells. The different viral proteins can be demonstrated in infected cell cultures as well as in infected tissue. These antibodies do not cross-react with adenoviruses or other herpes viruses.

Applications

These antibodies to CMV demonstrate the virus in infected cells producing a nuclear immunopositive reaction. However, at a later stage, both nuclear and cytoplasmic immunoreaction with the early CMV antigen is seen. Antibodies to CMV have a wide application to diagnostic surgical pathology, especially when characteristic CMV inclusions are not clearly evident. CMV infection (latent or active) may be seen in salivary glands, lungs, kidneys, gastrointestinal tract, and lymph nodes. Awareness of CMV as an opportunistic infection in the context of immunosuppression invokes the use of CMV immunohistochemistry for definitive diagnosis. Chemotherapy toxicity may mimic CMV gastritis, necessitating CMV immunohistochemistry to exclude false-positives. Antibodies to CMV may also be applied for the identification of atypical CMV inclusions in gastrointestinal mucosal biopsy specimens, where classic inclusions are rarely found.

Interpretation

It has been shown that immunohistochemistry with CCH2 detects a higher number of CMV infected cells than in situ hybridization. Hence, for routine diagnostic purposes at least, CMV immunohistochemistry would appear to be the method of choice for a rapid, sensitive, and specific method of CMV detection.

Selected references

Swenson PD, Kaplan MH. Rapid detection of cytomegalovirus in cell culture by indirect immunoperoxidase staining with monoclonal antibody to an early nuclear antigen. *J Clin Microbiol* 1985;21:669–73.

Zweygberg WB, Wirgart B, Grillner L. Early detection of cytomegalovirus in cell culture by a monoclonal antibody. *J Virol Methods* 1986;14:65–9.

Cytotoxic molecules (TIA-1, granzyme B, perforin)

Background

Natural killer cells and cytotoxic T lymphocytes are characterized by the presence of cytoplasmic granules that are released in response to target cell recognition. Among the wealth of cytotoxic molecules found in cytotoxic cells, perforin and granzyme B are two well-characterized proteins involved in one major pathway leading to apoptosis in target cells. Perforin allows the entry of granzyme molecules into the target cells, which then activate the apoptotic protease CPP32. The genes for perforin and granzyme B have been cloned and antibodies directed against these molecules have been generated. T-cell-restricted intracellular antigen (TIA-1), another molecule found in cytotoxic cells, is recognized by the antibody. The exact function of TIA-1 has not been elucidated. Since it induces DNA fragmentation of digitonin-permeabilized thymocytes, it may be implicated in the killing induced by cytotoxic lymphocytes. TIA-1 has been demonstrated in many intestinal intraepithelial lymphocytes of normal proximal small intestine and a corresponding increase of TIA-1 positive cells in active celiac disease.

Applications

1. The expression of all the three cytotoxic molecules appears to be largely restricted to cytotoxic cells. Granzyme B, TIA-1, and perforin have been demonstrated in the majority of intestinal T-cell lymphomas but not in intestinal B-cell lymphomas and CD8-negative peripheral nodal T-cell lymphomas. Antibody 2G9, which recognizes TIA-1, proved to be the most sensitive immunohistological marker.
2. Anaplastic large-cell lymphomas of T cell (T-ALCL) have also been shown to express cytotoxic molecules with antibody GB9 to granzyme B whilst being absent in B-cell anaplastic large-cell lymphomas, proving that T-ALCL are derived from activated cytotoxic T cells.
3. Granzyme B-positive T-cell lymphomas have also been mainly found in mucosa-associated lymphoid tissue, being more often associated with angioinvasion: nasal, gastrointestinal tract, and lung.
4. It has also been shown that immunohistochemical staining with anti-TIA-1 can be used to identify cytolytic T lymphocytes in epidermal lesions of human graft versus host disease.
5. Cutaneous CD8+ and CD56+ lymphomas appear to show different expressions of cytotoxic molecules, with the former expressing only one or two of the cytotoxic proteins compared with the latter, which expresses the entire panel of cytotoxic antigens.
6. Primary CD30+ cutaneous lymphomas and lymphomatoid papulosis frequently express at least one of the cytotoxic proteins.
7. Sinonasal lymphomas of CD3+ CD56+ phenotype invariably express all three cytotoxic antigens and Epstein–Barr viral RNA but not CD57.

Interpretation

Until recently, it was impossible to differentiate most functional T-cell subsets, e.g., suppressor and cytotoxic T cells, by membrane characteristics on paraffin-embedded tissue. The production of monoclonal antibodies against cytotoxic molecules has enabled the identification of the major components of the cytotoxic granules found in the cytoplasm of activated cytotoxic and natural killer cells. Intestinal T-cell lymphomas provide an ideal positive control for antibodies to cytotoxic molecules.

Selected references

Anderson P, Nagler-Anderson C, O'Brien C, et al. A monoclonal antibody reactive with a 15-kDa cytoplasmic granule associated protein defines a subpopulation of CD8+ T lymphocytes. *J Immunol* 1990;144:574–82.

D2-40

Background

Podoplanin or D2-40 clone reacts with a transmembrane O-linked sialoglycoprotein (mol. wt. 40 kilodaltons), found on lymphatic endothelium, ovarian and testicular germ cells, placenta (endothelium), lung (alveolar epithelium), brain, reticular cells, follicular dendritic cells, and myoepithelial cells. D2-40 clone does not react with vascular endothelium. It is functionally suggested to be involved in cell migration and actin cytoskeletal organization. This antibody is useful to differentiate between choroid plexus carcinoma and metastatic carcinoma, as well as for differentiating mesothelioma from adenocarcinoma.

Applications

1. Expressed in endothelial cells of tumors of lymphatic origin (100%), Kaposi's sarcomas (95–100%), and hemangioendothelioma (95%).
2. Mesotheliomas (85%) and brain tumors such as cerebellar hemangioblastoma, anaplastic ependymomas (100%), some medulloblastomas, glioblastoma, pineal germinoma (100%), craniopharyngioma (100%), choroid plexus papilloma (100%), choroid plexus carcinoma (100%), and meningioma (90%).
3. Other tumors: Squamous cell carcinoma of head and neck region, uterine cervix, breast carcinoma, skin adnexal tumors, seminomas, dysgerminomas, adrenal cortical carcinoma, schwannoma, epithelioid malignant peripheral nerve sheath tumor, distal epithelioid sarcoma, skeletal myxoid chondrosarcoma, and chondroid and chordoid tumors.

Interpretation

It is a membrane stain.

Selected references

Kahn HJ, Bailey D, Marks A. Monoclonal antibody D2-40, a new marker of lymphatic endothelium, reacts with Kaposi's sarcoma and a subset of angiosarcomas. *Mod Pathol* 2002;15:434–40.

Chu AY, Litzky LA, Pasha TL, et al. Utility of D2-40, a novel mesothelial marker, in the diagnosis of malignant mesothelioma. *Mod Pathol* 2005;18:105–10.

Kalof AN, Cooper K. D2-40 immunohistochemistry – so far! *Adv Anat Pathol* 2009;16: 62–4.

DBA.44 (hairy cell leukemia)

Background

DBA.44 recognizes an unknown fixation-resistant B-cell differentiation antigen expressed by mantle zone lymphocytes, reactive immunoblasts, monocytoid B cells, and a small proportion of high- and low-grade lymphomas. The monoclonal antibody was one of four generated against a B-lymphoma cell line (DEAU-cell line) grafted in athymic nude mice. Within the group of low-grade B-cell lymphomas, DBA.44 reacted principally with hairy cell leukemia. Among node-based lymphomas, the strongest membrane staining was observed in centroblastic, immunoblastic, and monocytoid B-cell lymphomas.

Applications

1. Hairy cell leukemia shows strong positive staining of the "hairy" surface membranes in routinely fixed and decalcified bone marrow biopsies. Also, proven usefulness of DBA.44 in the detection of minimal residual disease following treatment. DBA.44 appears to be a more sensitive marker of hairy cells than the traditional tartrate-resistant acid phosphatase (TRAP) activity.
2. Mantle zone lymphocytes and their corresponding lymphoma are DBA.44 positive.
3. Monocytoid B-cell lymphoma: DBA.44 observed in only occasional cases.

Selected references

Cordone I, Annino L, Masi S, et al. Diagnostic relevance of peripheral blood immunocytochemistry in hairy cell leukaemia. *J Clin Pathol* 1995;48:955–60.

Hounieu H, Chittal SM, al Saati T, et al. Hairy cell leukaemia: Diagnosis of bone marrow involvement in paraffin-embedded sections with monoclonal antibody DBA.44. *Am J Clin Pathol* 1992;98:26–33.

Deleted in pancreatic cancer locus 4 (DPC4/SMAD4)

Background

DPC4, also known as *SMAD4*, is a tumor suppressor gene that encodes a member of the Smad family of signal transduction proteins. DPC4 acts as a cofactor that binds transforming growth factor-beta (TGFβ) receptor-activated serine threonine receptor kinases, Smad2 and Smad3, thereby generating transcriptional complexes. These complexes then translocate to the nucleus, bind to a specific sequence of DNA, and regulate the transcription of target genes. Consequently, DPC4 plays a pivotal role in SMAD-mediated transcriptional activation.

Defects in *SMAD4* are a cause of juvenile polyposis syndrome (JPS), an autosomal dominant gastrointestinal hamartomatous polyposis syndrome in which patients are at risk for developing colonic and other gastrointestinal cancers. Defects in SMAD4 are also a cause of juvenile polyposis/ hereditary hemorrhagic telangiectasia syndrome (JP/HHT).

Inactivation or deletion of *DPC4* is a late event in the neoplastic progression of pancreatic cancer and is found in about half of cases.

Applications

1. Immunohistochemical expression of DPC4 recapitulates the genetic status of *DPC4* in pancreatic adenocarcinoma. Pancreatic cancer patients with retained DPC4 expression have been shown to have significantly longer survival as compared with those lacking DPC4 expression, and loss of DPC4 expression by immunohistochemistry may be used as a marker of poorer prognosis.
2. Loss of Dpc4 expression in colonic adenocarcinomas also correlates with the presence of metastatic disease and is associated with lymph node metastases in gastric cancer.

Selected references

Lagna G, Hata A, Hemmati-Brivanlou A, et al. Partnership between DPC4 and SMAD proteins in TGF-beta signalling pathways. *Nature* 1996;383:832–6.

Maitra A, Molberg K, Albores-Saavedra J, et al. Loss of Dpc4 expression in colonic adenocarcinomas correlates with the presence of metastatic disease. *Am J Pathol* 2000;157:1105–11.

Wilentz RE, Iacobuzio-Donahue CA, Argani P, et al. Loss of expression of Dpc4 in pancreatic intraepithelial neoplasia: Evidence that DPC4 inactivation occurs late in neoplastic progression. *Cancer Res* 2000;60:2002–6.

Wilentz RE, Su GH, Dai JL, et al. Immunohistochemical labeling for dpc4 mirrors genetic status in pancreatic adenocarcinomas: A new marker of DPC4 inactivation. *Am J Pathol* 2000;156:37–43.

Xia X, Wu W, Huang C, et al. SMAD4 and its role in pancreatic cancer. *Tumour Biol* 2015;36:111–19.

NOTES

Desmin

Background

Desmin belongs to the class of "intermediate" (10 nm) filaments and is a cytoplasmic protein, which is characteristically found in myogenic cells. It has a molecular weight of 53 kDa and is composed of an N-terminal "headpiece" and a C-terminal "tailpiece," both of which are nonhelical in conformation. The two pieces bracket an α-helical middle domain of about 300 amino acid residues, which is highly conserved from species to species, with striking interspecies homology. This homology is even higher than that exhibited between intermediate filament proteins in the same species, with cytokeratin, vimentin, glial fibrillary acidic protein, neurofilaments, and desmin exhibiting sequence homology of about 30%. In smooth muscle cells, desmin is associated with cytoplasmic dense bodies and subplasmalemmal dense plaques, and in striated muscle it is linked to sarcomeric Z disks. Muscle cells depleted of desmin (skeletin) are still able to contract in response to adenosine triphosphate and calcium, suggesting that desmin plays no role in contractility but, rather, serves to maintain the relationship and orientation of actin and myosin filaments and to anchor them to the plasmalemma. Desmin also serves a nucleic acid–binding function, is susceptible to processing by calcium-activated proteases, and is a substrate for cyclic adenosine monophosphate–dependent protein kinases. With its shared structural homology to laminins, the proteins of the nuclear envelope, desmin may also serve as a modulator between extracellular influences governing calcium flux into the cell and may have a role in nuclear transcription and translation. These newer roles of the intermediate filaments, including desmin, relegate the supportive cytoskeletal function of intermediate filaments to a secondary role.

Applications

1. Smooth muscle tumors: Desmin is widely used to support the diagnosis of smooth muscle differentiation. Leiomyomas from all sites and histologic variants (such as angio-, myo-, and lipoleiomyomas) all show consistent desmin positivity.
   In leiomyosarcomas, desmin positivity is variable, ranging from 59% to 86% of cases, and degree/extent of expression decreased in high-grade leiomyosarcoma cases.
   Desmin, along with CD10 and h-caldesmon, is used to separate uterine smooth muscle tumors from endometrial stromal neoplasms (ESN). Typically, ESN are negative for desmin and when positive show weak or focal positivity.
2. Myofibroblastic lesions: Focal staining for desmin can be seen in tumors of myofibroblastic differentiation, such as fibromatosis, dermatofibrosarcoma protuberans, inflammatory pseudotumor, and postoperative spindle cell nodule Skeletal muscle tumors: Desmin is seen in rhabdomyomas and 100% of rhabdomyosarcomas (RMS) and does not help to distinguish between various RMS types.
3. Fibrohistiocytic tumors: Desmin can be expressed in fibrohistiocytic tumors, including benign fibrous histiocytomas, and up to approximately 50% of angiomatoid fibrous histiocytomas are diffusely or patchily desmin positive.
4. Mesothelial cells: Reactive/benign mesothelial cells have been shown to be strongly positive for desmin in cell block preparations of serous fluids but not expressed by malignant mesothelioma and adenocarcinoma, suggesting that desmin may be a useful marker to separate these three entities. Other muscle markers, including actin, myoglobin, and myogenin, are not expressed by the reactive mesothelial cells.
5. Other miscellaneous tumors: Desmin expression is also seen in other tumors with polyphenotypic expression, including desmoplastic small round cell tumor, atypical teratoid/rhabdoid tumor, and other tumors including anaplastic plasmacytoma, melanoma, and a very small percentage (2%) of GIST. Other tumors that can occasionally express desmin include PEComa, mammary

myofibroblastoma, myofibroblastic sarcoma, ossifying fibromyxoid tumor, and biphenotypic sinonasal sarcoma.

6. Vulvovaginal mesenchymal tumors: Most tumors show desmin positivity, such as angiomyofibroblastoma, aggressive angiomyxoma, and fibroepithelial stromal polyp. Tumors that are typically desmin negative include cellular angiofibroma and superficial angiomyxoma.

Selected references

Azumi N, Ben-Ezra J, Battifora H. Immunophenotypic diagnosis of leiomyosarcomas and rhabdomyosarcomas with monoclonal antibodies to muscle-specific actin and desmin in formalin-fixed tissue. *Mod Pathol* 1988;1: 469–74.

Li Z, Colucci E, Babinet C, Paulin D. The human desmin gene: A specific regulatory program in skeletal muscle both in vitro and in transgenic mice. *Neuromuscul Disord* 1993;3: 423–7.

Nagai J, Capetanaki YG, Lazarides E. Expression of the genes coding for the intermediate filament proteins vimentin and desmin. *Ann N Y Acad Sci* 1985;455:144–55.

Pollock L, Rampling D, Greenwald SE, et al. Desmin expression in rhabdomyosarcoma: Influence of the desmin clone and immunohistochemical method. *J Clin Pathol* 1995;48: 535–8.

Desmoplakins

Background

Epithelial cells contain complexes of cytokeratin filaments (tonofilaments) associated with specific domains of the plasma membrane that appear as symmetrical junctions known as desmosomes or as asymmetrical hemi-desmosomes. These regions of filament–membrane attachment are characterized by 14–20 nm thick dense plaque; these desmosomal plaques comprise a dense mixture of intracellular attachment proteins including plakoglobin and desmoplakins. Transmembrane linker proteins, which belong to the cadherin family of cell–cell adhesion molecules, bind to the plaques and interact through their extracellular domains to hold the adjacent membranes together by a Ca^{2+}-dependent mechanism. Desmoplakins I and II (DPI and DPII) are two polypeptides that make up the desmoplakins and are of molecular mass 46 and 24 kD, respectively, suggesting that DPI may be a dimer in solution and DPII a monomer.

Applications

1. The widespread presence of desmosomes in epithelial cells and their corresponding tumors makes the presence of desmoplakins a specific marker of epithelial differentiation. Unfortunately, these proteins are fixative sensitive, restricting the use of antibodies to desmoplakins to fresh cellular preparations or frozen sections. Applications in diagnostic pathology have therefore been limited to some studies in bullous skin diseases. In autoimmune acantholytic diseases such as pemphigus vulgaris and pemphigus erythematosus, desmoplakins are intact even in acantholytic cells, whereas in Hailey-Hailey's disease and Darier's disease the normal plasma membrane localization of desmoplakins is lost and the protein is internalized and present diffusely in the cytoplasm.

2. Desmoplakins have been demonstrated in follicular dendritic cells and their corresponding tumors. More recent studies employing anti-desmoplakins have included the progression of squamous intraepithelial lesions of the uterine cervix, where the assembly of desmosomes has been shown to be affected during progression of atypia with a dramatically decreased expression of desmoplakins and desmogleins.

Comments

Acetone fixation followed by plastic embedding allows the immunostaining of the desmoplakins in permanent sections. Trypsin digestion needs to be employed.

Selected references

O'Keefe EJ, Erickson HP, Bennett V. Desmoplakin I and desmoplakin II: Purification and characterization. *J Biol Chem* 1989;264:8310–18.

DOG-1

Background

Discovered on GIST-1 (DOG-1) was identified initially by gene expression profiling of sarcomas and is a chloride channel protein. In other contexts, DOG-1 was named as the tumor amplified and overexpressed sequence 1 (TAOS2), ORA cancer OVerexpressed 2 (ORAOV2), FLJ10261, and TMEM16A/Anoctamin-1 (ANO1). FLJ10261 was identified by analysis of chromosomal region 11q13 and was demonstrated to be expressed in silico in carcinomas of the esophagus, bladder, head and neck, breast, pancreas, and stomach and parathyroid tumors. TMEM16A/ANO1 has been demonstrated to be a Ca2+-activated chloride conductance channel.

DOG-1 is a marker of interstitial cells of Cajal. Normal tissue DOG-1 reactivity has been reported in the gastric foveolar epithelium, basilar cells of squamous epithelia, breast duct epithelium, endometrium, epithelia of the bile duct, dermal eccrine gland, and salivary acinar and intercalated ducts.

Applications

1. Antibodies to DOG-1 are useful for diagnosing gastrointestinal stromal tumors (GIST), and it exhibits a high sensitivity for GIST. DOG-1 combined with KIT (CD117) detects up to 95% of GISTs. DOG-1 is often positive in KIT-negative cases that often have *PDGFRA* mutations. Aside from occasional smooth muscle tumors, most tumors in the differential diagnosis of GIST are DOG-1 negative, including desmoid tumor, endometrial stromal sarcoma, inflammatory fibroid polyp, inflammatory myofibroblastic tumor, Kaposi sarcoma, liposarcoma, malignant peripheral nerve sheath tumor, melanoma, PEComa, schwannoma, solitary fibrous tumor, and undifferentiated sarcoma. Areas of dedifferentiation within GIST can lose DOG-1 expression.
2. A subset of benign and malignant smooth muscle tumors of the uterus and gastrointestinal tract are DOG-1 positive.

3. DOG-1 is positive in chondroblastoma, and focal reactivity is seen in synovial sarcoma and solid pseudopapillary neoplasms of the pancreas.
4. DOG-1 reactivity has been demonstrated in carcinoma of the head and neck, esophagus, and adenocarcinoma (stomach, lung, colon, and endometrium) and is detected in salivary gland acinic cell carcinomas.

Interpretation

DOG-1 immunopositivity is cytoplasmic and membrane in location.

Selected references

Chênevert J, Duvvuri U, Chiosea S, et al. DOG1: A novel marker of salivary acinar and intercalated duct differentiation. *Mod Pathol* 2012;25:919–29.

Choi JJ, Sinada-Bottros L, Maker AV, et al. Dedifferentiated gastrointestinal stromal tumor arising de novo from the small intestine. *Pathol Res Pract* 2014; 210:264–6.

Espinosa I, Lee CH, Kim MK, et al. A novel monoclonal antibody against DOG1 is a sensitive and specific marker for gastrointestinal stromal tumors. *Am J Surg Pathol* 2008;32:210–18.

Hemminger J, Iwenofu OH. Discovered on gastrointestinal stromal tumours 1 (DOG1) expression in non-gastrointestinal stromal tumour (GIST) neoplasms. *Histopathology* 2012;61:170–7.

Liegl B, Hornick JL, Corless CL, et al. Monoclonal antibody DOG1.1 shows higher sensitivity than KIT in the diagnosis of gastrointestinal stromal tumors, including unusual subtypes. *Am J Surg Pathol* 2009;33:437–46.

Miettinen M, Wang ZF, Lasota J. DOG1 antibody in the differential diagnosis of gastrointestinal stromal tumors: A study of 1840 cases. *Am J Surg Pathol* 2009;33:1401–8.

Sah SP, McCluggage WG. DOG1 immunoreactivity in uterine leiomyosarcomas. *J Clin Pathol* 2013;66:40–3.

E-cadherin/N/97-cadherin

Background

The cadherin family includes several distinctive members, two of which are E (epithelial)-cadherin, a 120 kD protein expressed in epithelial cells and concentrated in cell–cell adherens junctions, and N (nerve)-cadherin, a 135 kD protein expressed in nerve cells, developing skeletal muscle, embryonic and mature cardiac muscle cells, and pleural mesothelial cells. The *E-cadherin* gene (CDH1) is located on chromosome 16q22.1, a region frequently affected with loss of heterozygosity in sporadic breast carcinoma. During embryonic development, expression of distinctive members of the cadherin family determines the aggregation of cells into specialized tissues as they interact with identical cadherins within the same tissue. Hence, the mesoderm-derived mesothelial cells that form the pleura express N-cadherin, whilst epithelial cells of the lung express E-cadherin.

Applications

1. High level of expression of N-cadherin in all mesotheliomas and E-cadherin in all pulmonary adenocarcinomas.
2. Ovarian epithelial tumors: Both E- and N-cadherins are expressed in serous and endometrioid tumors, whilst mucinous tumors strongly express E-cadherin only. The expression of N-cadherin in serous and endometrioid tumors traces their origin to the mesoderm-derived ovarian surface epithelium.
3. Reduction in E-cadherin expression has been associated with lack of cohesiveness, high malignant potential, and invasiveness in epithelial neoplasms of the colon, ovary, stomach, pancreas, lung, breast, and head/neck.
4. N-cadherin has also been demonstrated in astrocytomas/glioblastomas and rhabdomyosarcomas.
5. Breast cancer: Downregulation of E-cadherin has been suggested to be a predictive marker of nodal metastasis in breast cancer, and loss of E-cadherin is considered to be a fundamental defect in diffuse-type gastric carcinoma and infiltrating lobular carcinoma of the breast. Invasive lobular breast carcinomas, which are typically completely E-cadherin negative, often show inactivating mutations in combination with loss of heterozygosity of the wild type *CDH1* allele. Ductal breast carcinomas in general show heterogeneous loss of E-cadherin expression, associated with epigenetic transcriptional downregulation.

Interpretation

Malignant mesothelioma and colonic adenocarcinoma tissue are recommended for use as positive controls for N- and E-cadherin, respectively. We have found trypsin predigestion followed by heat-induced epitope retrieval (HIER) to produce the greatest immunoreactivity for these antigens, particularly E-cadherin.

Selected references

Hedrick L, Cho KR, Vogelstein B. Cell adhesion molecules as tumor suppressors. *Trends Cell Biol* 1993;3:36–9.

Madhavan M, Srinivas P, Abraham E, et al. Cadherins as predictive markers of nodal metastasis in breast cancer. *Mod Pathol* 2001;14:423–7.

Matsuura K, Kawanishi J, Jujii S, et al. Altered expression of E-cadherin in gastric cancer tissues and carcinomatous fluid. *Br J Cancer* 1992;66:1122–30.

Epidermal growth factors: TGF-α and EGFR

Background

Transforming growth factors (TGF) were discovered due to their ability to transform fibroblasts to a malignant phenotype. Two distinct polypeptides were subsequently isolated: TGF-α and TGF-β. TGF-α is a polypeptide of 50 amino acids and is acid and heat stable. TGF-α belongs to the epidermal growth factor family, members of which share a common amino acid sequence and biological activities. They also bind to a common receptor, epidermal growth factor receptor (EGFR), on target cells.

EGFR is a 170 kD protein comprising a cell surface ligand-binding transmembrane domain and a highly conserved cytoplasmic tyrosine kinase domain. When TGF-α binds to EGFR, tyrosine kinase of the receptor is activated. This is followed by phosphorylation and an increase in cytosolic calcium ions within target cells. The resultant effect is increased DNA synthesis with proliferation and differentiation of the cell.

TGF-α is a potent growth stimulator and is distributed in both fetal and adult tissues, playing a role in the physiological regulation of normal growth and differentiation.

Applications

1. TGF-α is an important growth factor for transformation of various cell types to a malignant phenotype. The coexpression of both the ligand (TGF-α) and its receptor (EGFR) has been documented in a variety of carcinomas – both gastrointestinal and nongastrointestinal carcinomas.
2. The EGFR antibody reacts with the majority of squamous cell carcinomas arising from both squamous epithelium and metaplastic squamous epithelium. The expression of the EGF receptor may also be of prognostic value in breast cancer, although some studies showed no association with cancer-specific survival, tumor size, lymph node status, histologic grade, c-erbB-2, and hormone status.
3. EGFR is universally expressed in gastrinomas, and overexpression correlates with aggressive growth and lower curability.
4. In invasive thymoma EGFR has also been found to be strongly expressed, suggesting a potential therapeutic target.

Selected references

Carpenter G. Properties of the receptor for epidermal growth factor. *Cell* 1984;37:357–8.

Chen WS, Lazar CS, Lund KA, et al. Functional independence of the epidermal growth factor receptor from a domain required for ligand-induced internalization and calcium regulation. *Cell* 1989;59:33–43.

Epithelial membrane antigen

Background

Anti-epithelial membrane antigen (EMA) antibodies recognize a group of closely related high-molecular-weight transmembrane glycoproteins with high carbohydrate content. The *MUC1* gene, located on chromosome 1 in the 1q21–24 region, encodes EMA. EMA is very similar to the human milk fat globule (HMFG). A heterogeneous population of HMFG proteins can be recovered from the aqueous phase of skimmed milk following extraction in chloroform and methanol. EMA is related to the high-molecular-weight glycoproteins of HMFG, especially to HMFG2. Preparations of EMA reacted with polyclonal antibodies raised to delipidized HMFG with avid binding to wheat germ agglutinin and peanut agglutinin. A similar mucin-containing glycoprotein was solubilized from HMFG and labeled PAS-O because of reactivity for PAS. PAS-O and EMA represent closely allied glycoprotein moieties with common antigenic determinants on both proteins. From a practical standpoint, patterns of immunoreactivity for EMA and HMFG are very similar.

Applications

1. EMA can be used as a marker of epithelial cells, although there are other (better) markers available to demonstrate an epithelial origin of cells.
2. EMA has been used in mesenchymal tumors, including synovial sarcoma, anaplastic large cell lymphoma (CD30+), and perineurioma. Cytokeratin expression in monophasic (spindle) synovial sarcoma may be focal but EMA is often more extensively positive in such cases, even in the rare pleuropulmonary synovial sarcoma.
3. The expression of EMA in chordoma serves to distinguish it from chondroma and chondrosarcoma.
4. EMA is expressed in solitary fibrous tumors.
5. EMA immunostaining may help identify ovarian granulosa cell tumors from tumors that mimic their various histological patterns. While keratin may be expressed in granulosa cell tumors, the absence of EMA and immunoreactivity for smooth muscle actin allows distinction from primary and metastatic carcinomas.
6. While EMA is generally not expressed by germ cells, normal hemato-lymphoid, mesenchymal, neural, and neuroectodermal, it may be expressed by certain nonepithelial tissues such as fetal notochord, arachnoid granulations, ependyma, choroid plexus, epineurial and perineural fibroblasts, histiocytes, and plasma cells and their corresponding neoplasms.
7. EMA is normally expressed by plasma cells and is conserved and even increased in plasma cell neoplasms. Neoplasms from earlier-stage B-cell differentiation do not usually express EMA, and in lymph node–based B-cell lymphomas, EMA is found mainly in diffuse large cell lymphomas and T-cell-rich B-cell lymphomas. EMA is more frequently seen in T-cell neoplasms, occurring in about 20% of all T-cell lymphomas. EMA expression in Reed–Sternberg cells is unusual, although it is frequently found in the L & H cells of nodular lymphocyte-predominant Hodgkin's disease. EMA is also found in almost 50% of cases of anaplastic large cell lymphoma of CD30 phenotype.
8. EMA has also been demonstrated in nonsecretory epithelia such as urothelium, renal distal and collecting tubules, and syncytiotrophoblast.

Comments

EMA reactivity is usually limited to apical cell membranes in benign secretory epithelium and well-differentiated carcinomas such as those of the breast, but in poorly differentiated carcinomas, cytoplasmic staining is seen and there is loss of staining polarity in the cell membranes.

Selected references

Heyderman E, Strudley I, Powell G, et al. A new monoclonal antibody to epithelial membrane antigen (EMA) – E29: A comparison of its immunocytochemical reactivity with polyclonal anti-EMA antibodies and with another monoclonal antibody HMFG-2. *Br J Cancer* 1985;52:355–61.

Epstein–Barr virus, LMP

Background

The antibody (Isotype: IgG1, Kappa) has been raised against recombinant fusion protein containing sequences of bacterial β-galactosidase and the EBV-encoded latent membrane protein (LMP-1). LMP is one of the few viral proteins that are expressed in a latent infection. The antibody reacts with a 60 kD latent membrane protein encoded by the BNLF gene of the Epstein–Barr virus. Being a cocktail of clones CS1, CS2, CS3, and CS4, all four anti-LMP antibodies recognize distinct epitopes on the hydrophilic carboxyl region of LMP. These four epitopes are present on the internal aspect of the membrane-associated viral LMP. Therefore, the antibody does not react with viable cells but with fixed cells in paraffin sections, cytological preparations, and cryostat sections, and in immunoblotting.

Applications

The antibody is characterized by its strong positivity with EBV-positive lymphoblastoid cell lines and EBV-infected B-cell immunoblasts in infectious mononucleosis.

1. Although EBV is consistently present in nasopharyngeal undifferentiated carcinoma among Oriental patients, LMP-1 antibody is only positive in about 60% of cases. LMP protein expression is especially useful in identifying these cancers in cervical lymph node metastases. This antibody may also be useful in the diagnosis of lymphoepithelioma-like carcinoma of the lung, mediastinum, stomach, and paranasal.
2. Post-transplantation lymphoproliferative disorders arising in patients treated with a variety of immunosuppressive regimens after organ transplantation usually show a type III latency pattern with LMP-1 expression. The EBV-positive AIDS-associated B-cell lymphomas usually demonstrate a latency type III in the large cell lymphomas, permitting the use of antibody to LMP-1.
3. Nasal T-/NK cell lymphoma is strongly associated with EBV.
4. LMP-1 expression has also been associated with an aggressive clinical course and hepatosplenomegaly in nodal T-cell lymphomas. About 20–30% of CD30 (Ki-1)-positive anaplastic large cell lymphomas show LMP-1 immunoreaction.
5. Approximately 50% of Hodgkin's disease is associated with EBV. In almost all these positive cases, nearly all the Reed–Sternberg cells are positive for EBV.

Interpretation

A note of caution with respect to antibodies against LMP is advised: strong staining of normal early myeloid and erythroid precursors may be seen despite a total absence of evidence of EBV by polymerase chain reaction (PCR). LMP is localized to the cytoplasm and cell membrane.

Selected references

Bruin PCD. Detection of Epstein-Barr virus nucleic acid sequences and protein in nodal T-cell lymphomas: Relation between latent membrane protein-1 positivity and clinical course. *Histopathology* 1993;23:509–18.

Delecluse H-J, Kremmer E, Rouault J-P, et al. The expression of Epstein-Barr virus latent proteins is related to the pathological feature of post-transplant lymphoproliferative disorders. *Am J Pathol* 1995;146:1113–20.

Hording U, Nielsen HW, Albeck H, et al. Nasopharyngeal carcinoma: Histopathological types and association with Epstein-Barr virus. *Eur J Cancer Clin Oncol* 1993;29B:137–9.

Kanavaros P, Lecsc M-C, Briere J, et al. Nasal T-cell lymphoma: A clinicopathologic entity associated with peculiar phenotype and with Epstein-Barr virus. *Blood* 1993;81:2688–95.

NOTES

ERG (avian v-ets erythroblastosis virus E26 oncogene homolog)

Background

ERG (avian v-ets erythroblastosis virus E26 oncogene homolog) is a member of the *ETS* family of transcription factors characterized by the 98–amino acid sequence containing a basic helix–turn–helix structure of DNA binding proteins. ERG is constitutively expressed in endothelial cells regulating angiogenesis and endothelial apoptosis. ERG expression is detected in endothelial cells, subsets of hematopoietic stem cells and myeloid progenitors, and fetal mesoderm-derived cells, including endothelium and cartilage.

Applications

1. Identification of endothelium of normal tissue and in vascular lesions. ERG is positive in malignant vascular neoplasms including nearly all (>95%) cases of angiosarcoma, epithelioid hemangioendothelioma, and Kaposi sarcoma. Essentially all benign vascular proliferations and neoplasms, including hemangioma, lymphangioma, and papillary endothelial hyperplasia, are positive for ERG.
2. Sarcomas: ERG immunoreactivity has been demonstrated in 40–50% of epithelioid sarcomas, and nuclear immunoreactivity is detected in most Ewing sarcoma cases with *EWSR1:ERG* translocations and less commonly with *EWSR1:FLI1* or *EWSR1:NFAT2*. In addition, ERG nuclear positivity is seen in the *EWSR1-SMAD3* rearranged fibroblastic tumor.
3. Prostatic adenocarcinoma subsets containing the *TMPRSS2-ERG* and *SLC45A3-ERG* and *NDRG1-ERG* translocations. The *TMPRSS2:ERG* gene translocation is the most frequent large chromosomal aberration in prostatic adenocarcinoma and is present in about half of total prostatic adenocarcinoma cases. The *TMPRSS2:ERG* translocation causes increased expression of ERG that can be detected immunohistochemically with high sensitivity. In *TMPRSS2:ERG* prostatic adenocarcinoma,

benign prostatic tissue and low- and high-grade prostatic intraepithelial neoplasia demonstrate ERG reactivity in addition to the prostatic adenocarcinoma.
4. ERG is also detected in blastic extramedullary myeloid proliferations and acute myeloid leukemias with the *FUS-ERG* rearrangement.
5. ERG is negative in almost all other tumor types with rare examples of pulmonary large cell undifferentiated carcinoma and malignant mesothelioma showing positivity.
6. Nonnuclear, cytoplasmic, or membrane ERG immunoreactivity has been noted in some nonendothelial tumors, including gastrointestinal stromal tumors, ductal carcinoma of the breast, and papillary carcinoma of the thyroid.

Interpretation

ERG is a nuclear stain. Clone (9FY) produces the best results. Immunoreactivity appears not to be enhanced by boiling or proteolytic digestion and is best demonstrated by following retrieval at 120°C in EDTA buffer at pH 9.0.

Selected references

Birdsey GM, Dryden NH, Amsellem V, et al. Transcription factor ERG regulates angiogenesis and endothelial apoptosis through VE-cadherin. *Blood* 2008;111:3498–506.

Falzarano SM, Zhou M, Carver P, et al. ERG gene rearrangement status in prostate cancer detected by immunohistochemistry. *Virchows Arch* 2011;459(4):441–7.

Kumar-Sinha C, Tomlins SA, Chinnaiyan AM. Recurrent gene fusions in prostate cancer. *Nat Rev Cancer* 2008;8: 497–511.

Miettinen M, Wang ZF, Paetau A, et al. ERG transcription factor as an immunohistochemical marker for vascular endothelial tumors and prostatic carcinoma. *Am J Surg Pathol* 2011;35:432–41.

Miettinen M, Wang Z, Sarlomo-Rikala M, et al. ERG expression in epithelioid sarcoma: A diagnostic pitfall. *Am J Surg Pathol* 2013;37:1580–5.

Sun C, Dobi A, Mohamed A, et al. TMPRSS2-ERG fusion, a common genomic alteration in prostate cancer activates C-MYC and abrogates prostate epithelial differentiation. *Oncogene* 2008;27:5348–53.

Wang WL, Patel NR, Caragea M, et al. Expression of ERG, an Ets family transcription factor, identifies ERG-rearranged Ewing sarcoma. *Mod Pathol* 2012;25:1378–83.

Erythropoietin

Background

Erythropoietin (EPO) is a glycoprotein hormone that stimulates erythropoiesis in mammals. Its synthesis is increased in the anemic and hypoxic state. Although the liver is the major source of EPO production in the fetus, the kidney is the major organ of EPO production in adults. The EPO antibody is an immunoglobulin G antibody that binds to an epitope within the first 26 amino acids at the NH_2 terminus of human urinary and recombinant EPO.

The production of EPO is responsible for stimulating polycythemia in various malignancies: renal cell carcinoma, nephroblastoma, hepatocellular carcinoma, and cerebellar hemangioblastoma.

EPO has been reported to be synthesized in the normal brain, placenta, and capillary endothelium, glandular and surface epithelial cells of the normal cervix and endometrium, and oocytes, granulosa, theca interna, and lutein cells of the ovary. A case of uterine myoma with erythropoietin synthesis by tumor tissue and erythrocytosis has been reported.

High levels of EPO and EPO receptor expression have been reported in malignant cells and tumor vasculature in breast cancer but not in normal breast tissue.

Applications

1. EPO immunopositivity is useful in the identification of both primary and metastatic renal cell carcinoma. This is useful to distinguish them from other carcinomas but not from hemangioblastoma, which may also be EPO positive.

Selected references

Acs G, Acs P, Beckwith SM, et al. Erythropoietin and erythropoietin receptor expression in human cancer. *Cancer Res* 2001;61:3561–5.

Estrogen receptor (ER)

Background

The first monoclonal antibodies to the estrogen receptor (ER) protein (estrophilin) were produced from a human breast cancer cell line, MCF-7, subjected to affinity column processing and elution. The antibodies were produced by immunization of rats with this partially purified estradiol–estrophilin complex. Fusion of splenic lymphocytes from the immunized animals with myeloma cells yielded three hybridoma cells lines after cloning by limited dilution techniques; the antibodies thus produced recognized estrogen-occupied as well as unoccupied receptors.

The human ER is a member of a family of nuclear receptors for small hydrophobic ligands such as thyroid hormone, vitamin D, retinoic acid, and the steroid hormones. Each receptor has a ligand-binding domain, a hinge region, a DNA binding domain, and a variable or regulatory domain. The ER gene is located on the long arm of chromosome 6 (q24–27) and comprises 8 exons and intervening introns spanning at least 140 kilobases. Binding of the ligand to the receptor is thought to result in an allosteric alteration that allows the hormone–receptor complex to bind to its DNA response element in the promoter region of a target gene. In the absence of hormone binding, the domain appears to be inhibitory in function, preventing transcriptional activation. Studies demonstrating cytoplasmic localization of ER protein in addition to nuclear localization have mostly employed fluorescein-tagged estrogen analogs, whereas modern immunoenzyme techniques utilizing monoclonal antibodies to ER protein have shown only nuclear reactivity.

Applications

1. Breast cancer: It has been suggested that ER may be used to identify metastatic breast carcinoma, but a variety of other lesions with epithelioid features may also express ER. These include epithelioid smooth muscle tumors, malignant melanoma, meningioma, sclerosing hemangioma, desmoid tumors, thyroid neoplasms, and cervical, endometrial, and ovarian cancers, rendering the marker less useful as a diagnostic discriminant.
2. The demonstration of ER in 56% of primary pulmonary carcinoma of bronchiolar alveolar type and 80% of adenocarcinoma of no special type emphasizes further the dangers of using ER as a marker of breast carcinoma, especially in the metastatic setting. Interestingly, nuclear staining was obtained in these cases with clone 6F11 and not 1D5, confirming that the clones may detect different epitopes of the ER antigen.

Comments

It is possible to obtain consistent staining of ER in cytologic preparations by employing clone 1D5 with heat-induced epitope retrieval (HIER) on smears, which are initially completely air-dried before fixation in 10% buffered formalin.

It is important, as with most other antibodies employed for immunohistology, that each laboratory determines its optimal time for epitope retrieval and should not purely rely on the procedures developed for other laboratories.

Computerized image analysis has been claimed to produce increasing specificity and sensitivity relative to biochemical assays; however, other studies have shown identical results by image analysis and visual examination, and significantly similar agreement between the two and biochemical values. It is clear, however, that there is significant interlaboratory variation in sensitivity to warrant caution when comparing results between laboratories; much of this may be due to differences in antibody clones, duration of fixation, and, importantly, antigen retrieval techniques.

While the antigen is largely nuclear in location, one form of ER is localized to the cell membrane, and it appears that Her2/neu interacts with the latter. Tamoxifen resistance was found to be associated with Her2/neu downregulation and ER upregulation in breast cancer cell lines. Tamoxifen-induced

E

apoptosis occurred immediately after dissociation of Her2/neu from cell membrane ER.

Selected references

Allred DC, Harvey JM, Berardo M, et al. Prognostic and predictive factors in breast cancer by immunohistochemical analysis. *Mod Pathol* 1998;11:155–68.

Balaton AJ, Mathieu M-C, Le Doussal V. Optimization of heat-induced epitope retrieval for estrogen receptor determination by immunohistochemistry on paraffin sections: Results of a multicentric comparative study. *Appl Immunohistochem* 1996;4:259–63.

Taylor CR. Paraffin section immunocytochemistry for estrogen receptor: The time has come. *J Histotechnol* 1997;20:97–100.

Factor VIII RA (von Willebrand factor)

Background

Factor VIII-related antigen is more appropriately known as the von Willebrand factor. Factor VIII is a glycoprotein and is complexed with Factor VIII-related antigen in plasma. Factor VIII is also present in endothelial cells, where it shows a granular pattern of reactivity. It is also present in the cytoplasm of megakaryocytes.

Applications

1. Factor VIII-related antigen or von Willebrand factor was one of the first markers employed for endothelial cell differentiation in angiosarcomas, but it soon became apparent that the von Willebrand factor is seldom expressed in poorly differentiated vascular tumors. There is also considerable overlap between the expression of von Willebrand factor in vascular and lymphatic endothelium.
2. Von Willebrand factor remains a sensitive marker of benign blood vessels and has been used for the study of angiogenesis in neoplasms such as breast cancer, although other markers of endothelial cells, including CD34 and CD31, serve this purpose better, particularly CD31, which is more sensitive and more specific.

Selected references

Jiric G, Zarkovic N, Nola M, et al. The value of cell proliferation and angiogenesis in the prognostic assessment of ovarian granulose cell tumors. *Tumori* 2001;87:47–53.

Marder VJ, Mannucci PM, Firkin BG, et al. Standard nomenclature for factor VIII and von Willebrand factor: A recommendation by the International Committee on Thrombosis and Haemostasis. *Thromb Haemost* 1985;54:871–2.

Sehested M, Hou-Jensen K. Factor VHI-related antigen as an endothelial cell marker in benign and malignant diseases. *Virchows Arch* 1981;391:217–25.

Factor XIIIa

Background

Factor XIIIa is a blood proenzyme found in plasma and platelets. The reaction of Factor XIIIa with fibrin is the last enzyme-catalyzed step on the coagulation cascade, leading to the formation of a normal blood clot stabilized as a result of fibrin cross-linkage. This transglutaminase exists in two forms, as an extracellular or plasma Factor XIIIa subunit attached to a dimer of the carrier protein, or Factor XIIIb, and an intracellular Factor XIII, which is exclusively the dimer of subunit "a" only. Intracellular Factor XIIIa has been identified in a variety of cells, including human dendritic reticulum cells in reactive lymphoid follicles, fibroblast-like mesenchymal cells in connective tissue, and neoplastic fibroblastic and fibrohistiocytic lesions. The dermal dendrocytes have been characterized as Factor XIIIa-positive dendritic cells of bone marrow origin that are typically found in the adventitia of dermal blood vessels and in the interstitial dermal connective tissues. In one study of dermal dendritic cells using CD34 and Factor XIIIa, it was found that antigenic profiles differed among the dendritic cell types.

Applications

1. The current diagnostic applications of Factor XIIIa pertain largely to the identification of dermal dendritic cells and their presence and role in various cutaneous and soft tissue tumors. Factor XIIIa has been described in various fibrohistiocytic tumors, including aneurysmal fibrous histiocytoma, dermatofibroma, and dermatofibrosarcoma protuberans. In the latter two conditions, Factor XIIIa expression appears to be associated with early lesions, with loss of expression in late or "mature" lesions.
2. Has been used as a diagnostic discriminator for hepatocellular carcinoma from its morphologic mimics cholangiocarcinoma and metastatic carcinoma in the liver.
3. Other tumors that are positive include calcifying fibrous pseudotumor, dermatofibroma, solitary fibrous tumor, xanthoma, xanthogranuloma, pigmented villonodular synovitis, fibroblastic reticular cell tumor, atypical fibroxanthoma, and epithelioid histiocytic proliferations.
4. Glomus tumor, meningioma, neurothekoma, inflammatory pseudotumor, and cerebellar hemangioblastoma also express this antigen, albeit less frequently.

Selected references

Alawi F, Stratton D, Freedman PD. Solitary fibrous tumor of the oral soft tissues: A clinicopathologic and immunohistochemical study of 16 cases. *Am J Surg Pathol* 2001;25:900–10.

Busam KJ, Granter SR, Iversen K, et al. Immunohistochemical distinction of epithelioid histiocytic proliferations from epithelioid melanocytic nevi. *Am J Dermatopathol* 2000;22:237–41.

Hill KA, Gonzalez-Crussi F, Chou PM. Calcifying fibrous pseudotumor versus inflammatory myofibroblastic tumor: A histological and immunohistochemical comparison. *Mod Pathol* 2001;14:784–90.

Kraus MD, Haley JC, Ruiz R, et al. "Juvenile" xanthogranuloma: An immunophenotypic study with a reappraisal of histiogenesis. *Am J Dermatopathol* 2001;23:104–11.

Mentzel T, Kutzner H, Rutten A, et al. Benign fibrous histiocytoma (dermatofibroma) of the face: Clinicopathologic and immunohistochemical study of 34 cases associated with an aggressive clinical behaviour. *Am J Dermatopathol* 2001;23:419–26.

Nestle FO, Nickoloff BJ. A fresh morphological and functional look at dermal dendritic cells. *J Cutan Pathol* 1995;22:385–93.

Nestle FO, Nickloff BJ, Burg G. Dermatofibroma: An abortive immunoreactive process mediated by dermal dendritic cells? *Dermatology* 1995;190:265–8.

Takata M, Imai T, Hirone T. Factor XIIIa-positive cells in normal peripheral nerves and cutaneous neurofibromas of type-1 neurofibromatosis. *Am J Dermatopathol* 1994;16:37–43.

Zelger BW, Zelger BG, Steiner H, et al. Aneurysmal and hemangiopericytoma-like fibrous histiocytoma. *J Clin Pathol* 1996;49:313–18.

Fas (CD95) and Fas-ligand (CD95L)

Background

Fas (CD95) is a cell surface protein that belongs to the tumor necrosis factor family. Cross-linking of Fas and Fas-ligand (FasL) transduces signals, which culminate in apoptosis in sensitive cells. These proteins, therefore, have a role in the genesis of neoplasms and have been extensively studied in this context. Their expression in certain malignancies has been implicated as a possible key mechanism in the immune privilege of such tumors. FasL is also expressed in immunologically privileged sites in the nonneoplastic state. The induction of apoptosis by FasL in invading lymphocytes acts as a mechanism of immune privilege and is important in preventing graft rejection. The placenta, another immune privileged site, has also been shown to express high levels of FasL.

Applications

1. Interest in immunostaining for Fas and FasL centers around their role in tumor destruction. Macrophages and lymphocytes express high levels of Fas, and it has been thought that expression of FasL by tumor cells allows destruction of Fas-positive lymphocytes.
2. With the discovery that tumors may express both FasL and Fas, it was realized that tumors like melanoma may induce their own apoptosis in an autocrine and/or paracrine fashion and that the decline of tumor apoptosis rather than the apoptosis of infiltrating lymphocytes may affect prognosis.
3. Macrophages heavily infected by tuberculosis or leprosy bacteria have been shown to be induced to express high levels of FasL, which may protect them from destruction by Fas-expressing lymphocytes.

Selected references

Bamberger AM, Schulte HM, Thuneke I, et al. Expression of the apoptosis-inducing Fas ligand (FasL) in human first and third trimester placenta and choriocarcinoma cells. *J Clin Endocrinol Metab* 1997;82:3173–5.

Ciccocioppo R, D'Alo S, Di Sabatino A, et al. Mechanisms of villous atrophy in autoimmune enteropathy and coeliac disease. *Clin Exp Immunol* 2002;128:88–93.

De la Monte SM, Sohn YK, Wands JR. Correlates of p53- and Fas (CD95)-mediated apoptosis in Alzheimer's disease. *J Neurol Sci* 1997;152:73–83.

Fine A, Anderson NL, Rothstein TL, et al. Fas expression in pulmonary alveolar type II cells. *Am J Physiol* 1997;273:(1 Part 1):L64–L71.

Hellquist HB, Olejnicka B, Jadner M, et al. Fas receptor is expressed in human lung squamous cell carcinomas, whereas bcl-2 and apoptosis are not pronounced: A preliminary report. *Br J Cancer* 1997;76:175–9.

Kazufumi M, Sonoko N, Masanori K, et al. Expression of bcl-2 protein and APO-1 (Fas antigen) in the lung tissue from patients with idiopathic pulmonary fibrosis. *Microsc Res Tech* 1997;38:480–7.

Lee J, Richburg JH, Younkin SC, et al. The Fas system is a key regulator of germ cell apoptosis in the testis. *Endocrinology* 1997;138:2081–8.

Nichans GA, Brunner T, Frizelle SP, et al. Human lung carcinomas express Fas ligand. *Cancer Res* 1997;57:1007–12.

Nonomura N, Mild T, Yokoyama M, et al. Fas/APO-1-mediated apoptosis of human renal cell carcinoma. *Biochem Biophys Res Commun* 1996;229:945–51.

Shukuwa T, Katayama I, Koji T. Fas-mediated apoptosis of melanoma cells and infiltrating lymphocytes in human malignant melanomas. *Mod Pathol* 2002;15:387–96.

Strater J, Wellisch I, Riedl S, et al. CD95 (APO-l/Fas)-mediated apoptosis in colon epithelial cells: A possible role in ulcerative colitis. *Gastroenterology* 1997;113:160–7.

Fascin

Background

Human fascin is a highly conserved 55 kD actin-bundling protein. Fascin is encoded by the human homolog for *hsn* gene and is thought to be involved in the formation of microfilament bundles. Strong immunoreactivity has been observed in dendritic cells of the thymus and spleen. Histiocytes, smooth muscle cells, endothelial cells, and squamous mucosal cells may also express fascin. Fascin immunoexpression has been demonstrated in interdigitating reticulum cells, follicular dendritic cells, and interstitial dendritic cells in lymph nodes.

Applications

1. Fascin-expressing dendritic cells are decreased or absent in the neoplastic follicles of germinal centers compared with hyperplastic follicular centers. In contrast, reactive centers reveal tight syncytial networks of fascin-positive follicular dendritic cells.
2. Fascin has been demonstrated in the cytoplasm of most Reed–Sternberg cells and their variants in Hodgkin's disease; whilst only a minority of non-Hodgkin's lymphomas are immunoreactive. Fascin immunopositivity has highlighted Reed–Sternberg cells in follicular Hodgkin's lymphoma.
3. Follicular dendritic cell tumors and juvenile xanthogranulomas have demonstrated uniform immunopositivity with fascin; 75% of interdigitating dendritic cell sarcomas were fascin positive.

Fascin immunoreactivity in Hodgkin's disease may serve to complement CD 15 and CD30 to identify Reed–Sternberg cells. Similarly, addition of fascin to CD21 and CD35 would be useful to identify follicular dendritic cell tumors.

Selected references

Biddle DA, Ro JY, Yoon GS, et al. Extranodal follicular dendritic cell sarcoma of the head and neck region: Three new cases, with a review of the literature. *Mod Pathol* 2002;15:50–8.

Gaertner EM, Tsokos M, Derringer GA, et al. Interdigitating dendritic cell sarcoma: A report of four cases and review of the literature. *Am J Clin Pathol* 2001:115:589–97.

Kansal R, Singleton TP, Ross CW, et al. Follicular Hodgkin lymphoma: A histopathologic study. *Am J Clin Pathol* 2002;117:29–35.

Kraus MD, Haley JC, Ruiz R, et al. "Juvenile" xanthogranuloma: An immunophenotypic study with a reappraisal of histogenesis. *Am J Dermatopathol* 2001;23:104–11.

Mosialos G, Birkenbach M, Ayehunie S, et al. Circulating human dendritic cells differentially express high levels of 55-kd actin-bundling protein. *Am J Pathol* 1996;148:593–600.

Pinkus GS, Pinkus JL, Langhoff E, et al. Fascin, a sensitive new marker for Reed-Sternberg cells of Hodgkin's disease: Evidence for a dendritic or B-cell derivation? *Am J Pathol* 1997;150:543–62.

Ferritin

Background

Ferritin, the iron storage protein, plays a key role in iron metabolism, and its ability to sequester iron gives ferritin the dual functions of iron detoxification and iron reserve. The distribution of ferritin is ubiquitous among living species and its three-dimensional structure is highly conserved. All ferritins have 24 protein subunits arranged in 432 symmetry to give a hollow shell with an 80 A diameter cavity capable of storing up to 45 000 Fe (III) atoms as an inorganic complex. Subunits are folded as four-helix bundles, each having a fifth short helix at roughly 60 degrees to the bundle axis.

Applications

1. Ferritin was one of the first markers employed for the identification of hepatocytes and their neoplastic counterparts but it proved to be of low sensitivity and low specificity, being found in a wide range of benign and neoplastic tissues.
2. Ferritin is expressed in hepatoid tumors such as those in the ovary.
3. Ferritin is employed as a marker of hemorrhage in the brain and as a marker of microglia.
4. In bone marrow biopsies, ferritin has been found to correlate with marrow hemosiderin as detected by the Perls' stain and is advocated as a more sensitive tool for the evaluation of body iron stores.
5. In the skin, ferritin is localized to the outer layer of the eccrine duct, and in sweat gland neoplasms, two distinct patterns were noted. In syringoma the antibody decorated the outermost layer of cells in the epithelial cords of the tumor so that a characteristic ring was produced in cross sections, whereas only sparse staining was observed with other eccrine duct tumors such as dermal duct tumor and eccrine poroma. Syringoma showed diffuse staining, as did acrospiroma and a number of other adnexal carcinomas.
6. The presence of ferritin in epithelial cells often indicates increased cell permeability, and this property has been exploited in the demonstration that hyaline globules associated with a variety of tumors are the product of apoptotic cell death; the name "thanatosomes" has been recently proposed for such hyaline globules.

Comments

The diagnostic applications of this marker are limited, and except perhaps for the assessment of bone marrow iron stores, ferritin immunostaining is never employed alone.

Selected references

Abenoza P, Manivel JC, Wick MR, et al. Hepatoblastoma: An immunohistochemical and ultrastructural study. *Hum Pathol* 1987;18:1025–35.

Harrison PM, Arosio P. The ferritins: Molecular properties, iron storage function and cellular regulation. *Biochem Biophys Acta* 1996;1275:161–203.

Imoto M, Nishimura D, Fukuda Y, et al. Immunohistochemical detection of alpha-fetoprotein, carcinoembryonic antigen, and ferritin in formalin-fixed sections from hepatocellular carcinoma. *Am J Gastroenterol* 1985;80:902–6.

Kaneko Y, Kitamoto T, Tateishi J, et al. Ferritin immunohistochemistry as a marker for microglia. *Acta Neuropathol* 1989;79:129–36.

Momotani E, Wuscger N, Ravisse P, et al. Immunohistochemical identification of ferritin, lactoferrin and transferrin in leprosy lesions of human skin biopsies. *J Comp Pathol* 1992;106:213–20.

Navone R, Azzoni L, Valente G. Immunohistochemical assessment of ferritin in bone marrow trephine biopsies: Correlation with marrow hemosiderin. *Acta Haematol* 1988;80:194–8.

Papadimitriou JC, Drachenberg CB, Brenner DS, et al. "Thanatosomes": A unifying morphogenetic concept for tumor hyaline globules related to apoptosis. *Hum Pathol* 2000;31:1455–65.

Penneys NS, Zlatkiss I. Immunohistochemical demonstration of ferritin in sweat gland and sweat gland neoplasms. *J Cutan Pathol* 1990;17:32–6.

Fibrin

Background

Proteolytic conversion of fibrinogen to fibrin results in self-assembly to form a clot matrix that subsequently becomes cross-linked by factor XIIIa to form the main structural element of the thrombus in vivo. The roles of fibrin and its precursor have been extensively studied both in vitro and in vivo.

Applications

Diagnostic applications of fibrin are mainly limited to the study of glomerulopathy with sporadic use of anti-fibrin to identify fibrin deposits and thrombi in extrarenal sites.

Comments

The diagnostic applications of anti-fibrin are limited to specific situations. Applications in nephropathology, particularly with immunofluorescence techniques, are still extensive.

Selected references

Dowling JP. Immunohistochemistry of renal diseases and tumours. In: Leong AS-Y, ed. *Applied immunohistochemistry for surgical pathologists*. London: Edward Arnold, 1993, pp. 210–59.

Gaffhey PJ. Structure of fibrinogen and degradation products of fibrinogen and fibrin. *Br Med Bull* 1997;33:245–51.

Imokawa S, Sato A, Hayakawa H, et al. Tissue factor expression and fibrin deposition in the lungs of patients with idiopathic pulmonary fibrosis and systemic sclerosis. *Am J Respir Crit Care Med* 1997;156(2 Pt 1):631–6.

Takahashi H, Shibata Y, Fujita S, et al. Immunohistochemical findings of arterial fibrinoid necrosis in major and lingual minor salivary glands of primary Sjogren's syndrome. *Anal Cell Pathol* 1996;12:145–57.

Fibrinogen

Background

Fibrinogen is a 340 kD multi-subunit glycoprotein present in plasma and tissue of all classes of vertebrates. Fibrinogen has a variety of physiologically important functions, most of which, if not all, are assigned to certain structures of fibrin, including double-stranded fibrin protofibrils and highly cross-linked fibrin. Its role in hemostasis and thrombosis has been extensively studied.

Applications

Immunostaining for fibrin/fibrinogen deposits is employed for the detection of microthrombi. Diagnostic applications of fibrinogen are largely limited to the identification of fibrinogen deposition and breakdown products in glomerular diseases.

Selected references

Dowling JP. Immunohistochemistry of renal diseases and tumours. In: Leong AS-Y, ed. *Applied immunohistochemistry for the surgical pathologist*. London: Edward Arnold, 1993, pp. 210–59.

Stewart FA, Te Poele JA, Van der Wal AF, et al. Radiation nephropathy & the link between functional damage and vascular mediated inflammatory and thrombotic change. *Acta Oncol* 2001;40:952–7.

Fibronectin

Background

Fibronectin is a noncollagenous connective tissue glycoprotein found in association with both basement membranes and interstitial connective tissue. Fibronectin is a β-glycoprotein with a molecular weight of 44 kD comprising two nearly identical subchains. It is widely distributed throughout many normal tissues including connective tissues, blood vessel walls, and basement membranes. Some of the properties of fibronectin include forming cross-links with fibrin in blood clots through factor XIII and binding to heparin and collagen. It is also thought to play a role in cellular adhesion, wound healing, and tissue repair.

Applications

1. Fibronectin (and laminin) has been demonstrated to line cystic lumina and surround tumor islands in adenoid cystic breast and salivary gland carcinomas. Fibronectin immunoreactivity in breast adenoid cystic carcinomas is also useful to distinguish them from cribriform carcinoma, the latter being negative.
2. In soft tissue tumors, fibronectin was found to be most abundant in the stroma, both benign and malignant.

Selected references

D' Arderme AJ, Burns J, Skyes BC, et al. Fibronectin and type III collagen in epithelial neoplasms of gastrointestinal tract and salivary gland. *J Clin Pathol* 1983;36:756–63.

D'Ardenne AJ, Kirkpatrick P, Sykes BC. The distribution of laminin, fibronectin and interstitial collagen type III in soft tissue tumors. *J Clin Pathol* 1984;37:895–904.

D'Ardenne AJ, Kirkpatrick P, Wells CA, et al. Laminin and fibronectin in adenoid cystic carcinoma. *J Clin Pathol* 1986;39:138–144.

NOTES

FLI-1 protein

Background

Approximately 90% of Ewing's sarcomas (ES)/primitive neuroectodermal tumor (PNET) are characterized by a reciprocal translocation t(11;22) (q24;q12), which results in the fusion of the *EWS* gene on chromosome 22 to the *FLI-1* (Friend leukemia virus integration site 1) gene on chromosome 11. *FLI-1* gene on 11p23-q24 and its translocation in ES results in a chimeric transcription factor belonging to the avian Erythroblastosis virus transforming sequence (ETS) family of DNA-binding transcription factors, which are involved in cellular proliferation and tumorigenesis. The FLI-1 protein is a member of the DNA-binding transcription factor family, is associated with cellular proliferation, and is normally expressed in endothelial cells and hematopoietic cells. FLI-1 is frequently expressed in vascular neoplasms but is also expressed in hematopoietic cells.

Applications

1. Ewing sarcoma: FLI-1 is expressed in most cases of ES (71–100%) that have the *EWSR1-FLI1* translocation but also other fusions.
2. FLI is expressed in several other small round blue cell tumors such as lymphoblastic lymphomas (90%), synovial sarcoma, desmoplastic small round cell tumor, and Merkel cell carcinoma. Hence, most often FLI-1 is used along with a panel of other immunohistochemical markers in this scenario, with the diagnosis of ES established usually by fluorescence in situ hybridization testing.
3. Vascular tumors: there is high sensitivity (94%) among vascular tumors that stain with FLI-1, including hemangiomas, hemangioendotheliomas, angiosarcoma, Littoral cell angioma, and Kaposi's sarcoma.
4. There is now an expanded spectrum of FLI-1 immunoreactive tumors: carcinomas, lymphomas, sex cord–stromal tumors, malignant melanoma, solid pseudopapillary neoplasm of pancreas, phosphaturic mesenchymal tumors, and the majority of epithelioid sarcomas.

Comments

These observations and the availability of more specific markers of endothelial cells limit the utility of FLI-1 in the diagnosis of poorly differentiated angiosarcoma.

FLI-1 is a nuclear stain.

Selected references

Cuda J, Mirzamani N, Kantipudi R, et al. Diagnostic utility of Fli-1 and D2-40 in distinguishing atypical fibroxanthoma from angiosarcoma. *Am J Dermatopathol* 2013;35:316–18.

Folpe AL, Chand EM, Goldblum JR, et al. Expression of Fli-1, a nuclear transcription factor, distinguishes vascular neoplasms from potential mimics. *Am J Surg Pathol* 2001;25:1061–6.

Folpe AL, Hill CE, Parham DM, et al. Immunohistochemical detection of FLI-1 protein expression: A study of 132 round cell tumors with emphasis on CD99-positive mimics of Ewing's sarcoma/primitive neuroectodermal tumor. *Am J Surg Pathol* 2000;24:1657–62.

Nilsson G, Wang M, Wejde J, et al. Detection of EWS/FLI-1 by immunostaining: An adjunctive tool in diagnosis of Ewing's sarcoma and primitive neuroectodermal tumor on cytological samples and paraffin-embedded archival material. *Sarcoma* 1999;3:25–32.

Stockman DL, Hornick JL, Deavers MT, et al. ERG and FLI1 protein expression in epithelioid sarcoma. *Mod Pathol* 2014;27(4):496–501.

Tajima S, Takashi Y, Ito N, et al. ERG and FLI1 are useful immunohistochemical markers in phosphaturic mesenchymal tumors. *Med Mol Morphol* 2016;49(4):203–9.

Turc-Carel C, Aurias A, Mugneret F, et al. Chromosomes in Ewing's sarcoma. I: An evaluation of 85 cases of remarkable consistency of t(11; 22)(q24; q12). *Cancer Genet Cytogenet* 1988;32:229–38.

Zucman J, Delattre O, Desmaze C, et al. Cloning and characterization of the Ewing's sarcoma and peripheral neuroepithelioma t(11; 22) translocation breakpoints. *Genes Chromosomes Cancer* 1992;5:271–7.

FOXL2

Background

FOXL2 is a forkhead transcription factor that is active in multiple tissues including the eyelid, ovary, and pituitary gland. It is expressed as a nuclear protein mainly in the adult ovary and is important for the development of granulosa cells in the ovary. Testing for FOXL2 mutation (*402G-C*) is not widely available at present, and therefore FOXL2 immunostaining, which gives a nuclear pattern of staining, is useful.

Applications

1. Ovarian sex cord–stromal tumors (SCSTs) are a heterogeneous group of tumors that have varied appearances, which can lead to difficulties in diagnosis. FOXL2 staining is present in almost all SCSTs (80–90%) with a *FOXL2* mutation and also in a majority of SCSTs without a mutation. Absence of FOXL2 immunostaining suggests lack of a *FOXL2* mutation.
2. In granulosa cell tumors (GCTs), 70–95% harbor a missense point mutation in the *FOXL2* gene (*402 C>G*). The mutation is occasionally present in a very small proportion of thecomas, juvenile granulosa cell tumors, and Sertoli–Leydig cell tumors (SLCT). Regardless of growth pattern (solid, cystic, trabecular, gyriform, cystic, or pleomorphic), FOXL2 expression is present in all adult GCTs (95% positive). Juvenile GCTs also show consistent FOXL2 expression.
3. However, FOXL2 immunoexpression is present in **all** SCSTs, except in SLCT, in which FOXL2 expression is seen in only 50% of cases. Within SLCT, the retiform and poorly differentiated variants are typically negative.
4. FOXL2 staining can help distinguish tumors of sex cord origin from other mesenchymal tumors. In the fibrothecoma group, FOXL2 immunoexpression is seen in 90% of cases, in contrast to no reactivity in nonovarian mesenchymal lesions. FOXL2 stains sex cord–stromal cells in a gonadoblastoma.
5. Of note, female adnexal tumors of probable Wolffian origin (FATWO), which usually occur in the broad ligament and may be confused with SCSTs, are also immunoreactive for FOXL2.
6. Steroid cell tumors (rare) have also been shown to show weak FOXL2 expression.
7. FOXL2 is also positive in a subset of pituitary adenomas.
8. Surface epithelial and germ cell ovarian tumors are FOXL2 negative.

Comments

FOXL2 is more sensitive than the more widely used markers such as inhibin and calretinin.

Selected references

Al-Agha OM, Huwait HF, Chow C, et al. FOXL2 is a sensitive and specific marker for sex cord–stromal tumors of the ovary. *Am J Surg Pathol* 2011;35:484–94.

Buza N, Wong S, Hui P. FOXL2 mutation analysis of ovarian sex cord-stromal tumors: Genotype-phenotype correlation with diagnostic considerations. *Int J Gynecol Pathol* 2018;37(4):305–15.

Shah SP, Kobel M, Senz J, et al. Mutation of FOXL2 in granulosa-cell tumors of the ovary. *N Engl J Med* 2009;360:2719–29.

Stewart CJ, Alexiadis M, Crook ML, et al. An immunohistochemical and molecular analysis of problematic and unclassified ovarian sex cord–stromal tumors. *Hum Pathol* 2013;44:2774–81.

GATA 3 binding protein 3 (GATA3)

Background

The name GATA is given to a family of transcription factors whose members bind the DSA sequence (A/T) GATA (A/G) via two zinc- finger domains with consensus sequence CX2C17-18CX2 C. The family is comprised of six members, which are divided into two subgroups on the basis of their tissue distribution, structure, and function. Group one members include GATA1, GATA2, and GATA3, which have an overwhelming association with hematopoietic lineage and the development of the nervous system. The second group is composed of GATA4, GATA5, and GATA 6 and is associated with a large variety of mesoderm- and endodermal-derived tissues, including parts of the genitourinary system, lungs, parts of the gastrointestinal tract organs including stomach and intestine, and vasculature. The GATA family (with the exception of GATA5) plays an obligatory developmental role. They influence cell fate specification, differentiation, proliferation, and movement.

GATA3, also known as endothelial nuclear transcription factor 3, is a ~48 kDa protein comprised of 443 amino acids encoded by a gene located on chromosome 10p15. It is expressed in early-stage erythrocytes and T cells. While it is extensively expressed in embryonic tissues such as brain, parathyroid, skin, inner ear, adrenal glands, liver, and placenta, normal adult tissues, including lung, parotid gland, stomach, small intestine, colon, pancreas, liver, thyroid, prostate, seminal vesicle, ovary, and endometrium, are negative. In normal adult cells GATA3 is expressed in T lymphocytes, luminal glandular epithelial cells of breast, parathyroid glands, and urothelium. In the kidney GATA3 has been reported to be expressed in distal tubules but absent in proximal tubules.

Applications

1. Urothelial carcinoma: GATA3 is positive in 80–90% of typical urothelial carcinomas. Among the variants of urothelial carcinoma, micropapillary and plasmacytoid are positive in 60% and 45% of cases, respectively. Sarcomatoid and small cell variants express GATA3 weakly and only in 15% and 5% of cases, respectively. Thus, while GATA3 expression is helpful in identifying the urothelial origin of micropapillary and plasmacytoid urothelial carcinoma, it has very limited, if any, usefulness in the workup of sarcomatoid and small cell carcinoma variants of urothelial carcinoma. However, 41% of primary urothelial signet ring carcinomas and 8% of signet ring cancers with extracellular mucin are GATA3 positive.

2. Distinguishing high-grade prostatic adenocarcinoma from high-grade urothelial carcinoma. While the majority of prostate cancers can be clinically and morphologically distinguished from urothelial carcinoma, this distinction may be difficult if not impossible in poorly differentiated tumors that involve the bladder neck.

    Urothelial carcinoma tends to show a more nested growth pattern with atypical pleomorphic cells. Subtle cribriforming can be seen in prostatic adenocarcinoma as well. Additionally, rarely, prostate cancers may appear to grow in a nested pattern with pleomorphic cells: the so-called "pleomorphic giant cell adenocarcinoma."

3. In cases where both prostate-specific antigen and prostate-specific membrane antigen (PSA and PSMA) are lost in high-grade prostatic adenocarcinoma, additional prostatic adenocarcinoma markers and GATA3 are helpful in teasing out the differences.

4. High-grade urothelial carcinoma and spread from anal squamous cell carcinoma (SCC) or spread from a uterine cervical squamous carcinoma.

5. Primary SCC of the urinary bladder is rare and associated with specific etiologic events. The differential diagnosis of SCC in bladder includes primary urothelial SCC or a secondary involvement of bladder via extension from SCC of the uterine cervix or anus. In such cases GATA3 is only seen in about 7% of primary SCC of bladder; on the other hand, SCC arising from uterine cervix or anus can be positive for GATA3 in approximately 6% and 7%

of cases, respectively. The use of GATA3 may therefore spuriously suggest urothelial origin.

6. High-grade, poorly differentiated urothelial carcinoma of the renal pelvis that extensively invades the renal parenchyma may be difficult to distinguish from a poorly differentiated primary renal cell carcinoma. An immunohistochemical panel with GATA3 (65% to 90%), S100P (another marker commonly expressed in urothelial carcinoma), and PAX 8 (expressed in all subtypes of renal cell carcinomas but absent in urothelial carcinoma) will help differentiate the two.

7. GATA3 is highly expressed in breast carcinomas across all histological subtypes, and GATA3 has been found to be a more sensitive immunohistochemical marker for breast cancer. GATA3 therefore is a useful marker when the differential diagnosis of metastatic breast cancer does not include urothelial carcinoma, e.g., in separating a breast lobular carcinoma from a metastatic gastric signet cell carcinoma. Additionally, low expression of GATA3 has been associated with a poorer prognosis for invasive carcinoma.

8. It is positive in SCC of skin, while SCC of lung is negative.

9. GATA3 is positive in clear cell papillary and chromophobe renal cell carcinomas.

10. In salivary gland secretory carcinomas, 100% are positive.

11. Miscellaneous tumors: paraganglioma/ phaeochromocytoma (70–75% of cases), pancreatic ductal adenocarcinoma (40%), 100% of choriocarcinomas and gestational trophoblastic tumors, malignant mesotheliomas, basal cell carcinomas and adnexal tumors of skin, neuroblastoma, and peripheral T-cell lymphoma.

Interpretation

Nuclear staining.

Selected references

Chang A, Amin A, Gabrielson E, et al. Utility of GATA3 immunohistochemistry in differentiating urothelial carcinoma from prostate adenocarcinoma and squamous cell carcinomas of the uterine cervix, anus, and lung. *Am J Surg Pathol* 2012;36:1472–6.

Ellis CL, Chang AG, Cimino-Mathews A, et al. GATA-3 immunohistochemistry in the differential diagnosis of adenocarcinoma of the urinary bladder. *Am J Surg Pathol* 2013;37:1756–60.

Liu H, Shi J, Prichard JW, et al. Immunohistochemical evaluation of GATA-3 expression in ER-negative breast carcinomas. *Am J Clin Pathol* 2014;141:648–55.

Liu H, Shi J, Wilkerson ML, et al. Immunohistochemical evaluation of GATA3 expression in tumors and normal tissues: A useful immunomarker for breast and urothelial carcinomas. *Am J Clin Pathol* 2012;138:57–64.

Ordonez NG. Value of GATA3 immunostaining in tumor diagnosis: A review. *Adv Anat Pathol* 2013;20:352–60.

Simon MC. Gotta have GATA. *Nat Genet* 1995;11:9–11.

Yoon NK, Maresh EL, Shen D, et al. Higher levels of GATA3 predict better survival in women with breast cancer. *Hum Pathol* 2010;41:1794–801.

Glial fibrillary acidic protein (GFAP)

Background

GFAP is an intermediate filament (IF) protein of astroglia and belongs to the type III subclass of IF proteins. Like other IF proteins, GFAP is composed of an amino-terminal head domain, a central rod domain, and a carboxy-terminal tail domain. GFAP, with a molecular mass of 50 kD, has the smallest head domain among the class III IF proteins. Despite its insolubility, GFAP is in dynamic equilibrium between assembled filaments and unassembled subunits. As with other IF proteins, assembly of GFAP is regulated by phosphorylation–dephosphorylation of the head domain by alteration of its charge. The frequent copolymerization of GFAP with vimentin IF in immature, reactive, or radial glial indicates that vimentin has an important role in the build-up of the glial architecture. The human *GFAP* gene is localized to chromosome 17. GFAP or a GFAP-like protein is also found in Schwann cells, enteric glia, cells in all portions of the pituitary, cartilage, the iris and lens epithelium, and the fat-storing cells of the liver.

Applications

1. In the central nervous system, astrocytes, rare ependymal cells, and cerebellar radial glia express GFAP. Mature oligodendrocytes do not express GFAP. Immunohistochemical staining of GFAP has proven use in the identification of benign astrocytes and neoplastic cells of glial lineage.
2. While it was initially thought that the GFAP expression in salivary gland tissues and pleomorphic adenomas was in myoepithelial cells, in fact, GFAP is expressed in both epithelial and myoepithelial cells.
3. GFAP has been demonstrated in chordomas.
4. Choroid plexus tumors and ependymomas can express GFAP. In the setting of vacuolated clear cell tumors occurring in the retroperitoneal space, GFAP positivity would serve to distinguish chordoma and ependymoma from other mimics, including renal cell carcinoma and colorectal carcinoma.

Selected references

Inagaki M, Nakamura Y, Takeda M, et al. Glial fibrillary acidic protein: Dynamic property and regulation by phosphorylation. *Brain Pathol* 1994;4:239–43.

NOTES

Glut-1

Background

A 38–55 kD erythroid/brain type carboxy terminal of hexose transporter Glut-1 protein (member of the sodium independent glucose transporter gene superfamily) was originally reported by immunofluorescence studies in rat brain and liver tissues, and later in normal rat kidney cells with increased expression in glucose-deprived cells.

Applications

Increased expression in breast cancer, glioblastoma, pancreatic neoplasms, small cell and non-small-cell lung cancer, head and neck squamous cell carcinoma, gastric carcinomas, rhabdomyosarcoma, choriocarcinoma, invasive urothelial carcinoma, embryonal neoplasms of the central nervous system, borderline and malignant ovarian neoplasms, Fallopian tube carcinoma, uterine carcinoma, cervical carcinoma, colorectal adenomas and carcinomas, malignant thyroid nodules, cholangiocarcinoma, juvenile hemangioma, renal cell carcinoma, perineurioma, epithelioid and sarcomatoid mesotheliomas, and thymic carcinoma.

Selected references

Haber RS, Weiser KR, Pritsker A, et al. GLUT1 glucose transporter expression in benign and malignant thyroid nodules. *Thyroid* 1997;7:363–7.

Lyons LL, North PE, Mac-Moune Lai F, et al. Kaposiform hemangioendothelioma: A study of 33 cases emphasizing its pathologic, immunophenotypic, and biologic uniqueness from juvenile hemangioma. *Am J Surg Pathol* 2004;28:559–68.

Mentzel T, Kutzner H. Reticular and plexiform perineurioma: Clinicopathological and immunohistochemical analysis of two cases and review of perineurial neoplasms of skin and soft tissues. *Virchows Arch* 2005;447:677–82.

Glypican-3

Background

Glypican-3 is a glycosylphosphatidylinositol-anchored heparan sulfate cell surface proteoglycan. One of the six glypicans, glypican-3, regulates several developmental signaling pathways by acting as a coreceptor for many heparin-binding growth factors, such as fibroblast growth factors, Hedgehog, and Wnt. *GPC3* is mutated in Simpson–Golabi–Behmel syndrome, which is characterized by tissue overgrowth and an increased risk of embryonal malignancies. It is widely expressed in a variety of tissues during development, including fetal liver and placenta, but is suppressed in most adult tissues. It is also involved in the modulation of growth in predominantly mesodermal tissues and organs.

Applications

1. Glypican 3 is overexpressed in hepatocellular carcinoma (HCC). Benign liver lesions, including cirrhotic nodules, are negative for glypican 3.
2. Glypican 3 is also a sensitive but not a specific marker for testicular and ovarian yolk sac tumors.
3. It is expressed in placental site nodules and placental site trophoblastic tumors.
4. Glypican-3 is expressed in rhabdomyosarcomas but not adult spindle cell and pleomorphic sarcomas.
5. Also expressed in ovarian clear cell carcinoma, gastric hepatoid adenocarcinoma, pancreatic acinar cell carcinoma, Merkel cell carcinoma, small cell neuroendocrine carcinoma, squamous cell carcinomas from various primary sites, and urothelial carcinoma.

Selected references

Capurro MI, Xiang YY, Lobe C, et al. Glypican-3 promotes the growth of hepatocellular carcinoma by stimulating canonical Wnt signaling. *Cancer Res* 2005;65:6245–54.

Capurro M, Wanless IR, Sherman M, et al. Glypican-3: A novel serum and histochemical marker for hepatocellular carcinoma. *Gastroenterology* 2003;125:89–97.

Ou-Yang RJ, Hui P, Yang XJ, et al. Expression of glypican 3 in placental site trophoblastic tumor. *Diagn Pathol* 2010;5:64.

Shafizadeh N, Kakar S. Diagnosis of well-differentiated hepatocellular lesions: Role of immunohistochemistry and other ancillary techniques. *Adv Anat Pathol* 2011;18:438–45.

Maeda D, Ota S, Takazawa Y, et al. Glypican-3 expression in clear cell adenocarcinoma of the ovary. *Mod Pathol* 2009;22:824–32.

Ushiku T, Uozaki H, Shinozaki A, et al. Glypican 3-expressing gastric carcinoma: Distinct subgroup unifying hepatoid, clear-cell, and alpha-fetoprotein-producing gastric carcinomas. *Cancer Sci* 2009;100:626–32.

Gross cystic disease fluid protein-15 (GCDFP-15, BRST-2)

Background

Gross cystic disease fluid protein-15 (GCDFP-15) is one of four major component proteins found in the cystic fluid obtained from patients with fibro-cystic changes of the breast. GCDFP-15 is a marker of apocrine glandular differentiation in both benign and malignant mammary epithelium. This protein has widespread distribution in apocrine glands elsewhere in the axillary and perianal tissues as well as in the sublingual and submaxillary salivary glands. The GCDFP-15 protein is a 15 kD glycoprotein shown to be prolactin inducible, the GCDFP-15 gene having been recently cloned. Ultrastructurally, the GCDFP-15 protein has been localized in Golgi vesicles and cytoplasmic granules. The protein is released by exocytosis at the apices of the mammary epithelial cells.

Applications

1. GCDFP-15 stains 55–75% of cases of primary and secondary breast carcinoma. The expression of GCDFP-15 varies among the histologic subtypes of breast carcinoma, with highest incidence in infiltrating lobular carcinoma with signet ring cell differentiation (90%) compared with 70% in ordinary infiltrating ductal carcinoma and 75% in those subtypes showing apocrine differentiation. Expression of the GCDFP-15 gene was significantly associated with relapse-free survival and was suggested to represent a marker of prognostic relevance.
2. Salivary glands, sweat glands, bronchial glands, prostate, and seminal vesicle are also positive.
3. It is also a marker of apocrine differentiation in the skin and can be applied in the separation of cutaneous adnexal tumors.

Selected references

Fiel MI, Cernainu G, Burstein DE, et al. Value of GCDFP-15 (BRST-2) as a specific immunocytochemical marker for breast carcinoma in cytologic specimens. *Acta Cytol* 1996;40:637–41.

Haagensen DE Jr, Dilley WG, Mazoujian G, et al. Review of GCDFP-15: An apocrine marker protein. *Ann N Y Acad Sci* 1990;586:161–73.

NOTES

H3K27M

Background

New genetic alterations in diffuse gliomas include histone *H3* genes encoding H3.3 and H3.1 proteins. Molecular studies have shown that mutations leading to Lys27Met substitution (K27M) lead to inhibition of H3K27me trimethylation. Such mutations are seen in midline gliomas in children but rarely seen in adults. H3K27me antibody can detect K27M and is helpful in establishing the diagnosis of midline diffuse gliomas, which often have aggressive behavior.

H3K27me immunohistochemical (IHC) loss reflects loss of trimethylation at lys27 in histone H3, which leads to inactivation in components of polycomb repressor 2 (PRC2) of chromatic regulation. Chromatin modifying proteins (EED and SUZ12) maintain trimethylation and hence, mutations are associated with H3K27M IHC loss.

Applications

1. H3K27M expression is seen in most glioma tumor cells (>80%) in samples with the H3K27M genotype, while tumors that are wild-type H3K27M do not show nuclear staining. So this IHC marker is very useful when dealing with the diagnosis of midline gliomas (which as referred to as H3K27-mutant diffuse midline gliomas).
2. Malignant peripheral nerve sheath tumors (MPNSTs) can be a challenging diagnosis to establish, and loss of H3K27me in tumor cells can be used to support such a diagnosis. However, loss is variable, ranging from 35% to 70% of cases. Sporadic MPNSTs show loss in up to 95% of cases. Post-radiation MPNSTs show loss in 90% of cases. In patients with NF-1, about 56–60% of MPNSTs show loss and a much smaller number (30%) in "low-grade" MPNST. Epithelioid MPNST usually has intact immunostaining. There does not appear to be a correlation between expression of S-100 and loss of H3K27me in MPNST. In about 10% of MPNSTs, H3K27me is retained, and there can be cases showing partial loss occasionally (5%).
3. Other nerve sheath tumors seldom show loss of H3K27me, including neurofibromas (no loss seen in either sporadic tumors or ones associated with NF-1 as well as "atypical" and plexiform neurofibromas), schwannoma (loss seen in a rare case, 2%), and perineurioma (no loss).
4. Complete loss of H3K27me can be seen in 40% of melanomas, including up to 25% of spindle cell melanomas and nodular malignant melanoma of childhood.
5. Synovial sarcoma, which is another morphologic differential diagnosis of MPNST, has been reported to show loss from 60% of cases to no loss, and fibrosarcomatous areas of dermatofibrosarcoma protuberans in 40% of cases.
6. Undifferentiated sarcomas, myxofibrosarcoma, rhabdomyosarcoma and leiomyosarcomas, spindle cell rhabdomyosarcoma, monophasic synovial sarcoma, and gastrointestinal stromal tumor show no loss.
7. Dedifferentiated liposarcoma (5%) and angiosarcoma (10%) can occasionally show complete loss of H3K27me.
8. Another tumor that has been described with H3K27me loss is post-radiation sarcoma (20%).

Interpretation

H3K27me loss is typically reported as complete when seen as a loss of the majority (>95%) of tumor cells. In many tumors a small percentage of tumor cells (<5%) can show loss of H3K27me, which is considered a nonspecific finding.

Selected references

Lee W, Teckie S, Wiesner T, et al. PRC2 is recurrently inactivated through EED or SUZ12 loss in malignant peripheral nerve sheath tumors. *Nat Genet* 2014;46:1227–32.
Le Guellec S, Macagno N, Velasco V, et al. Loss of H3K27 trimethylation is not suitable for distinguishing malignant peripheral nerve sheath tumor from melanoma: A study of 387 cases including mimicking lesions. *Mod Pathol* 2017;30:1677–87.

Preito-Granada CN, Wiesner T, Messina JL, et al. Loss of H3K27me3 is a highly sensitive marker for sporadic and radiation-induced MPNST. *Am J Surg Pathol* 2016;40: 479–89.

Schaefer IM, Fletcher CD, Hornick JL. Loss of H3K27 trimethylation distinguishes malignant peripheral nerve sheath tumors from histologic mimics. *Mod Pathol* 2016;29:4–13.

H

H3K27M

HAM56 (macrophage marker)

Background

Human alveolar macrophage-56 (IgM, Kappa) is a monoclonal antibody developed against human alveolar macrophages. The antigen being recognized by HAM56 has not yet been identified. This antibody was developed specifically for the study of human atherosclerotic plaques to identify tissue macrophages and monocyte-derived cells.

Applications

1. HAM56 has wide immunoreactivity, including tissue macrophages, germinal center macrophages, interdigitating reticulum cells, a subset of monocytes, a small population of lymphocytes, and endothelial cells.

2. Variable reactivity with a small number of B-cell lymphomas has also been reported. Inflammatory pseudotumors of lymph node have been shown to contain spindle-shaped macrophages resembling fibroblasts or myofibroblasts that have immunoreactivity for HAM56, CD68, HLA-DR, and CD45.

Selected references

Cheung ANY, Chiu P-M, Khoo U-S. Is immunostaining with HAM56 antibody useful in identifying ovarian origin of metastatic adenocarcinomas? *Hum Pathol* 1997;28:91–4.

NOTES

HBME-1 (mesothelial cell marker)

Background

The antibody reacts with an antigen present in the membrane of mesothelial cells and their neoplastic counterparts, particularly epithelioid mesotheliomas. In initial testing the antibody failed to decorate epithelial cells of the kidney, lung, liver, ovary, and pancreas. The antibody was derived from human epithelioid mesothelioma cells.

Applications

1. The antibody was designed primarily for the identification of normal and neoplastic mesothelial cells and separation from metastatic carcinoma. Absence of staining for HBME-1 makes the diagnosis of mesothelioma unlikely. However, HBME-1 is not specific: 24% of metastatic carcinomas and as many as 85% of ovarian carcinomas can be positive, especially in cytology preparations. HBME-1 does not label sarcomatoid malignant mesothelioma.

Interpretation

HBME-1 produces a "thick pattern of immunoreactivity of the cell surfaces, often including the intracytoplasmic lumina"

and is said to show excellent correlation with the presence of abundant long microvilli with electron microscopy. There is usually no cytoplasmic labeling, and although adenocarcinoma cells may show membrane staining, they do not display the characteristic "thick" membranes and may show cytoplasmic staining. As with epithelial membrane antigen (EMA), immunostaining with HBME-1 is aimed at highlighting the cell membranes and the long microvilli characteristic of mesothelioma.

Selected references

Ascoli V, Carnovale-Scalzo C, Taccogna S, et al. Utility of HBME-1 immunostaining in serous effusions. *Cytopathology* 1997;8:328–35.

Attanoos RL, Goddard H, Gibbs AR. Mesothelioma-binding antibodies: Thrombomodulin, OV 632 and HBME-1 and their use in the diagnosis of malignant mesothelioma. *Histopathology* 1996;29:209–15.

h-Caldesmon

Background

Caldesmon is a protein that binds to calmodulin, tropomyosin, and actin. It is thought to play an important role in the regulation of smooth muscle contraction. It exists in two isoforms: 1-CD (70–80 kDa) and high-molecular-weight caldesmon (h-CD: 120–150 kDa). Although 1-CD is present in many cells, h-CD is exclusively expressed in vascular and visceral smooth muscle cells and in myoepithelial cells. Although nonneoplastic myoepithelial cells are immunopositive for h-CD, tumors with a myoepithelial cell component (pleomorphic adenomas, chondroid syringoma, myoepithelioma, and epimyoepithelial carcinoma) are negative for h-CD.

Applications

1. h-CD is most useful in confirming smooth muscle differentiation and typically leiomyomas. Leiomyosarcomas are positive for h-CD along with desmin. h-CD is consistently expressed in leiomyomas, but its expression is inconsistent in leiomyosarcomas of peripheral soft tissue, where it shows variable expression with loss in poorly differentiated leiomyosarcomas. Tumors in the differential diagnosis, such as myofibroblastic tumor and tumors of myoepithelial differentiation, are h-CD negative.
2. h-Caldesmon is usually negative in rhabdomyosarcoma (RMS) (rare variants such as epithelioid RMS can have desmin expression).

3. The other common application is in the differential diagnosis of uterine smooth muscle tumors (h-CD positive) from endometrial stromal tumors (usually h-CD negative).
4. h-CD expression has also been reported in GIST (gastrointestinal stromal tumor) and glomus tumors.
5. Other tumors with reported caldesmon positivity include PEComa, angiomyolipoma, rhabdomyoma, gastric plexiform fibromyxoma, and angiomatoid fibrous histiocytoma.

Comments

Unlike smooth muscle actin (SMA), caldesmon is not expressed by myofibroblastic and myofibroblastic tumors.

Selected references

Demicco EG, Boland GM, Brewer Savannah KJ, et al. Progressive loss of myogenic differentiation in leiomyosarcoma has prognostic value. *Histopathology* 2015;66:627–38.

Hisaoka M, Wei-Qi S, Jian W, et al. Specific but variable expression of h-caldesmon in leiomyosarcomas: An immunohistochemical reassessment of a novel myogenic marker. *Appl Immunohistochem Mol Morphol* 2001;9: 302–8.

Heat shock proteins (HSPs)

Background

When prokaryotic or eukaryotic cells are submitted to a transient rise in temperature or to other proteolytic treatments, the synthesis of a set of proteins called heat shock proteins (HSPs) is induced. The structure of these proteins has been highly conserved during evolution. The signal leading to the transcriptional activation of the corresponding genes is the accumulation of denatured and/or aggregated proteins inside the cells after being subjected to stress. The expression of a subset of HSPs is also induced during early embryogenesis and many differentiation processes. Two different functions have been ascribed to HSPs: a molecular chaperone function whereby they mediate the folding, assembly, or translocation across the intracellular membranes of other polypeptides, and a role in protein degradation.

Applications

1. Role as prognostic markers in various tumors and in tumor resistance to chemotherapy, overexpression of HSPs allowing tumor cells to resist stressful situations and agents including cytotoxic drugs. In endometrial cancers, expression of HSP27 has been correlated with the degree of tumor differentiation as well as with the presence of estrogen and progesterone receptors. In patients with cervical cancer, HSP27 is predominantly expressed in well-differentiated and moderately differentiated squamous cell carcinomas, but the expression of this protein seems to be a negative prognostic factor for gastric cancer.

2. Different isoforms of HSP27 have been found in lymphoid tissue of patients with acute lymphoblastic leukemia and the protein has been associated with viral infections.

3. The presence of HSP70 appears to be associated with breast cancers of high histological grades and it has been suggested that high levels of the protein identify a subset of patients with node-negative breast cancer who show a high risk for disease recurrence. Increased HSP70 expression has also been correlated with low levels of differentiation in colorectal cancer.

4. Immunostaining for HSP27 and HSP90 is indicative of prolonged survival from hypoxic attacks, whereas weak staining for excitatory amino acid transporter 2 was observed in almost all asphyxia deaths.

5. HSP27 immunoexpression has been reported to correlate inversely with survival in patients with oral squamous cell carcinoma.

Comments

The HSPs show immunolocalization in the cytoplasm as diffuse or finely granular staining. HSP70 appears to be selectively overexpressed in the blast cells of reactive germinal centers and paracortex of lymph nodes, the significance of which remains unknown.

Selected references

Ciocca DR, Oesterreich S, Chamness GC, et al. Biological and clinical implications of heat shock protein 27,000 (Hsp27): A review. *J Natl Cancer Inst* 1993;85:1558–70.

Helicobacter pylori

Background

Helicobacter pylori (HP) is a spiral bacillus that can colonize the human gastric mucosa and induce a specific humoral immunologic reaction in the host. Colonization of the gastric mucosa by HP is a very common finding in gastric ulcers and active chronic gastritis. HP is increasingly recognized as one of the most prevalent human pathogens worldwide and possibly plays a pathogenetic role in gastric carcinogenesis and primary gastric lymphogenesis. The details of the interaction between bacteria, epithelial cells, and inflammatory cells are currently being explored. As effective specific treatment for HP-associated gastroduodenal disorders emerges, surgical pathologists are requested to identify the organism in endoscopic biopsies. Histologic identification of HP (with special staining methods) has been shown to be as accurate as microbiologic culture techniques.

Applications

Bacteria lying within the mucus and on the epithelial surface can be seen on sections stained with hematoxylin–eosin (H&E). However, organisms closely adherent to cells, insinuated in intercellular spaces, or intimately associated with and perhaps phagocytosed by inflammatory cells are frequently difficult to identify.

Comments

Immunohistochemical methods for the detection of *H. pylori* are highly specific and play an important role in selected situations but cannot be advocated for the routine diagnosis of *H. pylori* gastritis. HP-infected gastric tissue is recommended as positive control tissue.

Selected references

Cartun RW, Kryzmowski GA, Pedersen CA, et al. Immunocytochemical identification of *H. pylori* in formalin-fixed gastric biopsies. *Mod Pathol* 1991;4:498–502.

Genta RM, Robason GO, Graham DY. Simultaneous visualization of *Helicobacter pylori* and gastric morphology: A new stain. *Hum Pathol* 1994;25:221–6.

Hep Par 1 (hepatocyte marker)

Background

Hep Par 1 (hepatocyte paraffin 1) is an IgGκ antibody to both normal and neoplastic hepatocytes raised at the Pittsburgh Cancer Institute. Hep Par 1 detects an antigen that is localized to the hepatocyte cytoplasm and produces no staining of bile ducts or other nonparenchymal cells. The staining is granular, occasionally ring-like, and is seen diffusely throughout the hepatocyte cytoplasm without canalicular accentuation. There is no apparent zonal preference in normal liver.

Applications

Its main diagnostic application would be for the distinction of hepatocellular carcinoma (HCC) from cholangiocarcinoma (CC) and metastatic adenocarcinoma in the liver. When employed with CK 19 and CK 20, it is able to provide useful diagnostic information to allow the separation of these three entities. CK 19 is largely limited to bile duct epithelium and its corresponding neoplasms, including CC, whereas CK 20 is a marker of gastrointestinal carcinomas, particularly those from the colon and less consistently the upper gastrointestinal tract and pancreas.

Comments

As the staining of Hep Par 1 is heterogeneous and may be focal within HCCs, caution should be exercised in interpretation as small biopsies such as needle cores may produce false negative results.

Selected references

Fasano M, Theise ND, Nalesnik M, et al. Immunohistochemical evaluation of hepatoblastomas with use of the hepatocyte-specific marker, hepatocyte paraffin 1, and the polyclonal anti-carcinoembryonic antigen. *Mod Pathol* 1998;11:934–8.

Leong AS-Y, Sormunen RT, Tsui WM-S, et al. Immunostaining for liver cancers. *Histopathology* 1998;33:318–24.

Hepatitis B core antigen (HBcAg)

Background

The complete HB virus (Dane particle) is a 42 nm double-stranded DNA virus (Hepadna virus), composed of a 27 nm core particle and envelope 7 nm in thickness, and is immunolocalized within endoplasmic reticulum of liver cells. The HB core protein of 183 amino acids is encoded by the gene C. It is self-assembling and has binding sites for HBV-RNA, which is encapsulated together with viral polymerase. Immunolocalization of HBcAg is cytoplasmic, cytoplasmic membranous, and nuclear. Antibodies are raised against HBcAg obtained from recombinant core DNA of HB virus purified from lysates of *Escherichia coli* clones. HBcAg is expressed predominantly in the nuclei of liver cells, although variable immunoreaction may also be seen in the perinuclear.

Applications

Antibody to HBcAg detects the replicative form of the virus found in the nucleus of HB-infected cells. Perinuclear cytoplasmic immunolocalization is sometimes observed. In very actively replicating infections, cells with cytoplasmic reactivity may outnumber those with nuclear labeling. The presence of HBcAg on immunohistochemistry is usually correlated with complete viral synthesis, as proved by positivity for viral DNA in both liver and blood as well as circulating Dane particles in blood. Demonstration of HBc in liver cells therefore reflects failure to eliminate cells with active viral replication. This is often associated with signs of active disease (piecemeal necrosis or chronic lobular hepatitis) with a membranous pattern of hepatitis B surface antigen (HBsAg). HBcAg is seen with the greatest frequency in immunosuppressed patients with chronic hepatitis. Excess accumulation of core particles can be recognized in an H & E stain in rare cases as "sanded" nuclei.

Comments

It is assumed that viral DNA active in HBcAg production is episomal and not integrated into the host genome.

Selected references

Burns J. Immunoperoxidase localization of hepatitis B antigen (HB) in formalin-paraffin processed liver tissue. *Histochemistry* 1975;44:133–5.

Hepatitis B surface antigen (HBsAg)

Background

The complete hepatitis B virus (Dane particle) is a 42 nm double-stranded DNA virus (Hepadna virus), composed of a 27 nm core particle and envelope 7 nm in thickness, and is immunolocalized within endoplasmic reticulum of liver cells. The glycosylated surface protein of hepatitis B (HB) virus is composed of three gene products: the small, middle, and large HBs-protein, governed by the S, pre-S2, and pre-S1 domain, respectively.

Applications

These antibodies react with antigen-positive cells in patients with type B viral hepatitis, cirrhosis, and hepatocellular carcinoma. Immunoreaction may occur in seropositive as well as seronegative patients. HBsAg in human liver biopsies has two expression patterns with apparently different biological implications:

Membranous HBsAg is strongly associated with HBcAg expression and is an indirect indication of replicative HBV infection.

Intracytoplasmic HBsAg in excess is visible by H & E staining as a homogeneous ground glass appearance of the cytoplasm and is an indicator of chronic elimination insufficiency for this antigen but is an unreliable marker of active replication. In contrast, membrane-associated HBsAg should always raise suspicion of active viral replication.

In patients with IgA nephropathy and HBV antigenemia, polyclonal antibodies have demonstrated HBcAg and HBsAg in the nuclei of glomerular mesangial cells, suggesting immune complex deposition as a possible mechanism of the nephropathy. In situ hybridization studies of HBV DNA in such patients showed coexpression of HBV DNA and HBsAg and/or HBcAg, suggesting the expression of HBsAg in situ in infected renal cells.

Selected references

Gudat F, Bianchi L. HGsAg: A target antigen on the liver cell? In: Popper H, Bianchi L, Reutter W, eds. *Membrane alterations as basis of liver injury*. Lancaster: MTP Press, 1977, pp. 171–8.

Herpes simplex virus I and II (HSV I and II)

Background

The antigens used in the production of these antibodies comprise detergent-solubilized HSV I and HSV II–infected whole rabbit cornea cell. The 302M antibody reacts with HSV I specific antigens, whilst the 303M antibody reacts with HSV II specific antigens. Both antibodies react with antigens common to HSV I and II, all major glycoproteins present in the viral envelope, and at least one core protein. There is no demonstrable cross-reactivity with Varicella zoster virus, cytomegalovirus, or Epstein–Barr virus.

Applications

Antibodies detect the presence of HSV I and HSV II in tissue sections, e.g., skin and brain. A diffuse intranuclear signal is produced, often coinciding with the ground glass intranuclear inclusions of HSV. Similar intranuclear inclusions associated with biotin accumulation have been observed in glandular epithelia of gestational endometrium. Hence, to the unwary, any attempt to demonstrate HSV in these biotin inclusions may produce a false-positive immunoreaction, especially when the avidin–biotin immunodetection system is utilized. The application of prewashing with 0.05% free avidin and 0.05% free biotin does *not* eliminate this cross-immunoreactivity. It is therefore recommended that the peroxidase anti-peroxidase (PAP) or alkaline phosphatase anti-alkaline phosphatase (APAAP) immunodetection system be used for any HSV immunohistochemical investigation of gestational endometrium.

Comments

Biotin-like activity has been observed in thyroid lesions as well. Hence, awareness of this interference is crucial to avoid misinterpretation of immunohistochemical investigations, especially with the ABC immunodetection system. Genital lesions with typical multinucleated giant cells with "ground glass" intranuclear inclusions should be used as positive control tissue.

Selected references

Miliauskas J, Leong AS-Y. Localized herpes simplex lymphadenitis: Report of three cases and review of the literature. *Histopathology* 1991;19: 355–60.

HHV-8 (human herpesvirus 8)

Background

Kaposi's sarcoma herpesvirus (KSHV) or human herpesvirus 8 (HHV-8) was isolated from Kaposi's sarcoma (KS) lesions from patients with the acquired immunodeficiency syndrome (AIDS). Differential expression analysis comparing lytic and latent stages of infection demonstrated that the HHV-8 open reading frame 73 encodes LNA-1, which is a useful marker for HHV-8 infection since it is constitutively expressed in all infected cells. The LNA-1 protein is predominantly expressed during viral latency and appears to play a role in viral integration into the host genome. HHV-8 is present in all cases of KS and in other diseases including primary effusion lymphoma and Castleman's disease. KS can be a challenging diagnosis and differential diagnostic considerations can be very broad depending on the morphology, i.e., vasoformative or spindled. Normal endothelial cells are HHV-8 negative.

Applications

HHV-8 is best known for its diagnostic utility in the identification of KS, which shows consistent expression of HHV-8 in all stages. Benign vascular proliferations and neoplasms that mimic the broad spectrum of KS, including stasis dermatitis, pyogenic granuloma, spindle cell hemangioma (and other vascular lesions/ neoplasms), lymphangioma, and vascular transformation of lymph node, are HHV-8 negative.

Spindle cell lesions such as dermatofibrosarcoma protuberans, myopericytoma, and spindle cell melanocytic lesions, which can be diagnostic considerations in diagnosis of KS with spindle cells, are HHV-8 negative.

Malignant lesions that can also be in the differential diagnosis of KS, including cutaneous angiosarcoma and spindle cell melanoma, are HHV-8 negative.

Interpretation

Not all nuclei in KS are positive and there can be variable positivity (less than 25% of more than 75% of tumor cells) amongst the lesional cells. Typically, fewer cells are positive in the patch/plaque stage of KS.

Selected references

Cheuk W, Wong KO, Wong CS, et al. Immunostaining for human herpesvirus 8 latent nuclear antigen-1 helps distinguish Kaposi sarcoma from its mimickers. *Am J Clin Pathol* 2004;121(3):335–42.

Patel RM, Goldblum JR, Hsi ED. Immunohistochemical detection of human herpes virus-8 latent nuclear antigen-1 is useful in the diagnosis of Kaposi sarcoma. *Mod Pathol* 2004;17(4):456–460.

Robin YM, Guillou L, Michels JJ, et al. Human herpesvirus 8 immunostaining: A sensitive and specific method for diagnosing Kaposi sarcoma in paraffin-embedded sections. *Am J Clin Pathol* 2004;121(3):330–4.

HLA-DR

Background

HLA molecules are highly polymorphic glycoproteins with a single binding site for immunogenic peptides. The complex formed by HLA-DR molecules and peptides is the entity specifically recognized by the antigen receptor of CD4+ helper T lymphocytes. This biological function has been linked to the constitutive cell surface expression of HLA molecules on antigen-presenting cells, which provide immunogenic peptides through denaturation or fragmentation of antigen.

The HLA-DR is a member of the 11β subclass of HLA (the other member is HLA-DQ). B cells of the germinal centers and mantle zones express the HLA-DR antigen. It is also expressed by macrophages, monocytes, and antigen-presenting cells like interdigitating reticulum cells and Langerhans cells of the skin. Activated T cells, but not inactive T cells, may express the HLA-DR antigen. Some endothelial and epithelial tissues may also express HLA-DR.

Applications

Anti-HLA-DR may be useful in distinguishing B-cell follicle center lymphomas from T-cell lymphomas. The antibody also detects Class II antigens, which may be expressed de novo or increased in certain pathological states, e.g., autoimmune diseases.

Similarly, it will demonstrate aberrant expression of Class II antigen in various malignant cell types. Expression of HLA-DR was demonstrated in bladder carcinoma and may have a role in the treatment of such tumors with intravesicle Bacillus Calmette–Guerin. The expression of HLA-DR molecules on crypt epithelial cells of jejunal biopsies of patients with Hashimoto's thyroiditis together with other signs of mucosal T-cell activation was interpreted to suggest the potential of developing celiac disease.

Comments

Tonsil or skin may be used as positive control tissue.

Selected references

Crumpton MJ, Bodmer JC, Bodmer WF, et al. Biochemistry of class II antigens: Workshop report. In: Albert ED, Mayr WR, eds. *Histocompatibility testing.* Berlin: Springer-Verlag, 1984, pp. 29–37.

Jendro M, Goronzy JJ, Weyand CM. Structural and functional characterization of HLA-DR molecules circulating in the serum. *Autoimmunity* 1991;8:289–96.

HMB-45 (melanoma marker)

Background

The HMB-45 monoclonal antibody was generated to a whole-cell extract of a heavily pigmented lymph node deposit of human melanoma and has been shown to be a highly specific and sensitive reagent for the identification of melanoma. The designation *HMB* is derived from the immunogen employed, i.e., Human Melanoma, Black. The antigen is intracytoplasmic, and ultrastructural studies suggest that the antibody reacts with melanosomes before melanin deposition with HMB-45 binding to stage 1 and 2 melanosomes and to the non-melanized portion of stage 3, whereas stage 4 melanosomes and melanosome complexes found in macrophages and keratinocytes have been negative. The antibody appears to label premature and immature melanosomes in retinal pigment epithelium from fetuses and neonates but not from adults, leading to the suggestion that this "oncofetal" pattern of expression may indicate a role in melanocytic cell proliferation. This thesis has not been confirmed and the sequential expression of the HMB-45 antigen in melanocytes may relate to the activation by specific growth factors, resulting in alterations in protein glycosylation during various ontogenic and pathologic states of melanocytes. The epitope recognized by HMB-45 appears to be, in part, the oligosaccharide side chain of a sialated glycoconjugate, as the immunoreactivity can be abolished with neuraminidase treatment.

The gene corresponding to the HMB-45 defined proteins has recently been cloned and designated gp 100-cl. This gene encodes the melanocyte lineage–specific antigens recognized by HMB-45 and HMB-50 (one of two other monoclonal antibodies to melanocytes initially obtained with HMB-45) as well as another monoclonal antibody, NKI-beteb. These three antibodies appear to recognize different epitopes of the same antigen, the melanosomal matrix protein or pmel 17 gene product, defined by their being apparently related by differential splicing.

Applications

1. The staining for HMB-45 in melanocytic nevi depends on their location within the skin. Junctional nevi and the junctional components of compound nevi are HMB-45 positive. In contrast, intradermal nevi and the dermal components of compound nevi are consistently negative. Thus, HMB-45 does not provide distinction between benign and malignant melanocytic proliferations, and the difference in reactivity supports the concept, based on differences in morphology, enzyme activity, and other immunological reactivity, that junctional and dermal cells are not identical. Junctional nevus cells are in an activated or proliferative state compared with their quiescent dermal counterparts and their immunoreactivity with HMB-45 is analogous to the proliferating fetal melanocytes that are positive for the antigen whilst quiescent, adult melanocytes are nonreactive.

   Dysplastic nevi, in contrast, usually express HMB-45 in both the junctional nevus cells as well as the dysplastic cells in the superficial dermis. Nevus cells within the deeper dermis do not usually react with HMB-45. In one study, minimally dysplastic nevi displayed intense immunolabeling of the junctional melanocytes but no staining of dermal nevus cells, whereas with moderately and severely dysplastic nevi, the dermal melanocytes showed focal cytoplasmic immunoreactivity. The likelihood of expression of HMB-45 paralleled the degree of dysplasia of the nevi. Common blue nevi and cellular blue nevi are generally HMB-45 positive, as are malignant blue nevi. Other nevi, such as spindle and epithelioid cell nevi, congenital nevi, and other nevi occurring in hormonally reactive sites, show immunostaining in nevus cells in the deep dermis as well as those near the dermal–epidermal junction. Less common benign melanocytic proliferations such as plexiform spindle cell nevi, Spitz nevi, and atypical melanocytic hyperplasias are also HMB-45 positive.

Malignant melanoma shows strong cytoplasmic positivity for HMB-45 in the majority of cases (65–95%), with the proportion of positive tumor cells ranging from a few to 100%. When the expression of the antigen is weak, staining may appear as a fine granularity similar to that seen in cytologic preparations. The positivity for HMB-45 is seen in almost all types of primary and metastatic melanoma, including amelanotic melanoma, spindle cell melanoma, and acral lentiginous melanoma. One important exception is desmoplastic malignant melanoma, which consistently displays a much lower rate of positivity and may be completely negative. When it is positive, reactivity is usually seen in the superficial epithelioid cells rather than the dermal spindle cells, which only rarely stain for HMB-45.

Attesting to the specificity of the antigen, HMB-45 reactivity has been demonstrated in malignant melanomas of diverse morphology, such as signet ring melanoma, myxoid melanoma, small cell melanoma, and balloon cell melanoma, and in melanomas of different anatomic sites, such as the gallbladder, urinary bladder, anorectal region, vulva, sinonasal region, uterine cervix, other mucosal sites, and bone. Melanomas and melanocytic proliferations occurring in complex tumors such as pulmonary blastoma have also been HMB-45 positive.

HMB-45 staining also has application in the separation of melanin-containing macrophages from melanoma cells, allowing the accurate determination of tumor thickness and depth of invasion. Similarly, labeling for the antigen helps the identification of recurrence or residual spindle melanoma cells from desmoplastic fibroblasts at resection sites.

2. As HMB-45 immunoreactivity is melanocyte specific, positivity can be encountered in lesions with melanin production, such as adrenal pheochromocytoma, melanotic neuroectodermal tumor of infancy (progonoma), melanin-containing hepatoblastoma, malignant epithelioid schwannoma of the skin, pigmented carcinoid tumor, and esthesioneuroblastoma.

3. HMB-45 positivity has been reported in PEComas. This group of tumors has been expanded to comprise angiomyolipoma, lymphangiomyoma, lymphangioleiomyomaosis, renal capsuloma, clear cell myomelanocytic tumor of the falciform ligament, and clear cell "sugar" tumor. These are known as PEComas because of their differentiation towards a putative perivascular epithelioid cells angiomyolipoma, lymphangiomyomatosis, and sugar tumor of the lung. While these tumors consistently manifest HMB-45 immunoreactivity, they do not display obvious pigmentation. The expression of this antigen in angiomyolipoma and lymphangioleiomyomatosis, both manifestations of the tuberous sclerosis complex, has been linked by the recent demonstration of HMB-45 immunoreactivity in cardiac rhabdomyoma, brain lesions, and other mesenchymal as well as neural lesions found in the tuberous sclerosis complex.

4. These include breast carcinoma and normal breast epithelium, sweat gland tumors and normal counterparts, phaeochromocytomas, hepatocellular carcinoma, chordoma, adenocarcinomas, lymphoma, plasmacytoma, and plasma cells. This spurious staining is usually apical or perinuclear in location and granular in nature.

Selected references

Bacchi C, Bonetti F, Pea M, et al. HMB-45: A review. *Appl Immunohistochem* 1996;4:73–85.

hMLH1 and hMSH2 (mismatch repair proteins)

Background

The deoxyribonucleic acid (DNA) mismatch repair system comprises six genes and is required for the correction of DNA mismatches that occur during replication. Inactivation of DNA mismatch repair (MMR) genes most commonly involve *hMLHl* (human *mutL* homologue 1) and *hMSH2* (human *mutS* homologue 2). Germline mutations of *hMLHl* or *hMSH2* result in loss of protein function, accounting for 80–90% of observed mutations in hereditary nonpolyposis colon cancer (HNPCC) patients with mismatch repair deficiency. *hMLH2* is localized to chromosome 3p21 and encodes a 756–amino acid protein, whilst *hMSH2* is localized to chromosome 2p21–22 and encodes a 935–amino acid protein. With the development of tumor, the second (wild-type) allele of these genes is also inactivated, resulting in mismatch repair deficiency. This leads to an increased rate of mutations in microsatellite regions, so-called microsatellite instability (MSI). Such mutations also affect crucial genes that regulate growth, differentiation, and apoptosis. The present definition of replication error (RER)-positive tumors is that 30–40% of MSI markers tested need to show rearrangements in order to justify the designation RER-positive tumor.

DNA mismatch repair genes also play a role in approximately 10–15% of sporadic colon cancers. However, these genes are inactivated by somatic hypermethylation rather than germline mutations, with the latter only identified occasionally in tumor DNA. Hence, it is not only the HNPCC cases but also a significant number of sporadic colorectal carcinomas that share the molecular mechanisms with the familial counterparts as well as pathologic, clinical, and, more importantly, prognostic features, these being "early onset" (<50 years), right-sided cancers with an improved survival rate. Further, similarly to HNPCC patients, the sporadic colorectal carcinomas with MMR defects have an increased incidence of synchronous and metachronous tumors.

MSI testing requires the services of a molecular diagnostic laboratory, but these tumors may alternatively be recognized with immunohistochemical staining. The absence of *hMLHl* or *hMSH2* nuclear expression may identify tumors with an MMR deficiency. Loss of MLH1 or MSH2 was detected in 90% of MSI-high carcinomas, whereas all MSI-low and MS-stable tumors showed normal expression of both proteins.

Applications

It is important to identify patients with HNPCC for genetic counseling, screening, and prevention. It is equally important to stratify sporadic MSI tumors for future chemotherapeutic protocols. This would also identify patients who may be at a higher risk of developing a second carcinoma, including those of the endometrium, ovary, and urinary bladder. The immunohistochemical detection of MMR gene proteins (*hMLHl* and *hMSH2*) places the pathologist at the center of this decision-making process.

Selected references

Jiricny J. Eukaryotic mismatch repair: An update. *Mutat Res* 1998;409:107–21.

Lanza G, Gafa R, Maestri I, et al. Immunohistochemical pattern of MLH1/MSH2 expression is related to clinical and pathological features in colorectal adenocarcinomas with microsatellite instability. *Mod Pathol* 2002;15:741–9.

NOTES

Human immunodeficiency virus (HIV)

Background

Kal-1 reacts with the HIV type 1 capsid protein p24 and its precursor p55 as demonstrated by immunohistochemistry, immunoprecipitation, enzyme-linked immunosorbent assay (ELISA), and immunoblotting using lysates of purified virus and lysates of HIV type 1–infected cells. The antibody detects an epitope of the p24 protein, which is resistant to fixation and paraffin embedding. It does not cross-react with HIV type 2 or simian immunodeficiency virus (SIV) as shown by immunoblotting. During the phase of persistent generalized lymphadenopathy and subsequent stages of disease leading to the development of AIDS, follicular dendritic cells (FDC) forming the framework of lymphoid follicles degenerate. The expression of HIV-1 proteins by FDC in germinal centers in situ, and the presence of HIV-1 mRNA–positive cells in germinal follicles, suggests that FDC are infected and able to produce HIV-1. Such infection may contribute significantly to the destruction of the FDC network during the lymphadenopathy phase after HIV-1 infection. Kal-1 reacts with the p24 protein in cells infected with HIV type 1, i.e., lymphocytes, monocytes and macrophages, Langerhans cells of the skin, follicular dendritic cells, and brain cells of monocyte/macrophage or microglia lineage.

Comments

Interpretation of a positive lymph node biopsy with this antibody should always be confirmed with a serological assay or western blot. In some countries an informed consent is required from the patient before testing for HIV status. Hence, histopathologists should be cautious in the reporting of p24 positive lymph node biopsies.

Selected references

Daugharty H, Long EG, Swisher BC, et al. Comparative study with in situ hybridization and immunocytochemistry in detection of HIV-1 in formalin-fixed paraffin-embedded cell cultures. *J Clin Lab Anal* 1990;4:283–8.

Kaluza G, Willems WR, Lohmeyer J, et al. A monoclonal antibody that recognizes a formalin-resistant epitope on the p24 core protein of HIV-1. *Pathol Res Pract* 1992;188:91–6.

Human milk fat globule (HMFG)

Background

The human milk fat globule (HMFG) is a complex secretory product of mammary epithelium. HMFG is a relatively pure cell membrane product and is partially covered by a typical unit membrane that is extruded from the luminal surface of breast epithelial cells by reverse pinocytosis. Besides the covering unit membrane, filamentous membrane structures, including cytoplasm-associated glycoproteins, can be detected on the inner coat of the HMFG. Similarly to the plasma membrane, HMFG expresses considerable enzymatic activity, including that of glucose-6-phosphate dehydrogenase, acid and alkaline phosphatases, magnesium-dependent ATPase, aldolase, galactosyl transferase, and xanthine oxidase.

A heterogeneous population of HMFG proteins can be recovered from the aqueous phase of skimmed milk following extraction in chloroform and methanol. This pool of solubilized glycoproteins is derived from a human epithelial membrane and referred to as epithelial membrane antigen (EMA). HMFG is thus very similar to EMA and from a practical standpoint antibodies to these proteins have very similar patterns of immunoreactivity. A polyclonal antibody was initially shown to react with EMA and related HMFG protein determinants in formalin-fixed, paraffin-embedded sections and has been extensively used in normal and neoplastic tissues.

Applications

1. The expression of HMFG is heterogeneous in both normal and neoplastic epithelium and its distribution bears no relationship to cellular morphology. The heterogeneity appears to be the result of normal cellular glycosylation patterns and appears to be reproducible in clonal proliferations of all epithelial cells. HMFG proteins are widely distributed in secretory epithelia and their corresponding tumors and fetal anlage. These include sweat glands, sebaceous, apocrine, and salivary glands, epithelium of the intestines, bile ducts, endometrium, and endosalpinx, pulmonary alveolar cells, and exocrine pancreas. HMFG is also expressed by some nonsecretory epithelia such as the distal and collecting tubules of the kidney and urothelium. Syncytiotrophoblasts and glandular cells of the endocervix, prostate, epididymis, rete testes, and thyroid may also be reactive for HMFG. Generally, hepatocytes and proximal tubular epithelia are negative.

2. HMFG-1 reacts with apocrine sweat glands but not with eccrine sweat glands and may be used with other markers to distinguish skin adnexal tumors. It is also immunoexpressed in extramammary Paget's disease, a tumor of apocrine differentiation. The antibody has been applied with limited success for the detection of aspirated milk in lung sections in infant death cases, anti-human alpha lactalbumin showing the greatest sensitivity and clearest reaction.

3. Some mesenchymal cells such as mesothelial cells, plasma cells, and their corresponding tumors may express HMFG/EMA. In addition, soft tissue tumors such as synovial sarcoma, epithelioid sarcoma, peripheral nerve sheath tumor, smooth muscle tumor, rhabdomyosarcoma, chordoma, ependymoma, and choroid plexus tumors may express HMFG/EMA.

Selected references

Edwards PAW. Heterogeneous expression of cell-surface antigens in normal epithelia and their tumours, revealed by monoclonal antibodies. *Br J Cancer* 1985;51:149–60.

Freudenstein C, Keenan TW, Eigel WN, et al. Preparation and characterization of the inner coat material associated with fat globule membranes from bovine and human milk. *Exp Cell Res* 1979;118:277–94.

Heyderman E, Steele K, Omerod MG. A new antigen on the epithelial membrane: Its immunoperoxidase localisation in normal and neoplastic tissue. *J Clin Pathol* 1979;32:35–9.

NOTES

Human papilloma virus (HPV)

Background

The most extensively studied area of HPV infection has been in epithelia of the anogenital tract, particularly the uterine cervix. Over 25 HPV genotypes have been isolated to date from the female genital tract. HPV genotypes have enabled specific types to be correlated with morphological lesions, e.g., HPV 6/11 being commonly associated with condylomata, whilst HPV 16/18 is frequently associated with high-grade cervical intraepithelial neoplasia (CIN) and invasive squamous cell carcinoma. It has recently been demonstrated that over 90% of cervical squamous cell carcinomas harbor a high-risk HPV, the genome of which is usually integrated into the host DNA. Hence, in conjunction with epidemiological data showing that HPV infection and cervical squamous cell carcinoma share several risk factors, the association between high-risk HPV and cervical cancer is now firmly established. Although only a small proportion of high-grade CIN progresses to invasive carcinoma, it is thought that HPV detection may assist in predicting the invasive potential of high-grade CIN.

Applications

The detection of HPV in clinical samples depends on the demonstration of viral components within cells and tissues. This entails the detection of either protein or nuclei acid. Viral proteins may be visualized with immunohistochemical techniques using either polyclonal or monoclonal antibodies. Antibodies directed to viral proteins are dependent on the expression/synthesis of the latter by the virus, which is dependent on transcription/translation of the viral genome within the nucleus. Polyclonal antibodies raised to bovine papillomavirus capsid protein are applicable to HPV types in human biopsy specimens as they cross-react with several human subtypes. The synthesis of bacterial fusion proteins used as immunogens in mice has led to the generation of monoclonal antibodies to specific viral proteins to achieve viral specificity. The use of the HPV 16 LI (capsid) protein has led to the production of several antibodies of varying specificity. The immunoreactivity of antibodies to HPV capsid protein is dependent on active viral replication, which is closely correlated with keratin production. This therefore produces an intranuclear signal in the upper third of the squamous epithelia harboring the virus. Apart from the cervix, the use of antibodies to HPV is applicable to the vulva, penis, anus, oral cavity, larynx, and esophagus.

Comments

With the advent of advanced in situ hybridization technology for the detection of HPV DNA, the demand for HPV immunohistochemistry has fallen. Nonisotope in situ hybridization techniques are easily accessible and readily applicable to the routine diagnostic histopathology laboratory. Squamous epithelium showing the typical morphological features of HPV infection is recommended for use as positive control. Staining should be mainly intranuclear with some perinuclear staining of koilocytes.

Selected references

Cooper K, McGee J O'D. Human papillomavirus, integration and cervical carcinogenesis: A clinicopathological perspective. *J Clin Pathol* 1997;50:1–3.

Patel D, Shepherd PS, Naylor JA, McCance DJ. Reactivities of polyclonal and monoclonal antibodies raised to the major capsid protein of human papillomavirus type 16. *J Virol* 1989;70:69–77.

Human parvovirus B19

Background

Human parvovirus B19 was accidentally discovered in 1975 in human serum being screened for hepatitis B surface antigen. Since discovery, this virus has been found to be the causative agent in erythema infectiosum, chronic anemia in immunosuppressed patients, fetal death associated with hydrops, and acute arthralgia/arthritis.

Parvovirus B19, which is cytotoxic to erythroid progenitor cells in vivo and in vitro, enters the erythroid precursor cell via the blood group P antigen. Human parvovirus B19 has been reported as a cause of severe and persistent anemia in patients immunocompromised from organ transplantation, autoimmune disease, hematologic malignancies, chemotherapy, and congenital or acquired immunodeficiency states, including HIV infection.

Applications

On bone marrow smears and trephine biopsies the presence of giant erythroblasts and small erythroid precursors with nuclear inclusions (Lantern cells) establishes the diagnosis. However, the inexperienced observer may easily overlook these cells, and the use of antibody to parvovirus B19 may be useful in establishing the diagnosis. A high index of suspicion when assessing bone marrow smear/biopsies in immunocompromised patients with chronic severe anemia is required.

Comments

Parvovirus B19 infection should be considered in any unexplained chronic persistent anemia in an immunocompromised patient.

Selected references

Brown KE, Anderson SM, Young NS. Erythrocyte P antigen: Cellular receptor of B19 parvovirus. *Science* 1993;262:114–17.

Liu W, Ittmann MD, Liu J, et al. Human parvovirus B19 in bone marrows from adults with acquired immunodeficiency syndrome: A comparative study using in situ hybridization and immunohistochemistry. *Hum Pathol* 1997;28:760–6.

Morey AL, O'Neill HJ, Coyle PV, et al. Immunohistological detection of human parvovirus B19 in formalin fixed paraffin embedded tissues. *J Pathol* 1992;166:105–8.

Human placental lactogen (hPL)

Background

Human placental lactogen (hPL) is a member of an evolutionarily related gene family that includes human growth hormone (hGH) and human prolactin. hPL, human chorionic gonadotropin (hCG), and pregnancy specific beta 1 glycoprotein (SP1) are the three major proteins produced by the placenta. Although its expression is limited to the placenta, its physiological actions are far reaching. hPL has a direct somatotropic effect on fetal tissues. It alters maternal carbohydrate and lipid metabolism to provide for fetal nutrient requirements and aids in the stimulation of mammary cell proliferation. Two hPL genes (hPL3 and hPL4) encoding identical proteins are responsible for the production of up to 1–3 g hPL hormone/day.

Applications

1. The presence of cytokeratin and hPL was found to be useful in identifying trophoblastic elements in endometrial curettings with a sensitivity of 75. hPL can also be employed in a panel for the distinction of trophoblastic proliferation.
2. Complete hydatidiform mole showed strong expression of hCG and weak expression of placental alkaline phosphatase (PLAP), whereas partial mole showed weak hCG and strong PLAP. Choriocarcinoma, on the other hand, showed strong hCG and weak hPL and PLAP.
3. hPL has also been employed as a marker of intermediate trophoblasts (IT). Extravillous trophoblasts are diffusely and strongly positive for hPL in contrast to the focal staining in villous trophoblasts. There appear to be three subpopulations of IT with distinct morphologic and immunohistochemical features, perhaps accounting for the differences in immunophenotype report for placental site tumors. Chorionic-type IT was found to comprise two populations – one with eosinophilic and the other with clear (glycogen-rich) cytoplasm. The former tended to be larger with more pleomorphic nuclei compared with the smaller, more uniform nuclei of the clear cell type. Both cell types were diffusely positive for PLAP but only focally positive for hPL, Mel-Cam (CD 146), and oncofetal fibronectin. These cells corresponded to those found in chorion laeve and placental site nodule and its neoplastic counterpart, epithelioid trophoblastic tumor. In contrast, implantation site IT cells were strongly positive for hPL, Mel-Cam, and oncofetal fibronectin, corresponding to cells in an exaggerated placental site and its neoplastic counterpart, placental site trophoblastic tumor.

Selected references

Brescia RJ, Kurman RJ, Main CS, et al. Immunocytochemical localization of chorionic gonadotropin, placental lactogen, and placental alkaline phosphatase in the diagnosis of complete and partial hydatidiform moles. *Int J Gynecol Pathol* 1987;6:213–29.

Cheah PL, Looi LM. Expression of placental proteins in complete and partial hydatidiform moles. *Pathology* 1994;26:115–18.

IDH1 and IDH2 (isocitrate dehydrogenase 1 and 2)

Background

IDH1 and IDH2 (isocitrate dehydrogenase 1 and 2) are enzymes that play a role in isocitrate decarboxylation in the citric acid (Krebs) cycle. Somatic mutations in isocitrate dehydrogenase (IDH) genes have been identified at the same codons, including position 132 of IDH1 and positions R172 and R140 of IDH2. In high-grade gliomas this finding has suggested the possible role of *IDH1* in progression of gliomas. More than 70% of Grade II/III astrocytomas and oligodendrogliomas carry *IDH* mutations, but they are usually not identified in pilocytic astrocytomas and other pediatric gliomas. This finding forms one of the bases of categorizing glioblastomas that arise from low-grade gliomas (secondary glioblastoma) or from de novo or primary glioblastoma. *IDH1* mutations have been described in 5.6% of primary and 76% of secondary glioblastomas, and mutation-positive gliomas have a longer survival compared with *IDH*-wild type gliomas. *IDH* mutation status is typically tested by IDH1 immunohistochemistry using IDH1 R132 H marker since this mutation accounts for the majority (about 90%) of the IDH mutations. When the IDH1 IHC is negative in tumor cells, molecular testing is performed to identify other *IDH1* and *IDH2* mutations in patients 55 years or younger (since *IDH* mutations are unusual in the older age group).

Applications

1. IDH1 immunohistochemistry (IHC) is useful in identifying gliomas (diffuse or infiltrating astrocytoma and oligodendroglioma) and secondary glioblastomas with *IDH* mutations. In routine practice IDH-1 IHC is performed in the diagnosis of diffuse astrocytoma and oligodendroglioma, and nearly all these tumors stain positively. Some exceptions include oligodendrogliomas in the pediatric age group, which lack *IDH1* mutations. In the testing algorithm, when such tumors are "IDH-1 IHC negative," *IDH-1/2* mutation analysis is performed to evaluate for other rare mutations.

2. When astrocytomas are *IDH*-wild type, their behavior is likely more aggressive (akin to a high-grade glioma). *IDH*-wild type tumors by IHC are typically followed up by molecular testing for *IDH1* and *IDH1* mutation analysis. This is reflected in the World Health Organization classification of brain tumors with diffuse gliomas being reported as "*IDH1* wild-type" or "*IDH1* mutant."

3. Mutations in *IDH* genes are uncommon but are seen in acute myeloid leukemia (IDH is of prognostic value), cholangiocarcinoma, and chondroid tumors.

Selected references

Dunn GP, Andronesi OC, Cahill DP. From genomics to the clinic: Biological and translational insights of mutant IDH1/2 in glioma. *Neurosurg Focus* 2013;34(2):E2.

Rodriguez FJ, Vizcaino MA, Lin MT. Recent advances on the molecular pathology of glial neoplasms in children and adults. *J Mol Diagn* 2016;18(5):620–34.

NOTES

IgG4

Background

Immunoglobulin gamma (IgG) is the most common of the immunoglobulins. Among the IgGs there are a variety of isotypes, including IgG1, IgG2a, IgG2b, IgG3, and IgG4. The rarest of the immunoglobulins is IgG4. However, despite its rarity, increased IgG4 production has been associated with a variety of pathologic processes over the last decade or so. A key clinical reason to have a low threshold for evaluating IgG4 in sclerotic lymphoplasmacytic infiltrates is the remarkable responsiveness of IgG4-related disease (IRD) to corticosteroid therapy.

Increased IgG4+ cells were first described in type 1 autoimmune pancreatitis, which shows the typical histologic features of IRD. Subsequently, IRD was found to encompass much more than autoimmune pancreatitis and now has been found to involve a large number of tissues, including secreting glands of other types (lacrimal, salivary), soft tissue (sclerosing mediastinitis, retroperitoneal fibrosis), and lung, kidney, and lymph node. IRD at any of these sites shows three major histologic features: 1) dense lymphoplasmacytic infiltration; 2) fibrosis, typically showing at least a focal storiform pattern; 3) obliterative phlebitis.

Applications

Because the histopathologic diagnosis of IRD requires comparison of the IgG4+ plasma cells with the total IgG+ plasma cells in the same section(s), evaluation for IRD requires staining for IgG4 and total IgG on sister sections. While the anti-IgG4 monoclonal antibody noted earlier is highly sensitive and specific for this isotype, poly-anti-IgG polyclonal antibodies tend to have lower sensitivity and specificity, leading to occasional difficulties in interpreting the total IgG stain. Therefore, in our laboratory, we routinely perform total IgG staining in two different concentrations of antibody in the hope that one of those two concentrations will prove relatively straightforward to quantify.

In terms of scoring IgG4/total IgG immunohistochemically (IHC), the typical thresholds required for the diagnosis of IRD are 1) greater than 40% IgG4+ forms among the total IgG+ cells or 2) greater than 50 IgG4+ cells per 400× field.

Selected references

Deshpande V, Sainani NI, Chung RT, et al. IgG4-associated cholangitis. *Mod Pathol* 2009;22:1287–95.

Kamisawa T, Takuma K, Anjiki H, et al. Sclerosing cholangitis associated with autoimmune pancreatitis differs from primary sclerosing cholangitis. *World J Gastroenterol* 2009;15:2357–60.

Immunoglobulins: Igκ, Igλ, IgA, IgD, IgE, IgG, IgM

Background

Surface membrane immunoglobulin (SIg) expression is the classical and specific marker of B lymphocytes and serves as the antigen recognition molecule for this lymphocyte population. Each of the heavy chain classes of Ig can be expressed on the B-cell membrane and more than one heavy chain class can be expressed on the same cell, the majority of peripheral B cells expressing IgM with or without IgD, and fewer than 10% expressing IgM or IgA.

IgM is the first heavy chain class to appear in B-cell ontogeny with the majority of immature B cells expressing IgM in high density. This decreases in density with maturation and increasing amounts of IgD appear on the cell membrane. The IgM and IgD molecules that coexist in the same membrane can exist independently but share the same idiotype and have the same light chain. Following B-cell activation and differentiation, there is loss of IgM and IgD as the result of a productive isotype gene rearrangement switch. With the progression to antibody-forming plasma cells, different subpopulations of SIgM- and/or SIgG-bearing memory B cells may appear.

Clonality of a given B-cell population can be inferred from the uniformity of light chain class expression, as an individual B cell can express either κ or λ light chains but not both; the ratio of κ-:λ-bearing B cells is 2:1. A vast predominance of κ or λ light chain–bearing B cells indicates monoclonality, generally implying a neoplastic proliferation, whereas a mixture of light chain–bearing cell types suggests polyclonality and a reactive or nonneoplastic proliferation of B cells.

Applications

1. About 80% of non-Hodgkin's lymphomas are of B-cell lineage and the majority express monotypic SIg. The SIg isotypes expressed by B-cell non-Hodgkin's lymphoma and lymphoid leukemias parallel those of normal B cells.
2. The most common heavy chain class is IgM, with or without associated IgD, and IgG and IgA are expressed much less frequently. The ratio of Igκ- to Igλ-bearing lymphomas is about 2:1.

Selected references

Merz H, Pickers O, Schrimel S, et al. Constant detection of surface and cytoplasmic immunoglobulin heavy and light chain expression in formalin-fixed and paraffin-embedded material. *J Pathol* 1993;170:257–64.

Leong AS-Y, Forbes IJ. Immunological and histochemical techniques in the study of the malignant lymphomas: A review. *Pathology* 1982;14:247–54.

Inhibin

Background

Inhibin is a peptide hormone produced by ovarian granulosa cells, which selectively inhibits the release of follicle-stimulating hormone (FSH) from the pituitary gland, acting as a modulator of folliculogenesis. Its peak serum level is reached during the follicular phase of the menstrual cycle; it is undetectable in the serum of menopausal women. It is produced and overexpressed by granulosa cell tumors, thus being an early marker for tumor growth. Hence, its usefulness pertains to being a marker of tumor recurrence before clinical manifestation. Several inhibin subunits can be detected by immunostaining in the granulosa cell layers of the human ovary and in neighboring theca cells. Clone R1 was raised against a synthetic peptide corresponding to the 1–32 peptide of the α-subunit of 32 kDa human inhibin and reacts specifically with this molecule (isotype IgG2b). Clone E4 was raised against a synthetic peptide corresponding to the 84–114 peptide sequence of the βA-subunit of 32 kDa human inhibin A and activin A (isotype 2b). E4 reacts with both the βA- and βB-subunits of human inhibin and activin.

Applications

1. Inhibin is a sensitive marker in the diagnosis of sex cord–stromal tumors of the ovary. The vast majority of adult and juvenile granulosa cell tumors, Sertoli cell tumors, Sertoli–Leydig cell tumors, and steroid cell tumors are positive for inhibin. The positivity is lower in fibromas and thecomas.
2. Inhibin can be expressed in some carcinomas, such as ovarian endometrioid carcinomas, mucinous tumors, and up to 10% of serous and 15% of poorly differentiated carcinomas.
3. Inhibin is expressed in the majority of adrenocortical adenomas and carcinomas and only rarely in phaeochromocytoma. Inhibin can also be useful in separating adrenocortical neoplasms from metastatic renal cell carcinomas, which are inhibin negative.
4. Inhibin is expressed in adult cystic nephroma (mixed epithelial stromal tumor) and not in pediatric cystic nephroma.
5. Inhibin is positive in all hemangioblastomas.
6. In testicular tumors, inhibin is expressed in Sertoli and Leydig cell tumors.
7. Inhibin is expressed in trophoblastic tumors but is of limited utility given the availability of more specific markers.
8. A variety of other tumors also express inhibin, including solid pseudopapillary neoplasm, serous cystic neoplasm of pancreas, non-small-cell lung carcinomas (20% of adenocarcinomas and 22% large cell undifferentiated carcinomas), and granular cell tumor of soft tissue.

Selected references

Li Y, Pawel BR, Hill DA, et al. Pediatric cystic nephroma is morphologically, immunohistochemically, and genetically distinct from adult cystic nephroma. *Am J Surg Pathol* 2017;41:472–81.

Sangoi AR, McKenney JK. A tissue microarray-based comparative analysis of novel and traditional immunohistochemical markers in the distinction between adrenal cortical lesions and pheochromocytoma. *Am J Surg Pathol* 2010;34:423–32.

Insulinoma-associated 1

Background

The **Ins**ulino**m**a-associated **1** (INSM1) gene was isolated using a subtraction library of insulinoma and glucagonoma samples and encodes a protein containing both a zinc finger DNA-binding domain and a putative prohormone domain. This protein is expressed in a variety of tumors and is thought to be a sensitive marker for neuroendocrine differentiation. INSM1 protein binds to DNA as well as proteins, especially cyclin D1, causing arrest of the cell cycle and mediating the transcriptional effects of INSM1. It is thought to play a late role in the development of neuroendocrine/neuroepithelial tumors.

Applications

1. Given its broad and widespread involvement with the greater neuroendocrine system, it is not surprising that INSM1 is implicated in a range of neuroendocrine/ neuroepithelial tumors: neuroendocrine tumors in any organ and location irrespective of tumor grade, pituitary adenoma, medullary thyroid carcinoma and C-cell hyperplasia, phaeochromocytoma, Merkel cell carcinoma, hypothalamic hamartoma, small-cell lung cancer, large cell neuroendocrine carcinomas, peripheral neuroblastic tumors (ganglioneuroblastoma, ganglioneuroma), medulloblastoma, central nervous system embryonal tumor, glioblastoma, and endocrine mucin producing sweat gland carcinoma. It can also be used to demonstrate neuroendocrine differentiation in carcinomas with a focal or not easily observed neuroendocrine component.
2. It should be noted that epithelial tumors of the thyroid and parathyroid are consistently negative; hence, follicular and papillary lesions of the thyroid and parathyroid adenoma/ carcinoma do **not** stain with INSM1.

INSM1 has demonstrated a sensitivity of 96.4% across all grades of thoracic neuroendocrine tumors, significantly more than the 87.4% using the panel of traditional markers comprising synaptophysin, chromogranin, and CD56.
3. Among extraskeletal myxoid chondrosarcomas, 90% are positive for INSM1.
4. Staining for INSM1 is also seen in occasional cases of chordoma, soft tissue myoepithelioma, ossifying fibromyxoid tumor, sinonasal SMARCB1 deficient BCOR-CCNB3 sarcoma, and Ewing sarcoma.

Interpretation of staining

As it is a transcription factor, strong nuclear labeling is encountered.

Selected references

Goto Y, De Silva MG, Toscani A, et al. A novel human insulinoma-associated cDNA, IA-1, encodes a protein with "zinc-finger" DNA-binding motifs. *J Biol Chem* 1992;267:15252–7.

Rooper LM, Sharma R, Li QK, et al. INSM1 demonstrates superior performance to the individual and combined use of synaptophysin, chromogranin and CD56 for diagnosing neuroendocrine tumors of the thoracic cavity. *Am J Surg Pathol* 2017;41:1561–9.

Rosenbaum JN, Guo Z, Baus RM, et al. A novel immunohistochemical and molecular marker for neuroendocrine and neuroepithelial neoplasms. *Am J Clin Pathol* 2015;144:579–91.

Xie J, Cai T, Zhang H, et al. The zinc-finger transcription factor INSM1 is expressed during embryo development and interacts with the Cbl-associated protein. *Genomics* 2002;80:54–61.

Islet1

Background

Islet1 is a 39 kD transcription factor that binds to the enhancer region of the insulin gene and is necessary for mesenchymal and endocrine cell formation in the dorsal bud of the pancreas during embryogenesis. Outside the gastrointestinal tract, it is also necessary in the development of cardiovascular progenitor cells and motor neuron development.

Applications

1. Islet1 is a nuclear stain, and expression is normally noted in the islet cells of the pancreas. It is useful diagnostically to assess the site of origin in cases of metastatic well-differentiated neuroendocrine tumors, as up to 15% of tumors may initially present as a metastasis. Determining site of origin is critically important, as pancreatic tumors may respond to chemotherapeutic agents that are less useful in tumors arising from the tubal gut. No differences were noted when the tumors were separated into syndromic and nonsyndromic, although gastrinomas from the pancreas were more likely to be Islet1 negative. While Islet1 is relatively sensitive, it is not specific for tumors of pancreatic origin. Positive staining can be seen in well-differentiated neuroendocrine tumors of the duodenum, rectum, and appendix; however, expression is rare in tumors from the ileum (which is often the main differential in liver metastases of unknown origin). High-grade neuroendocrine carcinomas, from sites within and outside the gastrointestinal tract, tend to be strongly positive for Islet1. Other tumors, such as medullary thyroid carcinoma, carcinoid tumors of the lung, neuroblastoma, paraganglioma, and olfactory neuroblastomas, may also stain strongly.

Selected references

Agaimy A, Erlenbach-Wünsch K, Konukiewitz B, et al. ISL1 expression is not restricted to pancreatic well-differentiated neuroendocrine neoplasms, but is also commonly found in well and poorly differentiated neuroendocrine neoplasms of extrapancreatic origin. *Mod Pathol* 2013;26:995–1003.

Ahlgren U, Pfaff SL, Jessell TM, et al. Independent requirement for ISL1 in formation of pancreatic mesenchyme and islet cells. *Nature* 1997;385(6613):257–60.

Bellizzi AM. Assigning site of origin in metastatic neuroendocrine neoplasms: A clinically significant application of diagnostic immunohistochemistry. *Adv Anat Pathol* 2013;20(5):285–314.

Graham RP, Shreshtha B, Caron BL, et al. Islet-1 is a sensitive but not entirely specific marker for pancreatic neuroendocrine neoplasms and their metastases. *Am J Surg Pathol* 2013;37(3):399–404.

Hermann G, Konukiewitz B, Schmitt A, et al. Hormonally defined pancreatic and duodenal neuroendocrine tumors differ in their transcription factor signatures: Expression of ISL1, PDX1, NGN3, and CDX2. *Virchows Arch* 2011;459:147–54.

Schmitt AM, Riniker F, Anlauf M, et al. Islet 1 (Isl1) expression is a reliable marker for pancreatic endocrine tumors and their metastases. *Am J Surg Pathol* 2008;32(3):420–5.

Ki-67 (MIB1, Ki-S5)

Background

The Ki-67 antibody was generated against a Hodgkin's disease cell line and was found to identify a nuclear antigen expressed in all non-G_0 phases of the cell cycle, i.e., all proliferating cells. The antigen recognized by Ki-67 is a 345–395 kD nonhistone protein complex, which is highly susceptible to protease treatment. The gene encoding the Ki-67 protein is localized on chromosome 10 and organized in 15 exons. The center of the gene is formed by an extraordinary 6845 bp exon containing 16 successively repeated homologous segments of 366 bp, the "Ki-67 repeats," each containing a highly conserved new motif of 66 bp, the "Ki-67 motif." The deduced peptide sequence of this central exon is associated with high turnover proteins such as other cell cycle–related proteins, oncogenes, and transcription factors. Like the last of these, the Ki-67 antigen plays a pivotal role in maintaining cell proliferation because Ki-67 protein antisense oligonucleotides significantly inhibit 3H-thymidine uptake in human tumor cell lines in a dose-dependent manner.

There is a good correlation between the percentage of Ki-67-positive cells in normal tissues and cell kinetic parameters such as ^{3}H-thymidine labeling indices, although generally, Ki-67 immunostaining gives a higher proliferative index than the S-phase fraction, as defined by flow cytometric analysis or by ^{3}H-thymidine incorporation.

Applications

1. Numerous studies have compared the Ki-67 proliferation indices in frozen sections with other prognostic parameters such as tumor grade, hormone receptor status, and p53 expression. In general, Ki-67 indices have been shown to be of prognostic relevance.

Comments

In many cells the Ki-67 antigen appears to be localized to the nucleoli or peri-nucleolar region with lighter diffuse nuclear staining in both frozen and fixed sections. When assessing proliferation indices, notable intratumoral heterogeneity will be observed and counts should be taken from the areas of highest proliferation, usually at the periphery of the tumor. MIB1 is the antibody of choice when assessing proliferation indices. A clone-dependent membrane staining pattern is seen in sclerosing pneumocytoma of lung and hyalinizing trabecular neoplasms of the thyroid.

Selected references

Brown DC, Gatter KC. Monoclonal antibody Ki-67: Its use in histopathology. *Histopathology* 1990;17:489–503.

Laminin

Background

Laminin, a glycoprotein of about 900 kD, is secreted by fibroblasts and epithelial, myoepithelial, endothelial, and smooth muscle cells. Laminin and type IV collagen form the two principal components of basal lamina. There are three genetically distinct chains of laminin, α-, β-, and γ-chains, which are held together by disulfide bonds and by a triple-stranded coiled-coil structure. Ultrastructurally, the basal lamina is composed of a lamina lucida of low electron density, adjacent to the parenchymal cells, and a basal lamina densa of high electron density, adjacent to the connective tissue matrix. By rotary shadowing, laminin has a cross-like shape consisting of three short arms of 200 kD and one long arm of 400 kD. Laminin is exclusively localized to the basal lamina, predominantly to the lamina lucida, and is invariably present in basal lamina surrounding muscle, nerve, fat, and decidua cells and separating epithelial and endothelial cells from adjacent connective tissues. Laminins are potent modulators of numerous biological processes in development, including cell proliferation, migration, and differentiation. In adult tissues, laminins influence the maintenance of specific gene expression and are involved in various pathological situations, including fibrosis, carcinogenesis, and metastasis.

Applications

1. Laminin has been shown to play a role in cell adhesion and attachment to the basal lamina both in vivo and in vitro. The basal lamina is generally extremely stable but in certain pathological states, may undergo local dissolution. This process is likely to play a crucial role in the invasiveness and progression of malignant tumors. In human breast carcinoma, there is a suggestion that overexpression of the *nm23-Hl* gene, a putative metastasis suppressor gene, leads to the formation of basal lamina and growth arrest.

   The majority of invasive carcinomas are recognized to synthesize varying amounts of basal lamina material, but the basal lamina surrounding the tumor nests is generally fragmented and in many cases, completely absent. Benign and in situ lesions appear to be circumscribed by intact basal lamina.

2. Diagnostic applications of collagen type IV immunostaining have mostly centered on the demonstration of basal lamina in invasive tumors, particularly epithelial tumors, and their changes with tumor invasion and metastasis. In particular, the demonstration of an intact basal lamina has been used to distinguish benign glandular proliferations such as microglandular adenosis and sclerosing adenosis from well-differentiated carcinoma like tubular carcinoma of the breast.

3. Distinctive patterns of basal distribution were recently demonstrated in various types of soft tissue tumors. While the presence of basal lamina cannot be used as an absolute discriminant for blood vessels and lymphatic spaces, the latter do not display the reduplication of the basal lamina characteristic of blood vessels and generally show thin and discontinuous staining of basal lamina.

4. The distinctive staining observed around blood vessels has been employed as a marker when performing capillary density measurements. Laminin immunostaining together with collagen type IV was employed to demonstrate frequent breaches in the basal lamina of the mucosa of patients with celiac disease, suggesting that interaction between gliadin and components of the extracellular matrix may have a role in the genesis of mucosal epithelial damage.

5. The presence of basal lamina as demonstrated with laminin immunostaining may be a clue to the identification of hepatocellular carcinoma, as nonmalignant hepatocytes lack basal lamina.

Selected references

Leong AS-Y, Vinyuvat S, Suthipintawong C, Leong FJ. Patterns of basal lamina immunostaining in soft-tissue and bony tumors. *Appl Immunohistochem* 1997;5:1–7.

Liotta LA. Tumor invasion and metastases: Role of the basement membrane. Warner-Lambert Parke-Davis Award Lecture. *Am J Pathol* 1984;117:339–48.

Lysozyme (muramidase)

Background

Lysozyme (muramidase) is a 14.5 kD strongly basic protein that is a mucolytic enzyme found in saliva, gastrointestinal secretions, tears, urine, and serum. Lysozyme has been localized in granulocytes, histiocytes, and some epithelial cells. The protein has been localized ultrastructurally in the secretory granules of Paneth cells and the brush border of granular mucous cells of the small intestine. It has also been localized to the granules of alveolar type II pneumocytes as well as the lysosomal granules of multinucleated histiocytes. In the lymph node, lysozyme is found in the tingible body macrophages of the germinal centers and in macrophages scattered in the paracortex. Dendritic reticulum cells, interdigitating reticulum cells, lymphocytes, and plasma cells generally lack lysozyme. Langerhans cells and sinus macrophages may show stainable lysozyme.

Applications

1. Lysozyme has been employed as a marker of histiocytes/macrophages and of myeloid differentiation.
2. It is a useful marker in both paraffin-embedded trephine biopsies and bone marrow clot preparations, allowing distinction of acute myeloid leukemia from acute lymphoblastic leukemia.
3. It is also useful in the identification of extramedullary myeloid cell tumors, where the combination of myeloperoxidase and lysozyme is a reliable marker of myeloid lineage.
4. Lysozyme has been described in Langerhans histiocytosis, follicular dendritic cell tumors, granular cell tumors, and various histiocytic tumors.
5. Lysozyme combined with GCDFP15 has great specificity for apocrine differentiation in adnexal tumors of the skin, whereas eccrine tumors stain only for GCDFP15.

Comments

While it is a useful marker of lysosomal inclusions in a variety of cell types, including histiocytes/monocytes, this marker is not specific and must be employed in the context of a panel that includes other histiocytic markers such as CD68, alpha-1-antitrypsin, and alpha-1-antichymotrypsin.

Selected references

Ansai S, Koseki S, Hozumi Y, Kondo S. An immunohistochemical study of lysozyme, CD15, (LeuM1), and gross cystic disease fluid protein-15 in various skin tumors: Assessment of the specificity and sensitivity of markers of apocrine differentiation. *Am J Dermatopathol* 1995;17:249–55.

MAC 387

Background

MAC 387 (IgG1, Kappa) was raised against purified peripheral blood monocytes. The antibody recognizes the leukocyte antigen L1 or calprotectin. The L1 antigen consists of three noncovalently bound polypeptide chains with a total molecular mass of 365 kD. This antigen is expressed in neutrophil granulocytes, monocytes, macrophages, squamous epithelia, and reactive epidermis. This antigen is also reputed to be expressed in early inflammation and is present only in cells of the mononuclear–phagocyte system and not the dendritic system.

Applications

1. Apart from identifying reactive macrophages, MAC 387 also highlights macrophages in several histiocytoses including hemophagocytic syndrome, Rosai–Dorfman disease, and Langerhans' cell histiocytosis. True histiocytic lymphomas should be MAC 387 positive, whilst a small number of large cell anaplastic lymphomas may show immunopositivity.
2. MAC 387 antibody produces a cytoplasmic labeling pattern in many myelomonocytic cells.
3. Squamous cell carcinomas of the skin, bronchus, bladder, and oral cavity may show immunoreactivity.

Interpretation

MAC 387 is a good broad-spectrum macrophage marker but is less specific for cells of the mononuclear–phagocyte system than other markers like CD68 and HAM56.

Selected references

Flavell DJ, Jones DB, Wright DH. Identification of tissue histiocytes on paraffin sections by a new monoclonal antibody. *J Histochem Cytochem* 1987;35:1217–26.

MART-1/Melan-A

Background

The Melan-A gene was cloned from the human melanoma cell line SK-Mel29. Independently, the same gene was found by using a different cell line and named MART-1 (melanoma antigen recognized by T-cells). Both clones are recognized by most HLA-A2-restricted tumor-specific tumor infiltrating lymphocytes harvested from patients with melanoma. MART-1 (clone M2–7C10) and Melan-A (clone A103) are two different antibody clones generated by separate groups but recognize the same antigen. The Melan-A/MART-1 protein comprises 118 amino acids with a molecular weight of 20–22 kD. Although not fully characterized regarding subcellular localization, it is nevertheless thought to be associated with melanosomes and endoplasmic reticulum.

In normal tissue, mRNA expression is limited to melanocytes in the skin and retina.

Applications

1. Melanocytic lesions: Immunopositivity for Melan-A/MART-1 has been demonstrated in both primary and metastatic malignant melanoma (especially with an epithelioid morphology) with a range of 81–90% positivity. These positive rates are slightly better than HMB-45 (75–80%). Unlike HMB-45, Melan-A/MART-1 shows a homogeneous cytoplasmic staining pattern in both melanomas and melanocytic nevi, with a stronger intensity and greater percentage of tumor cell immunopositivity. In contrast, HMB-45 stains mainly the intraepidermal and superficial dermal component of compound nevi. Melan-A/MART-1 has a limited role in the differential diagnosis of desmoplastic melanoma. Epithelioid melanomas (primary and metastatic) show a higher frequency of expression with Melan-A/MART-1 than in spindle cell and desmoplastic melanomas.

2. Strong, diffuse granular staining of Melan-A has been demonstrated in adrenocortical adenomas and carcinomas (primary and metastatic). Melan-A is useful in distinguishing adrenocortical carcinoma from renal cell and hepatocellular carcinomas. Melan-A is also a useful marker to separate adrenal cortical tumors from other primary adrenal tumors.

3. Leydig/Sertoli–Leydig cell tumors of the ovary and testes. Although regarded as nonspecific, steroid hormone–producing tumors staining with Melan-A is a consistent finding, but this is not the case with MART-1.

4. Immunopositivity with both Melan-A and MART-1 has been demonstrated in tumors of perivascular epithelioid cells (PEComas).

Selected references

Busam KJ, Jungbluth AA. Melan-A, a new melanocytic differentiation marker. *Adv Anat Pathol* 1999;6:182–7.

Maspin

Background

Maspin is a unique member of the serpin family, which inhibits tumor invasion and metastasis of human breast and prostate cancers. This inhibitory protease harbors tumor suppressor, tumor invasiveness suppression, and anti-angiogenic properties. Maspin has also been shown to inhibit cell motility and appears to be downregulated during cancer progression from benign to invasive and metastatic states. It is consistently expressed by mammary myoepithelial cells as well as many other human epithelial cells and is a cytoplasmic protein that associates with secretory vesicles and is present on the cell surface.

Applications

1. Maspin has been employed as a marker of myoepithelial cells producing no staining of stomal, neural, or vascular elements. It has been employed to distinguish radial scar from tubular carcinoma of the breast.
2. Maspin has also been demonstrated in mammary epithelial cells, the strongest immunoexpression being found in normal breast and fibrocystic change with a progressive decrease in staining from ductal carcinoma in situ to invasive cancer to lymph node metastasis. A subset of infiltrating carcinomas show strong maspin immunostaining and are significantly associated with a lower rate of nodal metastasis, independently of tumor size and grade.
3. Maspin immunostaining has been applied to distinguish pancreatic neoplasms with immunostaining in ductal adenocarcinomas, intraductal papillary mucinous tumors, and mucinous cystic tumors but not in acinar cell carcinomas, pancreatic endocrine tumors, solid-pseudopapillary tumors, and serous cystadenomas. It has been suggested that decreased immunoexpression of maspin may be a significant factor associated with the metastatic potential of stage I and stage II oral squamous cell carcinomas and may be of prognostic relevance also in prostatic carcinoma.

Interpretation

Antigen retrieval is necessary for immunoreactivity of this antibody in fixed sections. Myoepithelial cells show both nuclear and cytoplasmic staining; the protein is localized to the cytoplasm in epithelial cells.

Selected references

Lele SM, Graves K, Gatalica Z. Immunohistochemical detection of maspin is a useful adjunct in distinguishing radial sclerosing lesion from tubular carcinoma of the breast. *Appl Immunohistochem Mol Morphol* 2000;8:32–6.

MDM-2

Background

The MDM-2 protein encodes for a nuclear phosphoprotein that binds p53 and inhibits its ability to activate transcription by concealing the p53 activation domain. It has been suggested that MDM-2 overexpression might represent an alternative mechanism by which p53-mediated pathways are inactivated in human tumors, thus having a possible role in oncogenesis. The ability to stain for MDM-2 protein in fixed tissue sections has stimulated a great deal of interest in its expression in various neoplasms. The correlation of MDM-2 protein levels with p53 may provide insights into oncogenesis and has the potential of providing prognostic information. Several studies have included the detection of p21/WAF1 protein together with MDM-2, as both these oncoproteins are downstream effectors of p53, p21 playing a major role in negatively regulating cell cycle progression, while MDM-2 inhibits the effects of p53.

Results of immunohistochemical analyses of MDM-2 and p53 protein are far from conclusive, although many support an inverse correlation between the two oncoproteins. Such studies have included uterine sarcoma, breast carcinoma, thymoma, osteogenic sarcoma, glioblastoma, lung carcinoma, oral carcinoma, malignant melanoma, thyroid carcinoma, and rhabdomyosarcoma.

Other studies support the role of MDM-2 protein in tumorigenesis in tumors such as oral squamous cell carcinoma, malignant fibrous histiocytoma of the jejunum, well-differentiated and dedifferentiated liposarcoma, non-small-cell carcinoma of the lung, adult medulloblastoma, carcinoma of the breast, oral ameloblastoma, and carcinoma of the urinary bladder. Interestingly, MDM-2 protein was found to be confined to follicular adenomas of the thyroid, whereas p53 protein was not immunoexpressed in such tumors.

MDM-2 overexpression as a result of gene amplification is typically evaluated in most laboratories by fluorescence in situ hybridization (FISH). However, such increased expression can also be detected by immunohistochemical analysis.

Applications

1. MDM-2 has important applications in the workup of lipomatous tumors. There is nuclear positivity in atypical lipomatous tumors/well-differentiated liposarcoma with a small percentage (3%) being negative. However, often the extent of staining can be limited and the reported sensitivity and specificity are wide (45–100% and 59–100%, respectively). Other lipomatous tumors including lipoma, lipoma variants, and other variants of liposarcoma (myxoid, pleomorphic) are generally negative. Rare benign lipomas (2–5%) have been reported to be MDM-2 positive, suggesting that this limits the utility of MDM-2 immunohistochemistry in this setting.
2. Much like atypical lipomatous tumor (ALT)/well-differentiated liposarcoma (WD-LPS), MDM-2 immunohistochemical expression is seen in dedifferentiated (DD)-LPS. However the positivity is strong and diffuse, and this perhaps is one of the better uses of MDM-2 immunohistochemistry. MDM-2 is by no means specific; other spindle cell tumors such as MPNST (64%) and MFS (42%) can show MDM-2 positivity. In such cases evaluating for CDK4 coexpression is useful in supporting the diagnosis of DD-LPS.
3. Parosteal and central low-grade osteosarcoma and intimal sarcomas are also MDM-2 positive. MDM-2 and CDK4 immunochemical expression can be utilized in the differential diagnosis of osteosarcoma versus benign entities such as fibrous dysplasia in challenging cases.

Comments

MDM-2 positivity in ALT/WD-LPS usually is seen as scattered positive nuclei. CDK4 usually shows more diffuse positivity than MDM-2 in such tumors. Histiocytes in fat necrosis can be MDM-2 positive and to avoid this pitfall, concurrent CDK4 immunochemical testing can be performed or confirmed by FISH analysis. MDM-2 immunochemical positivity has also been reported in pleomorphic fibromas of skin, angiomyolipoma (14%), and gastrointestinal stromal tumor (GIST).

Amongst non-LPS, MDM-2 has been described in malignant peripheral nerve sheath tumors, myxofibrosarcoma, embryonal rhabdomyosarcoma, leiomyosarcoma, and synovial sarcoma. Hence, it has been suggested that CDK4 be used along with MDM-2, since combined positivity is much less common in non-LPS (8% of MPNST and 8% of MFS). Additionally, CDK4, while less sensitive, is more specific for the diagnosis of ALT/DD-LPS.

Others have suggested adding p16 to this panel to increase the sensitivity of the diagnosis, with the trio being expressed in 70% of WDL/DD-LPS cases. Only rare (2%) lipomas expressed all three markers. Some authors contend that such "lipomas" expressing all such markers require long-term follow-up to assess their clinical behavior.

Selected references

Gelsleichter L, Gown AM, Zarbo RJ, et al. P53 and mdm-2 expression in malignant melanoma: An immunocytochemical study of expression of p53, mdm-2, and markers of cell proliferation in primary versus metastatic tumors. *Mod Pathol* 1995;8:530–5.

Clay MR, Martinez AP, Weiss SW, et al.MDM2 and CDK4 immunohistochemistry: Should it be used in problematic differentiated lipomatous tumors? *Am J Surg Pathol* 2016;40:1647–52.

Measles

Background

The measles virion is composed of a central core of ribonucleic acid with a helically arranged protein coat surrounded by a lipoprotein envelope with spike-like structures. The virion is 120–200 nm in diameter and is classified as a morbillivirus in the paramyxovirus family.

Applications

Subacute sclerosing panencephalitis (SSPE) is a rare, fatal disease of children caused by a persistent measles virus infection of the central nervous system (CNS). Immunodetection of viral proteins using antibodies raised to measles is useful to confirm the diagnosis of SSPE in brain biopsies and postmortem CNS tissue.

Interpretation

Application of antibodies to measles virus would be useful in developing countries where SSPE is more frequently seen. Both polyclonal and monoclonal antibodies give good immunoreactivity following microwave pretreatment.

Selected references

Allen IV, McQuaid S, McMahon J, et al. The significance of measles virus antigen and genome distribution in the CNS in SSPE for mechanisms of viral spread and demyelination. *J Neuropathol Exp Neurol* 1996;55:471–80.

Mel-CAM (melanoma cell adhesion molecule, CD146)

Background

Melanoma cell adhesion molecule (Mel-CAM) is a cell adhesion molecule that belongs to the immunoglobulin supergene family. Mel-CAM was originally designated MUC18 and was discovered by differential screening of a cDNA library from a human melanoma cell line. Mel-CAM is a 113 kD single-chain molecule containing five immunoglobulin-like domains, a transmembrane stretch, and a short cytoplasmic tail with several potential phosphorylation sites. It functions by binding to an unidentified counter-receptor on the surface of adjacent cells. In addition to its action as a cell–cell adhesion molecule, the extracellular domain of Mel-CAM contains a potential proteoglycan-binding motif that may facilitate cell–extracellular matrix adhesion.

Applications

1. Mel-CAM expression has been detected in a variety of tissues, including hair follicles, cerebellar cortex, endothelium, and smooth muscle.
2. Mel-CAM is expressed in more than 90% of cutaneous melanomas.
3. It has also been detected in angiosarcomas, leiomyosarcomas, hematopoietic tumors, and glial tumors.
4. Mel-CAM has also been reported to be a specific cell surface marker for intermediate trophoblasts (ITs). In contrast, chorion-type ITs, endometrial glandular and surface epithelium, and inflammatory cells in the implantation site are Mel-CAM immunonegative or show only focal weak positivity. Hence, Mel-CAM is a specific and sensitive marker for IT differentiation in normal placentas, implantation sites, and gestational trophoblastic tumors.

Selected references

Albelda SM, Muller WA, Buck CA, et al. Molecular and cellular properties of PECAM-1 (endoCAM/CD31): A novel vascular cell-cell adhesion molecule. *J Cell Biol* 1991;114:1059–68.

Kuzu I, Bicknell R, Fletcher CDM, et al. Expression of adhesion molecules on the endothelium of normal tissue vessels and vascular tumors. *Lab Invest* 1993;69:322–8.

Mesothelin

Background

Mesothelin, a 40 kDa glycosylphosphatidylinositol-linked cell surface glycoprotein, was isolated by the monoclonal antibody (Mab K1) originally found to be reactive against ovarian carcinoma and mesotheliomas. It is on the surface of mesothelial cells, mesotheliomas, and ovarian carcinoma and plays a role in cellular adhesion.

Applications

1. Expressed in lung and mesothelial cells with low levels of expression in heart, placenta, and kidney. It is expressed in epithelioid mesotheliomas, ovarian carcinomas, and some squamous cell carcinomas. Though initially thought to be specific for mesotheliomas and ovarian carcinomas, it is positive in lung adenocarcinoma (40%), squamous cell carcinoma of lung (20%), esophagus (75%), and uterine cervix (25%) as well as in other adenocarcinomas (nonmucinous ovarian carcinoma – 100%, peritoneum – 100%, endometrium – 65%, pancreas – 90%, biliary tract – 45%, stomach – 50%, colon – 30%) but not in carcinomas of breast, kidney, thyroid, adrenal, or prostate, or in germ cell tumors, neuroendocrine tumors, or urothelial carcinoma.

2. Mesothelin is reported to be positive in desmoplastic small round cell tumor and epithelial component of biphasic synovial sarcoma.

3. Amongst nonmucinous ovarian carcinomas, mesothelin is expressed in serous, endometrioid, clear cell, and transitional carcinomas of the ovary as well as in Brenner tumor of ovary (100%). Approximately 50% of mucinous carcinomas of ovary are reported variably positive for mesothelin. Mesothelin positivity is reported in mature teratomas of ovary (100%).

Selected references

Chang K, Pastan I. Molecular cloning of mesothelin, a differentiation antigen present on mesothelium, mesotheliomas, and ovarian cancers. *Proc Natl Acad Sci USA* 1996;93:136–40.

Ordóñez NG. Value of mesothelin immunostaining in the diagnosis of mesothelioma. *Mod Pathol* 2003;16:192–7.

Metallothioneins

Background

Metallothioneins (MTs) are low-molecular-weight, heavy-metal-binding proteins whose expression is induced by heavy metals as well as other factors such as stress, glucocorticoids, lymphokines, and xenobiotics. MTs have been described in most vertebrate and invertebrate species. Two major isoforms, MT-I and MT-II, are distributed in most adult mammalian tissues. Recently, another isoform, MT-0, has been recognized, and genes for MT-III and MT-IV with restriction to brain neurons and stratified epithelium have been described. Interest in MTs has focused on their overexpression and susceptibility to carcinogenic and anticarcinogenic effects of cadmium, spontaneous mutagenesis and anti-cancer drugs, and tumor resistance to chemotherapeutics.

Applications

1. MT expression has been associated with the type and grade of some tumors, such as ductal breast carcinoma, skin carcinoma, cervical carcinoma, pancreatic carcinoma, prostatic carcinoma, melanoma, bladder carcinoma, renal cell carcinoma, small-cell carcinoma of the lung, and ovarian carcinoma. While overexpression of MTs appears to be mostly associated with locally invasive carcinomas of poor histological type and grade, reduced overall survival, and local recurrence of tumor (but not lymph node or distant metastases), this is not true of all tumors.

2. In colonic, bladder, and fibroblastic skin tumors, overexpression of MTs is associated with lower-grade, better-differentiated tumors. In squamous cell carcinoma of the esophagus, overexpression of MT appears to predict tumors that benefit from chemotherapy.

3. MT has been described as a marker of deep penetrating dermatofibroma, allowing its distinction from dermatofibrosarcoma protuberans, which was consistently negative by immunostaining.

4. Increased immunoexpression of MT has been demonstrated in fibroblasts of all ulcerative lesions of ulcerative colitis and Crohn's disease, suggesting a protective role for MT.

Interpretation

MT staining is found in nucleus, cytoplasm, and cell membrane, and the proliferating edges of tumors show most intense staining.

Selected references

Jasani B, Schmid KW. Significance of metallothionein overexpression in human tumors. *Histopathology* 1997;31:211–14.

Kagi JHR. Overview of metallothionein: Metallobiochemistry Part B: metallothionein and related molecules. *Meth Enzymol* 1993;205:613–26.

Microphthalmia transcription factor (MiTF)

Background

The microphthalmia (Mi) gene is located on chromosome 3p and encodes a basic–helix–loop–helix zipper protein. This DNA-binding protein regulates transcription of genes involved in melanin synthesis, such as tyrosinase. Studies in mice have shown that MiTF is essential for pigment synthesis and for embryogenesis and postnatal survival of melanocytes. In humans, MiTF comprises four isoforms that differ at their amino-termini and expression patterns. Isoforms A and B are present in retinal pigment epithelium, cervical cancer cells, and melanoma cells. Isoform H is present in the retinal pigment epithelium and cervical cancer cells but not in melanoma cells, whilst isoform M is present only in melanoma cells. Humans with heterozygous mutations of MiTF have Waardenburg syndrome 2a, which is characterized by the presence of a white forelock and deafness. All (100%) melanomas are positive with antibody D5, which recognizes both mouse and human MiTF.

Applications

1. The high sensitivity and specificity for melanocytic differentiation is seen in cutaneous nevi and in 88% of metastatic melanoma. MiTF is less helpful in the diagnosis of desmoplastic malignant melanoma with positivity ranging from 3% to 55%. This may be related to the diffuse nature of the tumor, as MiTF expression appears to be less common in small dermal desmoplastic melanomas than in those that form a distinct tumor mass.
2. MiTF immunoexpression has also been demonstrated in PEComas with an efficacy approximately equal to HMB-45 and Melan-A. An advantage of MiTF in small biopsies is that a greater number (>50%) of cells are positive.
3. Other soft tissue neoplasms with melanocytic differentiation have also been demonstrated to show MiTF expression, namely, melanotic schwannomas, cellular blue nevi, and clear cell sarcomas.

Interpretation

As a nuclear marker, MiTF is largely free of cytoplasmic staining.

Selected references

Busam KJ, Iversen K, Copian KC, et al. Analysis of microphthalmia transcription factor expression in normal tissues and tumors, and comparison of its expression with S-100 protein, gp100, and tyrosinase in desmoplastic malignant melanoma. *Am J Surg Pathol* 2001;25:197–204.

Mitochondria

Background

Monoclonal antibody clone 113–1 recognizes a 60 kD nonglycosylated protein component of mitochondria in human cells. This marker may be useful in the identification of mitochondria in cells, tissues, and biochemical preparations. It produces a cytoplasmic granular "spaghetti-like" staining pattern in the cytoplasm of human cells.

Applications

Antimitochondrial antibody clearly has a role in the identification of oncocytic tumors on both paraffin sections and cell preparations.

1. In the differential diagnosis of granular renal cell tumors. Distinctive staining patterns are observed: in chromophobe renal cell carcinoma (RCC) a peripheral accentuation of coarse cytoplasmic granules; a diffuse and fine granularity in renal oncocytomas; and an irregular cytoplasmic distribution of coarse granules in the granular variant of clear cell RCC. In addition, staining is most intense in the eosinophilic variant of papillary RCC with irregular cytoplasmic distribution of coarse granules.

2. In the salivary gland, immunohistochemistry using the antimitochondrial antibody proved to be a highly sensitive and specific method for light microscopic identification of mitochondria and superior to routine H&E or PTAH stains for the detection of normal and metaplastic oncocytic cells. This was also useful in the demonstration of neoplastic cells rich in mitochondria: Warthin's tumor, benign oncocytoma and oncocytic carcinoma, and deciduoid mesothelioma, all of which show an intense, finely granular immunoreactivity in the cytoplasm.

3. Antimitochondrial antibody is also useful in the confirmation/identification of poorly differentiated oxyphilic (Hurthle cell) carcinomas of the thyroid, showing selective marking of oxyphilic, mitochondria-rich cells.

4. Oncocytic (mitochondria-rich) differentiation identifying a subset of oncocytic meningiomas that behave aggressively may also be accomplished with the use of this antibody.

MLH1/MSH2 proteins

Background

hMLH1 is localized to chromosome 3p21 and encodes a 756–amino acid protein, while hMSH2 is localized to chromosome 2p21–22 and encodes a 935–amino acid protein. With development of tumor, the second (wild-type) allele of these genes is also inactivated, resulting in DNA mismatch repair (MMR) deficiency. This leads to an increased rate of mutations in microsatellite regions, so-called microsatellite instability (MSI). Such mutations also affect crucial genes that regulate growth, differentiation, and apoptosis. The present definition of replication error (RER)-positive tumors is that 30–40% of MSI markers tested need to show rearrangements in order to justify the designation RER+ tumor.

Colon cancers in HNPCC patients typically occur in right colon (in the absence of multiple polyps) and show poor differentiation with a cribriform pattern and a lymphoid inflammatory infiltrate but carry a better prognosis than "conventional tumors." DNA mismatch repair genes also play a role in approximately 10–15% of sporadic colon cancers. However, these genes are inactivated by somatic hypermethylation rather than germline mutations, with the latter only identified occasionally in tumor DNA. Hence, it is not only the hereditary nonpolyposis colorectal cancer (HNPCC) cases, but also a significant number of sporadic colorectal carcinomas, that share the molecular mechanisms with the familial counterparts as well as pathologic, clinical, and, more importantly, prognostic features – these being "early-onset" (<50 years) right-sided cancers with an improved survival rate. Further, similarly to HNPCC patients, the sporadic colorectal carcinomas with MMR defects have an increased incidence of synchronous and metachronous tumors.

MSI testing requires the services of a molecular diagnostic laboratory, but these tumors may alternatively be recognized with immunohistochemical staining. The absence of hMLH1 or hMSH2 nuclear expression may identify tumors with MMR deficiency. Immunohistology can discriminate accurately between MSI and microsatellite-stable tumors.

Loss of MLH1 or MSH2 is detected in 90% of MSI-high carcinomas, whereas all MSI-low and MS-stable tumors show normal expression of both proteins. Lack of MLH1 nuclear staining is observed more frequently than absence of MSH2. The finding of carcinomas on the left side of the colon with absence of staining for one MMR protein (some also later develop a second colorectal carcinoma) has resulted in the recommendation that all colorectal carcinomas be screened for loss of immunoexpression for hMLH1 and hMSH2, irrespective of the HNPCC status.

MSI is associated, among other cancers, with endometrial adenocarcinoma, which is the most common tumor after colorectal carcinoma in patients with HNPCC. Hence, some institutions are performing MMR protein evaluation on all women with endometrial adenocarcinomas. MSI is caused by DNA MMR deficiency (so-called "hypermutated phenotype") and tumors are divided into MSI-high, MSI-low and MS-stable (MSS), with MSI-H tumors being MMR deficient by immunohistochemistry (IHC). The majority of such MMR-deficient tumors are sporadic, caused by MLH1 promoter methylation leading to loss of MLH1 and PMS2. A minority of endometrial carcinomas are caused by somatic or germline mutations in MMR genes, and Lynch syndrome (LS) accounts for 2% to 6% of all endometrial carcinomas .

If clinical and pathologic criteria were solely used, a number of LS-associated endometrial carcinomas could be missed, suggesting support for universal screening in all patients with diagnosed endometrial carcinoma.

There is excellent correlation between MSI and MMR IHC testing in terms of concordance rates and in the MSH6 mutations, IHC is a more reliable method over MSI. IHC for MMR proteins is widely used in most institutions, using a four-antibody panel to obtain the greatest sensitivity as a way to screen for LS. Most institutions have developed criteria for MMR IHC testing in endometrial adenocarcinoma using recommended criteria, and these include patients 50 years of age or younger, associated morphologic criteria such as peritumoral lymphocytes, tumor-infiltrating lymphocytes (>40 lymphocytes/10 high power field), undifferentiated or dedifferentiated carcinoma, and synchronous ovarian clear cell carcinoma. Additionally, MMR IHC loss has been described in 6–7% of ovarian endometrioid and clear cell carcinomas, and many institutions include these tumors in universal testing for MMR IHC screening.

Applications

1. Immunohistochemical testing for MMR proteins using a panel of four markers (MLH1, PMS2, MSH2, and MSH6) is widely utilized as a screening methodology. Loss of MLH1 is associated with PMS2 loss, and such cases are tested for hypermethylation of MLH1 promoter by molecular testing. This is to exclude methylation as a sporadic event being a cause of MLH1/PMS2 IHC loss. However, there are those rare cases of LS with mutations in promoter methylation, and in such instances, when there is a strong family or personal history, further genetic testing is suggested. Other patients with loss of MSH2, MSH6, and isolated PMS2 loss are referred for genetic counseling and possible further molecular testing.

2. MMR IHC testing is also being performed to identify patients for treatment with immunotherapy.

3. Literature supports universal IHC-based MMR testing on all endometrial adenocarcinomas as a way to screen for LS. About 10% of LS patients can be missed, however, when using MMR as a way to screen.

4. Unusual patterns of IHC results in endometrial adenocarcinomas:

   a. Variable positivity for MLH1 and PMS2: There are some cases that can show abrupt loss of MLH1 and PMS2 expression. This has been shown to be as a result of heterogeneous promoter hypermethylation of MLH1 in various portions of the tumor. There does not appear to be an association with LS.

   b. Heterogeneous staining with MMR IHC markers: When there is variability in staining, including foci that are positive with other areas being weak or negative, this is usually attributed to technical reasons. However, more recently, subclonal losses of MMR IHC staining have been studied, showing that cases with subclonal loss are associated with MLH1 promoter methylation from a second-hit somatic mutation. Similarly, subclonal loss of

MSH6 also is likely explainable by somatic events rather than germline MSH6 mutations.

   c. Usually carcinomas with MLH1/PMS2 loss show concordant loss in the foci of atypical hyperplasia (EIN), but some cases can show discordant staining.

   d. When there is MMR IHC loss with no hypermethylation of MLH1 and no germline mutations, this has been referred to as "LS-like" and caused by "false positive IHC" due to interpretive errors or subclonal loss and sampling, undetected mutations, or last biallelic somatic mutations.

   e. Isolated loss of PMS2 IHC: PMS2 germline mutation is a rare cause of LS. About 50% of cases of isolated loss of PMS2 are associated with promoter hypermethylation of MLH1. In the other cases, PMS2 but no MLH1 germline mutations were found. Other literature suggests that MLH1 germline mutations can be identified in about 25% of such cases.

   f. POLE mutations can also lead to MMR IHC loss and in particular MSH6.

It is important to identify patients with HNPCC for genetic counseling, screening, and prevention. It is equally important to stratify sporadic MSI tumors for future chemotherapeutic protocols. This would also identify patients who may be at a higher risk of developing a second carcinoma, including those of the endometrium, ovary, and urinary bladder. The immunohistochemical detection of MMR gene proteins places the pathologist at the center of this decision-making process.

Comments

It is very important to avoid pitfalls in the performance and interpretation of MMR IHC markers. These include (a) overlooking patchy, weak, and focal positivity in tumor cells, in particular for MSH6; (b) not having a good positive control in the tissue, such as stromal cells and inflammatory cells; (c) occasional cases showing uninterpretable staining; and (d) subclonal regional loss of MMR proteins by IHC, including discrete areas of loss that correspond to portions of the tumor with MSI.

It has been suggested to test whether cost-effective MMR IHC screening can be performing by starting with MSH6 and PMS2 initially.

The ability to identify HNPCC with immunostaining has allowed the correlation of clinicopathological features of such tumors. MSI-high MLH1/MSH2+ carcinomas are more often located in the distal colon, are more frequently typed as ordinary adenocarcinoma, and are more likely to be well or moderately differentiated, p53+, and <7 cm in diameter than MLH1– and MSH2– carcinomas. Antibodies to other MMR gene proteins that are immunoreactive in fixed paraffin-embedded tissues include anti-PMS2 and anti-MSH6, but abnormalities of these proteins are less common in HNPCC.

Selected references

Jiricny J. Eukaryotic mismatch repair: An update. *Mutat Res* 1998; 409: 107–21.

Lanza G, Gafa R, Maestri I, et al. Immunohistochemical pattern of MLH1/MSH2 expression is related to clinical and pathological features in colorectal adenocarcinomas with microsatellite instability. *Mod Pathol* 2002; 15: 741–9.

MOC-31

Background

MOC-31 is a monoclonal antibody generated from a small-cell lung carcinoma cell line (GLS-1). The SCLC-cluster 2 antibodies detect a 38 kDa epithelial-associated transmembrane glycoprotein, which is also named "epithelial glycoprotein 2" or EGP-2, since it only occurs in epithelial cells. The latter was derived from the strong expression of EGP-2 in nonsquamous carcinomas and its absence in lymphomas, melanomas, and neuroblastomas. Hence, MOC-31 is a monoclonal antibody that recognizes a glycoprotein of unknown function present in the membrane of epithelial cells.

Applications

1. Adenocarcinomas from a variety of sites stain positively with MOC-31. MOC-31 reactivity was obtained in 100% of pulmonary adenocarcinomas and 85% of nonpulmonary adenocarcinomas but only in 5% of mesotheliomas. The latter were restricted to a few positive cells, in contrast to the adenocarcinomas, where positivity was strong and diffuse.
2. The role of MOC-31 has been expanded and shown to distinguish between hepatocellular carcinoma and adenocarcinoma (both metastatic and cholangiocarcinoma), MOC-31 being negative in primary hepatomas.
3. MOC-31 may be helpful as part of a panel of antibodies to distinguish between mesotheliomas and adenocarcinoma. There appears to be sufficient evidence to validate its inclusion in a panel to distinguish hepatomas from adenocarcinoma (both primary and secondary) in the liver.

Selected references

Edwards C, Oates J. OV 632 and MOC 31 in the diagnosis of mesothelioma and adenocarcinoma: An assessment of their use in formalin fixed and paraffin wax embedded material. *J Clin Pathol* 1995;48:626–30.

MSH6

Background

There are four main mismatch repair genes (MLH1, MSH2, MSH6, and PMS2). The products of these genes are necessary to identify and correct errors that occur during DNA replication at microsatellite loci, small repetitive sequences scattered throughout the genome. These areas are prone to DNA slippage, resulting in insertion and deletion loops. The mismatch repair proteins form heterodimers, with the MSH2–MSH6 complex recognizing the impaired bases while MLH1 and PMS2 excise the mismatched nucleotides. Germline mutations in these genes are associated with Lynch syndrome (hereditary nonpolyposis colorectal carcinoma [HNPCC]), an autosomal dominant disorder characterized by early-onset colorectal cancer and increased risk of cancer of the endometrium, stomach, ovary, skin, and other sites.

MSH6 (*mutS homolog 6*) is a mismatch repair gene located on chromosome 2p16.3 that is located within 1 megabase of its heterodimer partner, MSH2. It was first implicated as a cause of HNPCC in 1997, when a patient with HNPCC-like syndrome was found to have a *MSH6* mutation in both germline and tumor DNA. Numerous truncating mutations in MSH6 have been identified, although HNPCC secondary to an *MSH6* mutation is less common than mutations in MLH1 or MSH2 . Clinically, patients with germline *MSH6* mutations tend to have a lower incidence of colorectal carcinoma and tend to present at a later age. They also differ pathologically in that they are more likely to have a rectal tumor and may lack the typical histologic features associated with microsatellite instability (MSI)-high tumors.

Applications

MSH6 expression is normal in the proliferating epithelium of the gastrointestinal tract, so when assessing for MSI the pathologist should look for absence of staining in tumor nuclei. Loss of MSH6 is most commonly seen in two distinct scenarios: loss of both markers in the setting of a germline mutation of MSH2, or loss of MSH6 only, secondary to a germline mutation in MSH6. Variant staining patterns have been reported in the literature, most notably a "nucleolar" pattern and a "near-complete" loss pattern, which is felt to be related to prior chemotherapy or radiation therapy. Case reports have also suggested that somatic mutations in the MSH6 gene may be responsible for faint abnormal staining.

In practice, the MSH6 immunohistochemical stain is most commonly used in a panel with MLH1, MSH2, and PMS2. Although the four-stain panel is most commonly used, studies have shown that a panel consisting of MSH6 and PMS2 is equally sensitive with the added benefit of cost-effectiveness.

Immunohistochemistry to predict MSI can also be used to assess for MSI in extracolonic malignancies. Studies have confirmed its accuracy in detecting MSI in endometrial carcinomas, and it can also be used to screen for Lynch syndrome in patients with sebaceous neoplasms.

Selected references

Bedeir A, Krasinskas AM. Molecular diagnostics of colorectal cancer. *Arch Pathol Lab Med* 2011;135(5):578–87.

Bellizzi AM, Frankel WL. Colorectal cancer due to deficiency in DNA mismatch repair function: A review. *Adv Anat Pathol* 2009;16(6):405–17.

Garg K, Leitao MM Jr, Kauff ND, et al. Selection of endometrial carcinomas for DNA mismatch repair protein immunohistochemistry using patient age and tumor morphology enhances detection of mismatch repair abnormalities. *Am J Surg Pathol* 2009;33(6):925–33.

Hall G, Clarkson A, Shi A, et al. Immunohistochemistry for PMS2 and MSH6 can replace a four antibody panel for mismatch repair deficiency screening in colorectal adenocarcinoma. *Pathology* 2010;42(5):409–13.

Klarskov L, Holck S, Bernstein I, et al. Challenges in the identification of MSH6-associated colorectal cancer: Rectal location, less typical histology, and a subset with retained mismatch repair function. *Am J Surg Pathol* 2011;35(9):1391–9.

Radu OM, Nikiforova MN, Farkas LM, et al. Challenging cases encountered in colorectal cancer screening for Lynch syndrome reveal novel findings: Nucleolar MSH6 staining and impact of prior chemoradiation therapy. *Hum Pathol* 2011;42(9):1247–58.

Shia JR, Tang LH, Vakiani E, et al. Immunohistochemistry as first-line screening for detecting colorectal cancer patients at risk for hereditary nonpolyposis colorectal cancer syndrome: A 2-antibody panel may be as predictive as a 4-antibody panel. *Am J Surg Pathol* 2009;33(11):1639–45.

MUC2 (mucin 2)

Background

MUC2 (mucin2) is a high-molecular-weight glycoprotein consisting of a protein backbone with attached O-linked carbohydrate side chains that is involved in mucus gel formation in the small intestine and colon. It was the first human secretory mucin gene to be cloned and sequenced and is located on chromosome 11p15 within a gene complex that contains three other gel-forming mucins: MUC6, MUC5AC, and MUC5B .

MUC2 is strongly expressed by goblet cells of the small intestine and colon and is critical to the formation of the protective mucous barrier that separates the intestinal epithelium from the gut microbiota. Alterations of this mucous barrier are known to occur in inflammatory bowel disease as well as adenomas/carcinomas of the intestine.

Applications

1. MUC2 is a cytoplasmic stain. Its most common use is to assess the presence of goblet cells in gastroesophageal junction biopsies performed in the setting of suspected intestinal metaplasia.
2. Expression is also noted in a percentage of tumors of the gastrointestinal tract, although it lacks sensitivity. Positive staining is also commonly seen in nongastrointestinal mucinous carcinomas from sites such as breast, pancreas, and ovary, making it less useful in determining site of origin in cases of mucinous adenocarcinoma of unknown primary.
3. MUC2 may be diagnostically helpful in distinguishing site of origin in tumors originating in and around the ampulla of Vater. Tumors arising around the periampullary region/ duodenum were commonly positive for MUC2, whereas pancreatic ductal, ampullary carcinomas with ductal features, and intrahepatic cholangiocarcinomas lacked expression.
4. Other uses of MUC2 include use in cytology samples from the pancreas to highlight inadvertently sampled reactive duodenal epithelium, to stain the intestinal-type variant of intraductal papillary mucinous neoplasm, and in perianal Paget's disease to indicate a colorectal origin.

Selected references

Adsay NV, Merati K, Basturk O, et al. Pathologically and biologically distinct types of epithelium in intraductal papillary mucinous neoplasms: Delineation of an "intestinal" pathway of carcinogenesis in the pancreas. *Am J Surg Pathol* 2004;28(7): 839–48.

Chu PG., Schwarz RE, Lau SK, et al. Immunohistochemical staining in the diagnosis of pancreatobiliary and ampulla of Vater adenocarcinoma: Application of CDX2, CK17, MUC1, and MUC2. *Am J Surg Pathol* 2005;29(3): 359–67.

Kuan SF, Montag AG, Hart J, et al. Differential expression of mucin genes in mammary and extramammary Paget's disease. *Am J Surg Pathol* 2001;25(12): 1469–77.

Lau SK, Weiss LM, Chu PG. Differential expression of MUC1, MUC2, and MUC5AC in carcinomas of various sites. *Am J Clin Pathol* 2004;122(1): 61–9.

McIntire MG, Soucy G, Vaughan TL, et al. MUC2 is a highly specific marker of goblet cell metaplasia in the distal esophagus and gastroesophageal junction. *Am J Surg Pathol* 2011;35(7): 1007–13.

Rousseau K, Byrne C, Kim YS, et al. The complete genomic organization of the human MUC6 and MUC2 mucin genes. *Genomics* 2004;83(5): 936–9.

MUC4

Background

MUC4 is a transmembrane glycoprotein expressed on epithelial surfaces from the respiratory tract, colon, and vagina and in several carcinomas (pancreatico-biliary, breast, colon, ovary, lung, and prostate). The MUC4 gene is located on chromosome 3 (3q29) and has a role in proliferation of cells via interactions with the Erb/Her2 family. This was found by global gene expression analysis.

Applications

1. MUC4 immunochemical (IHC) utility has been best exploited in the diagnosis of low-grade fibromyxoid sarcoma (LGFMS); it is seen in virtually 100% of cases. LGFMS shows diffuse moderate to strong positivity in all cases. The vast majority of soft tissue tumors that are mimics of LGFMS are negative for MUC4.
2. Focal IHC positivity for MUC4 has been described in monophasic synovial sarcoma.
3. MUC4 expression is also seen in cases of sclerosing epithelioid fibrosarcoma (SEF) (80% of cases) when present in association with LGFMS. Expression of MUC4 in pure SEF is seen in 70% of cases. MUC4 expression, when present, is usually diffuse in distribution in the tumor cells.

   About 40% of MUC4-positive SEFs show FUS rearrangement, and these cases are likely related to LGFMS, which usually has FUS-CREBL2 rearrangements. MUC4 expression is also seen without FUS rearrangements and involves EWSR1-CREBL1 in more than half the cases. MUC4-negative SEF cases have been shown to have other more recently described rearrangements (YAP1 and/or KMT2A).

   Morphologic mimics of LGFMS such as myxofibrosarcoma, cellular myxoma, solitary fibrous tumors, and benign and malignant nerve sheath tumors are all MUC4 negative.
4. MUC4 expression has also been described in biphasic synovial sarcoma in the epithelial component in 20–30% of cases, but it is usually not the strong, diffuse pattern of staining as seen in SEF/LGFMS.
5. Focal MUC4 positivity has been described in a small number of other mesenchymal neoplasms that resemble SEF, including ossifying fibromyxoid tumor, epithelioid gastrointestinal stromal tumor, and rarely, myoepithelial carcinomas.
6. As well as mesenchymal tumors, MUC4 is expressed in a variety of adenocarcinomas from various sites (but not expressed in mesothelioma) and meningiomas.

Selected references

Doyle LA, Möller E, Dal Cin P, et al. MUC4 is a highly sensitive and specific marker for low-grade fibromyxoid sarcoma. *Am J Surg Pathol* 2011;35:733–41.

Doyle LA, Wang WL, Dal Cin P, et al. MUC4 is a sensitive and extremely useful marker for sclerosing epithelioid fibrosarcoma: Association with FUS gene rearrangement. *Am J Surg Pathol* 2012;36:1444–51.

Matsuyama A, Jotatsu M, Uchihashi K, et al. MUC4 expression in meningiomas: Under-recognized immunophenotype particularly in meningothelial and angiomatous subtypes. *Histopathology* 2019;74:276–83.

NOTES

MUC5AC

Background

MUC5AC is a human mucin produced by the surface epithelium of the stomach (as well as the respiratory tract) and is involved in cytoprotection and gel formation. The gene is found on chromosome 11 within a complex of other human mucins, including MUC2, MUC5B, and MUC6.

MUC5AC has been implicated in the clinical and biologic behavior of gastric carcinomas, with increased expression noted in diffuse/infiltrative tumors predominantly arising in the antrum (whereas MUC2 expression is more common in mucinous tumors arising from the cardia).

Applications

1. MUC5AC is a cytoplasmic stain. Expression is noted in foveolar-type dysplasia arising from the gastro-esophageal junction. This dysplasia lacks goblet cells (although it is often associated with intestinal metaplasia), and tends to be negative for markers of intestinal differentiation (MUC2, CDX2). Positive staining is also seen in foveolar-type dysplasia of the stomach, and when used in a panel with MUC6, can help distinguish pyloric gland adenoma (MUC6+, MUC5AC+) from gastrointestinal-type adenoma/foveolar-type dysplasia (MUC6−, MUC5AC+).
2. Within the gastrointestinal tract, expression of MUC5AC is also noted in most pancreatic ductal adenocarcinomas, intra- and extrahepatic cholangiocarcinomas, adenocarcinomas arising from the ampulla of Vater, small intestinal adenocarcinomas, and adenocarcinomas arising from the appendix, making it less helpful in determining site of origin in cases of metastases of unknown primary without additional immunostains. Hepatocellular carcinomas and colonic adenocarcinomas (non–signet ring type) tend to lack staining.

3. It may be helpful to use in tumors with signet ring differentiation, especially if a breast primary cannot be ruled out, as most breast tumors tend to lack expression, while gastric carcinomas are almost always positive.
4. Outside the gastrointestinal tract, endocervical adenocarcinomas, mucoepidermoid carcinomas, and extramammary Paget's disease often stain with MUC5AC. It may be useful in distinguishing high-grade mucoepidermoid carcinoma (MEC) from poorly differentiated squamous cell (SCC)carcinoma, as MEC tends to be positive.

Selected references

Brown IS, Whiteman DC, Lauwers GY. Foveolar type dysplasia in Barrett esophagus. *Mod Pathol* 2010;23(6):834–43.

Handra-Luca A, Lamas G, Bertrand J-C, et al. MUC1, MUC2, MUC4, and MUC5AC expression in salivary gland mucoepidermoid carcinoma: Diagnostic and prognostic implications. *Am J Surg Pathol* 2005;29(7):881–9.

Kuan SF, Montag AG, Hart J, et al. Differential expression of mucin genes in mammary and extramammary Paget's disease. *Am J Surg Pathol* 2001;25(12):1469–77.

Lau SK, Weiss LM, Chu PG. Differential expression of MUC1, MUC2, and MUC5AC in carcinomas of various sites. *Am J Clin Pathol* 2004;122(1):61–9.

O'Connell FP, Wang HH, Odze RD. Utility of immunohistochemistry in distinguishing primary adenocarcinomas from metastatic breast carcinomas in the gastrointestinal tract. *Arch Pathol Lab Med* 2005;129(3):338–47.

Pinto-de-Sousa J, David L, Reis CA, et al. Mucins MUC1, MUC2, MUC5AC and MUC6 expression in the evaluation of differentiation and clinico-biological behaviour of gastric carcinoma. *Virchows Arch* 2002. 440(3):304–10.

MUC6

Background

MUC6 is a gene that encodes a gastric mucin involved in gel formation and epithelial protection in the stomach. It is located within a complex including the *MUC2*, *MUC5AC*, and *MUC5B* genes on chromosome 11.

Applications

1. MUC6 is a cytoplasmic stain, with expression noted in cardiac glands, fundic neck cells, and pyloric glands of the stomach. Staining is also noted in Brunner's glands, the nonsurface glands of the gallbladder, the epithelium and periductular glands of the common bile duct, the centroacinar cells and ducts of the pancreas, and the seminal vesicles.
2. Focal patchy staining is often present in endocervical and endometrial glands as well.
3. Like MUC2, it may stain a wide variety of mucinous adenocarcinomas and by itself is not helpful in distinguishing site of origin for metastases of unknown primary. It is often positive in neoplasms with pyloric gland differentiation, including pyloric gland adenoma, intratubular gland adenoma of the pancreas (pyloric gland type), as well as the rare gastric carcinoma variant – gastric adenocarcinoma with chief cell differentiation.
4. Expression has also been noted in foveolar-type dysplasia in Barrett's esophagus (it is negative in intestinal metaplasia), serous neoplasms of the pancreas, and pyloric-type intracholecystic papillary neoplasms (pyloric gland type).

Selected references

Adsay V, Jang K-T, Roa JC, et al. Intracholecystic papillary-tubular neoplasms (ICPN) of the gallbladder (neoplastic polyps, adenomas, and papillary neoplasms that are ≥1.0 cm): Clinicopathologic and immunohistochemical analysis of 123 cases. *Am J Surg Pathol* 2012;36:1279–301.

Bartman AE, Buisine MP, Aubert JP, et al. The MUC6 secretory mucin gene is expressed in a wide variety of epithelial tissues. *J Pathol* 1999;186:398–405.

Chu PG, Chung L, Weiss LM, et al. Determining the site of origin of mucinous adenocarcinoma: An immunohistochemical study of 175 cases. *Am J Surg Pathol* 2011;35:1830–6.

Khor TS, Alfaro EE, Ooi EMM, et al. Divergent expression of MUC5AC, MUC6, MUC2, CD10, and CDX-2 in dysplasia and intramucosal adenocarcinomas with intestinal and foveolar morphology: Is this evidence of distinct gastric and intestinal pathways to carcinogenesis in Barrett esophagus? *Am J Surg Pathol* 2012;36:331–42.

Kosmahl M, Wagner J, Peters K, et al. Serous cystic neoplasms of the pancreas: An immunohistochemical analysis revealing alpha-inhibin, neuron-specific enolase, and MUC6 as new markers. *Am J Surg Pathol* 2004 28:339–46.

MUM-1 (interferon response factor 4, IRF4)

Background

MUM-1, or interferon response factor 4 (IRF4), is a nuclear transcription factor that is thought to be the master regulator of B-cell differentiation to plasma cells. MUM-1-deficient mice are without functional plasma cells, and MUM-1 has been shown to be required for immunoglobulin class switch recombination. As shown by RNA interference studies, MUM-1 is required for myeloma tumor cell viability irrespective of the underlying oncogenic mechanism and is therefore a putative target for therapeutic intervention. As an interferon response factor, MUM-1 also plays a role in response to viral infections; e.g., it is prominently expressed in Epstein–Barr virus (EBV)-infected B cells.

Applications

1. In normal B-cell differentiation, MUM-1 is expressed in late germinal center B cells, enabling them to differentiate to marginal zone–type B cells or plasma cells. Importantly, a variety of gene expression profiling studies on diffuse large B-cell lymphoma (DLBCL) have shown unequivocally that MUM-1 is an important marker of non-germinal center-type DLBCL/activated B-cell (ABC)-DLBCL.
2. In addition to post-germinal center B cells and plasma cells, as well as neoplasms derived from these cells, MUM-1 is expressed in other malignancies. It is perhaps the most sensitive marker of classical Hodgkin lymphoma, being strongly expressed in virtually 100% of Hodgkin and Reed–Sternberg (HRS cells). It is expressed to a more variable extent in nodular lymphocyte-predominant Hodgkin lymphoma.
3. A subset of follicular lymphomas, presumably those at the later stages of germinal center development, express MUM-1. In contrast, "early" germinal center–type neoplasms, such as Burkitt lymphoma, typically lack MUM-1 expression.
4. A subset of follicular helper T cells, particularly those that rosette the lymphocyte predominant (LP) cells of nodular lymphocyte-predominant Hodgkin lymphoma, express MUM-1.
5. Follicular helper-derived T-cell lymphomas, including angioimmunoblastic T-cell lymphoma, will show some degree of MUM-1 expression. Evaluation of MUM-1 expression, which is localized to the nucleus, is therefore of use in the diagnostic arena as part of the overall immunohistochemical evaluation for DLBCL, Hodgkin lymphoma, and T-cell lymphoma.

Selected references

Falini B, Fizzotti M, Pucciarini A, et al. A monoclonal antibody (MUM1p) detects expression of the MUM1/IRF4 protein in a subset of germinal center B cells, plasma cells, and activated T cells. *Blood* 2000; 95(6):2084–92.

Gualco G, Weiss LM, Bacchi CE. MUM1/IRF4: A review. *Appl Immunohistochem Mol Morphol* 2010; 18:301–10.

Klein U, Casola S, Cattoretti G, et al. Transcription factor IRF4 controls plasma cell differentiation and class-switch recombination. *Nat Immunol* 2006;7:773–82.

Shaffer AL, Emre NC, Lamy L, et al. IRF4 addiction in multiple myeloma. *Nature* 2008;454:226–31.

Muscle-specific actin (MSA)

Background

There are at least six different actin isotypes in mammals. Four isotypes are found exclusively in muscular tissues – α-skeletal, α-cardiac, and α- and γ-smooth muscle actins. Early anti-actin antibodies were polyclonal, did not distinguish among various actin isotypes, and were of low sensitivity and specificity. Various monoclonal antibodies have now been described, and the most widely used is clone HHF35, available commercially, which recognizes a common epitope of α-skeletal, α-cardiac, and α- and γ-smooth muscle actin isotypes. This antibody labels myoepithelial and smooth muscle cells as well as leiomyomas and leiomyosarcomas. Muscle-specific actins (MSAs) have also been described in pericytes, reactive myofibroblasts, and skeletal and cardiac muscle. Positive-staining cells have been reported in the deep ovarian cortical stroma and theca externa of secondary ovarian follicles, alveolar soft part sarcoma, epithelioid sarcoma, infantile digital fibromatosis, ovarian sclerosing stromal tumors, and Kaposi's sarcoma, representing either myofibroblasts or pericytes in these conditions. Glomus tumors stain positive for MSA, a finding that supports a smooth muscle derivation of these tumors. MSA has also been observed in the cells of the capsule of the liver, kidney, and spleen, and in decidual cells, some stromal cells of chorionic villi, and the so-called fibroblastic reticulum cells of lymph nodes and spleen.

Applications

1. Leiomyomas and leiomyosarcomas (LMS) are MSA positive. However, a broad range of other spindle cell tumors such as nodular fasciitis, myoepithelioma, and glomus tumors also express MSA, which greatly limits the specificity of use of MSA in this role.
2. MSA is positive in rhabdomyosarcomas (RMS), but its role in making a specific diagnosis is limited given the newer and more specific markers for RMS. Because of varying sensitivities, it is best to employ MSA with other myogenic markers such as desmin when examining tumors that can potentially be confused with RMS: leiomyosarcoma (LMS) and myofibroblastic tumors.
3. Myofibroblasts show a heterogeneous immunophenotype and may be positive for vimentin only; for vimentin and α-smooth muscle actin; for vimentin and desmin; or for vimentin, desmin, and α-smooth muscle actin. Myofibroblastic proliferations such as nodular fasciitis may display characteristic peripheral/subplasmalemmal staining for muscle actin, yielding a "tram-track" appearance. Other myofibroblastic lesions such as myofibroblastoma, including intranodal myofibroblastoma, show variable degrees of but consistent MSA positivity. Inflammatory pseudotumors can be MSA positive.
4. MSA is positive in a variety of other tumors, such as PEComa, postoperative spindle cell tumor, nodular fasciitis, desmoplastic fibroblastoma, glomus tumor, myoepithelioma, and myopericytoma.

Comments

The utility of MSA is limited by its lack of specificity. For example not all myofibroblastic lesions show diffuse MSA positivity, and other tumors, such as sarcomatoid carcinomas, can show MSA positivity occasionally.

There is significant overlap of lesions and tumors that mark with both MSA and SMA (smooth muscle actin). A few exceptions include RMS, which are MSA positive but usually not for SMA.

MSA can be expressed in tumors with rhabdoid features, such as atypical teratoid/rhabdoid tumor (AT/RT).

Selected references

Azumi N, Ben-Erza J, Battifora H. Immunophenotypic diagnosis of leiomyosarcomas and rhabdomyosarcomas with monoclonal antibodies to muscle specific actin and desmin in formalin-fixed tissue. *Mod Pathol* 1988;1:469–74.

NOTES

Mycobacterial antigen

Background

The identification of mycobacteria in tissue sections and smears is the most rapid method of detection compared with culture and polymerase chain reaction. This is underscored by the fact that mycobacterial infections carry significant morbidity and mortality, emphasizing the need for rapid identification in tissue sections. The yield of acid-fast stains for the detection of mycobacteria may be less than one organism per tissue section, and acid-fast stains require relatively intact organisms with retained capsular integrity.

The polyclonal rabbit anti-BCG (bacille Calmette–Guerin) was raised against an attenuated strain used to immunize against *Mycobacterium tuberculosis* infections, containing a substantial number of shared antigens with other mycobacterial species. Hence, this antibody is capable of detecting antigen in debris and fragmented organisms that retain their antigenicity and immunoreactivity. Using immunohistochemistry, it was demonstrated that fragments and wall components of BCG persisted in inoculation sites long after acid-fast stains could no longer detect bacilli. In clinical material, in 8 of 10 cases of culture-proven infection in which acid-fast stains were negative, immunoreactivity with anti-BCG was demonstrated in organisms and/or antigen. These authors detected immunoreactive clumps of mycobacterial debris, cells, and cell fragments in caseating granulomata. In histiocytic granulomata of mycobacterial infections, the cytoplasm of epithelioid cells contained both organisms and debris. Furthermore, this immunostaining reaction was evident at low-power (scanning) magnification.

However, immunohistochemical detection of mycobacterial antigen has limited utility in cases where many of the organisms are viable and abundant, having no advantage over established procedures (acid-fast stains) in these circumstances.

Applications

Anti-BCG has a role in detecting mycobacterial organisms/antigens in fixed paraffin-embedded sections, especially in cases in which acid-fast stains are negative and a high index of suspicion exists on morphological interpretation. Further, the cross-reactivity of polyclonal anti-BCG with a wide variety of mycobacterial species allows the detection of organisms in a wide range of clinical settings.

Selected references

Carabias E, Palenque E, Serrano R, et al. Evaluation of an immunohistochemical test with polyclonal antibodies raised against mycobacteria used in formalin-fixed tissue compared with mycobacterial specific culture. *APMIS* 1998;106:385–8.

NOTES

Myelin basic protein (MBP)

Background

Myelin basic protein (MBP) is found in the central and peripheral nervous system. It is found in oligodendrocytes and myelin of white matter in the brain and spinal cord and to a lesser extent in grey matter. It also is found in peripheral nerves.

Applications

MBP is useful in research but has limited applications in diagnostic immunohistochemistry, where its use is largely in the diagnosis of soft tissue tumors. It has been demonstrated in neuromas, neurofibromas, ganglioneuromas, and tumors with neural differentiation and neural elements but is not present in glial tissues. The protein has been employed in a panel of antibodies to identify palisaded encapsulated neuromas of the skin and is useful for the distinction of neurofibromas from neurotized melanocytic nevi. Neurofibromas showed focal staining for CD57 (Leu 7), glial fibrillary acidic protein, and MBP whereas neurotized nevi failed to express these markers. MBP (together with CD57) has also been demonstrated in some granular cell tumors, suggesting neural differentiation in some of these lesions. MBP is a useful marker of ganglioneuroblastomas, ganglioneuromas, and gangliocytic paraganglioma.

Interpretation

The use of MBP as a marker of schwannomas is well established, although some studies have failed to find MBP in Schwann cell neoplasms and both immunohistochemical and western blot analyses have failed to demonstrate MBP in oligodendrogliomas and Schwann cell tumors.

Selected references

Clark HB, Minesky JJ, Agrawal D, et al. Myelin basic protein and P2 protein are not immunohistochemical markers for Schwann cell neoplasms: A comparative study using antisera to S100, P2, and myelin basic proteins. *Am J Pathol* 1985;121:96–101.

Myeloperoxidase

Background

Myeloperoxidase is the major constituent of primary granules of myeloid cells. It therefore serves as a reliable marker for myeloid cells, including early (immature) and mature forms. The appearance of myeloperoxidase precedes neutrophil elastase during myeloid cell differentiation. Further, myeloperoxidase antibody does not react with lymphoid or epithelial cells. The myeloperoxidase immunogen was isolated from human granulocytes.

Other immunohistochemical markers for myeloid cells, e.g., lysozyme, CD15, MAC 387, and CD 68, despite being sensitive, lack specificity in that they also stain histiocytes and other cell types, including epithelium. CD43 and CD45RO also stain myeloid cells frequently but demonstrate T cells and histiocytes as well.

Applications

A positive immunoreaction excludes lymphoblastic leukemia and malignant lymphoma.

The advantage of myeloperoxidase over other markers in this area is reduced background staining.

Interpretation

Antimyeloperoxidase should be included in the immunohistochemical panel for lymphoma investigation. Any "lymphoma" that cannot be classified with confidence should raise the suspicion of a granulocytic sarcoma. Furthermore, tumor cells marking with only T-cell markers CD43 or CD45RO, but not the specific T-marker CD3, or staining only for histiocytic markers such as CD68 or CD15 should raise the alarm for a possible granulocytic sarcoma. Myeloperoxidase is not only specific but by far the most sensitive of the myeloid markers.

Selected references

Mason DY, Taylor CR. The distribution of muramidase (lysozyme) in human tissues. *J Clin Pathol* 1975;28:124–32.

Pinkus GS, Pinkus JL. Myeloperoxidase: A specific marker for myeloid cells in paraffin sections. *Mod Pathol* 1991;4:733–41.

MyoD1

Background

The differentiation of skeletal muscle at the molecular level requires activation and transcription of genes encoding muscle-specific proteins and enzymes such as desmin and creatine kinase. These activities are controlled by a set of genes including MyoD1, myogenin, myf-5, and myf-6. It is thought that MyoD1 activation is an early event that commits the cell to skeletal muscle lineage. Transfection of the MyoD1 gene into nonmuscle cells has been shown to induce conversion of fibroblasts into myoblasts. Similarly, muscle-specific genes in tumor cell lines may be activated by forced expression of exogenously introduced MyoD1. The MyoD1 gene has been localized to the short arm of chromosome 11. The activation of MyoD1 gene, as reflected in the detection of mRNA or protein product, represents a stage of skeletal muscle differentiation that is earlier than that of currently available immunohistochemical markers, such as desmin and myoglobin.

The MyoD1 protein is a 45 kD nuclear phosphoprotein (5.8A reacts with an epitope between amino acid residues 170 and 209) with nuclear expression restricted to skeletal muscle tissue. Monoclonal anti-MyoD1 strongly stains nuclei of myoblasts in developing skeletal muscle, whilst the majority of adult skeletal muscle has been found to be negative, including a wide variety of normal tissue. However, weak cytoplasmic staining has been observed in nonmuscle tissue, including glandular epithelium.

Applications

1. MyoD1 nuclear immunostaining has been demonstrated in the majority of rhabdomyosarcomas of various histological subtypes. It has been shown that the MyoD1 expression in rhabdomyosarcomas is inversely related to the degree of cellular differentiation of tumor cells. This phenomenon is useful to distinguish embryonal rhabdomyosarcomas from other small blue round cell tumors of childhood, i.e., Ewing's sarcoma/peripheral primitive neuroectodermal tumor, neuroblastoma, and childhood lymphomas. Wilm's tumors and ectomesenchymoma with rhabdomyosarcomatous foci also show nuclear expression of MyoD1. It has also been shown that the sensitivity and specificity of the MyoD1 antibody in the differential diagnosis of adult pleomorphic soft tissue sarcomas approach those in pediatric rhabdomyosarcomas. The demonstration of MyoD1 protein in four cases of alveolar soft part sarcoma was initially used as evidence for its rhabdomyosarcomatous differentiation; however, subsequent studies have not confirmed the presence of this regulatory protein in the tumor. Other evidence of myogenic differentiation in alveolar soft part sarcoma includes the demonstration of desmin and/or myoglobin.

Granular cytoplasmic immunoreactivity for MyoD1 has been demonstrated in most neuroblastomas and occasional Ewing's sarcomas/primitive neuroectodermal tumors (PNETs) and alveolar soft part sarcomas. Only nuclear staining should be considered as evidence of skeletal myogenic differentiation.

Interpretation

The cytoplasmic immunostaining with anti-MyoD1 has been suggested to represent cross-reactivity with an unknown cytoplasmic antigen. The cytoplasmic and nonspecific background staining and reactivity for nonmyoid tissues can hinder the practical utility in paraffin-embedded sections. Staining seems to be more consistent in alveolar rhabdomyosarcomas, especially in tumor cells lining fibrous septae and perivascular areas and embryonal rhabdomyosarcomas showing more variable staining.

Selected references

Cessna MH, Zhou H, Perkins SL, et al. Are myogenin and myoD1 expression specific for rhabdomyosarcoma? A study of 150 cases, with emphasis on spindle cell mimics. *Am J Surg Pathol* 2001;25:1150–7.

Wesche WA, Fletcher CDM, Dias E, et al. Immunohistochemistry of MyoD1 in adult pleomorphic soft tissue sarcomas. *Am J Surg Pathol* 1995;19:261–9.

Myogenin

Background

Myogenin belongs to a family of regulatory proteins essential for striated muscle development. Studies in mice indicate that myogenin is not required for the initial aspects of myogenesis, including myotome formation and the appearance of myoblasts, but late stages of embryogenesis are more dependent on myogenin. As a nuclear transcription factor, expression of myogenin is restricted to cells of skeletal muscle origin and is a useful marker for skeletal muscle differentiation in the identification and typing of round cell tumors in childhood. This makes myogenin a very useful marker in this setting, since other myoid markers such as desmin expression are not limited to skeletal muscle tumors. Normal adult skeletal muscle shows variable positivity, ranging from negative to being positive in some cases for myogenin, but damaged or regenerating skeletal muscle shows more consistent myogenin positivity.

Applications

1. The antibody to myogenin labels nuclei of the majority (90% or more) of rhabdomyosarcomas (RMS) and the extent of staining for myogenin has been reported to be inversely related to the degree of cellular differentiation in RMS tumor cells. Although all RMS show staining for myogenin, the alveolar variant shows the strongest nuclear staining even in cases with subtle alveolar architecture, in which myogenin highlights and enhances visualization of the alveolar pattern. Embryonal RMS, in contrast, show greater variability in staining pattern and some cases can show focal positivity. The intensity and pleomorphic RMS show the least immunoreactivity. Spindle cell RMS usually show diffuse myogenin positivity.
2. No reactivity has been reported in either round or spindle cell tumors in the differential diagnosis with RMS. This includes other small round cell tumors such as Ewing sarcoma and neuroblastoma, which are negative for myogenin, as are spindle cell tumors such

as nodular fasciitis, malignant peripheral nerve sheath tumor, inflammatory myofibroblastic tumor, leiomyoma, leiomyosarcoma, and the newly described entity low-grade sinonasal sarcoma. Alveolar soft part sarcomas are also myogenin negative.
3. Myogenin is useful in identifying heterologous RMS component in carcinosarcoma, adenosarcoma (such as of the gynecologic tract), and malignant peripheral nerve sheath tumors, teratoma, and dedifferentiated component of liposarcoma. This can have prognostic significance in some tumors, such as uterine carcinosarcoma.
4. Myogenin expression has been described in Wilm's tumor with myogenic differentiation and occasionally in stromal cells of benign fibroepithelial polyp of the lower female genital tract, although more recent literature suggests that they are negative.
5. Myogenin expression is seen in some recently characterized tumors, such as biphenotypic sinonasal sarcoma, round cell sarcoma with polyphenotypic differentiation with EWSR1-PATZ1 fusion.

Comments

Only nuclear staining should be regarded as positive, and cytoplasmic positivity, which has been described in some non-RMS, should be disregarded in interpreting this marker.

Selected references

Cessna M, Zhou H, Perkins S, et al. Are myogenin and MyoD1 expression specific for rhabdomyosarcoma? A study of 150 cases, with emphasis on spindle cell mimics. *Am J Surg Pathol* 2020;99:75–79. doi:10.1016/j.humpath.2020.03.006.

Flope AL. MyoD1 and myogenin expression in human neoplasia: A review and update. *Adv Anat Pathol* 2002;9:198–203.

Olson NJ, Fritchie KJ, Torres-Mora J, et al. MyoD1 expression in fibroepithelial stromal polyps. *Hum Pathol* 2020;99:75–79. doi: 10.1016/j.humpath.2020.03.006. Epub 2020 Mar 23.

Myoglobin

Background

Myoglobin, a 17.8 kD protein, is the oxygen carrier hemoprotein, a specific marker for striated muscle cells. It is also present in cardiac muscle. The antibodies do not cross-react with hemoglobin. Cross-reactivity with myoglobins of other mammalian species may occur with some antibodies.

Applications

1. Anti-myoglobin has been used to indicate early myocardium necrosis and skeletal muscle trauma and necrosis. Myoglobin was one of the earliest markers of striated muscle differentiation, but its expression appears to be linked to the differentiation of rhabdomyosarcoma cells, so that a sizeable number of such tumors, particularly the poorly differentiated ones, exhibit no staining. Morphologically recognizable rhabdomyoblasts express myoglobin, whereas poorly differentiated tumors fail to stain. Its application as a marker of early ischemic myocardium appears to be less reliable than cytoskeletal proteins such as vinculin, desmin, and alpha-actin.
2. Myoglobin immunostaining has been employed in the study of ragged-red fiber of patients with mitochondrial encephalomyopathy.

3. Staining for myoglobin can also be performed in renal biopsies of patients with myoglobin-containing casts due to conditions such as necrotizing myopathy or rhabdomyolysis.

Interpretation

Myoglobin is not a dependable marker of striated muscle differentiation, especially in poorly differentiated rhabdomyosarcoma. Other markers such as desmin, muscle-specific actin, and MyoD1 should be employed for the identification of striated muscle differentiation. The use of myoglobin as a marker of skeletal muscle tumors has been supplanted by myogenin. Protein released from necrotic muscle may be phagocytosed by macrophages, which are myoglobin positive but should not be mistaken for rhabdomyoblasts.

Selected references

Kunishige M, Mitsui T, Akaike M, et al. Localisation and amount of myoglobin and myoglobin mRNA in ragged-red fiber of patients with mitochondrial encephalomyopathy. *Muscle Nerve* 1996;19:175–82.

Zhang JM, Piddick L. Cytoskeleton immunohistochemical study of early ischemic myocardium. *Forensic Sci Int* 1996;80:229–38.

Napsin-A

Background

Napsin, an aspartic proteinase belonging to the class of endopeptidases, was originally discovered in two isoforms (Napsin-A and Napsin-B), of which Napsin-A was noted to be the functional isoform predominantly found in human kidney and lung. Napsin-A is a 38 kD single-chain protein. Type II pneumocytes, alveolar macrophages, subset of type I pneumocytes, respiratory epithelium of terminal and respiratory bronchioles, plasma cells, cells of distal convoluted tubule, collecting duct, loop of Henle, and subset of lymphocytes stain positive for this marker immunohistochemically.

Applications

1. Napsin-A positivity is reported in primary lung adenocarcinomas (80–85%), large-cell carcinoma of lung (30%), sarcomatoid carcinoma (20%), sclerosing hemangioma (100%), papillary renal cell carcinoma (79%), clear cell renal cell carcinoma (34%), chromophobe renal cell carcinoma (3%), and papillary thyroid carcinoma with tall cell morphology (5%), as well as in anaplastic (15%), poorly differentiated (13%), and micropapillary (100%) pattern thyroid carcinomas.
2. Napsin-A expression has also been reported in clear cell carcinoma of endometrium as well as clear cell and endometrioid adenocarcinomas of ovary and metastatic adenoid cystic carcinoma to lung.

Selected references

Hirano T, Gong Y, Yoshida K, et al. Usefulness of TA02 (napsin A) to distinguish primary lung adenocarcinoma from metastatic lung adenocarcinoma. *Lung Cancer* 2003;41:155–62.

Schauer-Vukasinovic V, Bur D, Kling D, et al. Human napsin A: Expression, immunochemical detection, and tissue localization. *FEBS Lett* 1999;462:135–9.

Suzuki A, Shijubo N, Yamada G, et al. Napsin A is useful to distinguish primary lung adenocarcinoma from adenocarcinomas of other organs. *Pathol Res Pract* 2005;201:579–86.

Neurofilaments

Background

Neurofilaments (NFs) differ from other intermediate filaments (IFs) in that they are composed of three different subunits of distinct but related proteins of 70, 150, and 200 kDa, whereas other IFs range from 40 to 70 kDa in molecular weight. The antigenic determinants of each of the subunits may be unique or shared, and each NF protein is a separate gene product. NFs are found in neurons and the neuronal processes of the central and peripheral nervous tissue. It is likely that nearly all neurons can constitutively express all three NF genes, and reports of absence of subunits of NF in certain neurons probably reflect technical limitations, as the proteins are fixation dependent. It is likely that NFs play an important role in the health of the neuron, with evidence that overexpression of NF 200 kDa results in severe neurological disorder, while elimination of this IF appears to impart resistance to some neurotoxic agents. The antibodies to NFs stain all neurons and axonal processes of the central and peripheral nervous system. The only exception seems to be the olfactory sensory neurons, which contain only vimentin IFs and are unique in that they die and are replenished throughout the lifespan of the mammal. The immunostaining of NF can be employed for the study of neuronal distribution and enervation in normal and abnormal tissues, although it plays a limited role in the workup of central nervous system tumors.

Applications

NFs are found in a variety of tumors. Among soft tissue tumors, they are expressed in neurofibroma, ganglioneuroma, neuroblastoma, ganglioglioma, medulloblastoma, retinoblastoma, and pineal parenchymal tumors, neuroendocrine and neuroepithelial tumors such as Merkel cell carcinoma, carcinoid, esthesioneuroblastoma, ganglioneuroblastoma, oat cell carcinoma, paraganglioma, pheochromocytoma, and teratomas with neuronal differentiation. NFs may also be expressed in primitive/peripheral neuroectodermal tumors (PNETs).

Comments

While NF is expressed in several tumors, it plays a somewhat limited role in surgical pathology with more specific markers available in the workup of soft tissue and central nervous system tumors.

Selected references

Gotow T. Neurofilaments in health and disease. *Med Electron Microscopy* 2000;33:173–99.

Neutrophil elastase

Background

Neutrophil elastase is a neutral protease, which plays a major role in the killing of micro-organisms and in the initiation of tissue injury during inflammatory reactions. The enzyme is present in the primary (azurophilic) granules of myeloid cells. Neutrophil elastase consists of three isoenzymes with similar molecular masses (approximately 30 kD). Monoclonal anti-neutrophil elastase (NP57) was raised against human neutrophil granule proteins. This antibody labels neutrophils in routinely processed histological specimens and also reacts (although more weakly) with a minor population of normal blood monocytes. Other cell types, including epithelial cells, are NP57 negative.

Applications

1. Acute myeloid leukemia is NP57 positive.
2. Among extramedullary myeloid cell tumors, 55% are positive. Leukemias of lymphoid origin are not stained.

Comments

The detection of elastase with monoclonal NP57 forms a useful supplement to other immunohistochemical markers for myeloid disorders. However, a recent study that compared a variety of markers for myeloid precursors in granulocytic sarcoma concluded that CD43, lysozyme, myeloperoxidase, and CD15 were the most sensitive markers, staining a large proportion of the cells of the majority of well-differentiated tumors and a smaller proportion of poorly differentiated/blastic tumors. Neutrophil elastase was the least sensitive of the markers of myeloid differentiation, including chloroacetate esterase histochemical staining.

Selected references

Ohlsson K, Olsson I. The neutral proteases of human granulocytes: Isolation and partial characterization of granulocyte elastases. *Eur J Biochem* 1974;42:519–27.

Pulford KAF, Erber WN, Crick JA, et al. Monoclonal antibody against human neutrophil elastase for the study of normal and leukaemic myeloid cells. *J Clin Pathol* 1988;41:853–60.

NKX2.2

Background

NKX2.2 belongs to the NK2 transcription factor family. It plays a role in development and differentiation of the central nervous system and endocrine cells (pancreas and gastrointestinal tract). NKX2.2 gene has been shown as a target of EWS-FLI-1 and upregulated in Ewing sarcoma. It is expressed in most Ewing sarcoma cases and not expressed in other sarcomas by gene expression data. By immunohistochemistry, the vast majority of Ewing sarcoma cases are positive for NKX2.2 (more than 90%). A small number of other tumors can show NKX2.2 expression, and these include olfactory neuroblastoma (consistently), small cell carcinoma, synovial sarcoma, mesenchymal chondrosarcoma, and malignant melanoma.

Applications

1. In Ewing's sarcoma NKX2.2 can be potentially useful along with other markers such as ETV4 and BCOR. NKX2.2 is positive in Ewing sarcoma with EWSR1-FLI1 and EWSR1-ERG fusions. *CIC* rearranged tumors are NKX2.2 negative.

2. Among other small round cell tumors that show consistent diffuse positivity for NKX2.2, olfactory neuroblastoma is the most consistent.

3. It is rarely expressed in other sarcomas, including desmoplastic small round cell tumor and soft tissue myoepithelial tumors.

Selected references

Hung YP, Fletcher CD, Hornick JL. Evaluation of NKX2-2 expression in round cell sarcomas and other tumors with EWSR1 rearrangement: Imperfect specificity for Ewing sarcoma. *Mod Pathol* 2016;29:370–80.

Machado I, Yoshida A, Lopez-Guerrero JA, et al. Immunohistochemical analysis of NKX2.2, ETV4, and BCOR in a large series of genetically confirmed Ewing sarcoma family of tumors. *Pathol Res Pract* 2017;213: 1048–53.

Yoshida A, Sekine S, Tsuta K, et al. NKX2.2 is a useful immunohistochemical marker for Ewing sarcoma. *Am J Surg Pathol* 2012;36: 993–9.

nm23/*NME1*

Background

The *nm23* gene family was originally identified in a murine melanoma cell-line and nm23 HI was found to be transcribed at a 10-fold higher rate in cells of lower metastatic potential. Two highly homologous human genes have subsequently been identified – *nmEl* and *nmE2*, located on chromosomes 17q and coding for the 18.5 and 17 kD proteins nm23 HI and nm23 H2, respectively. nm23 is mainly cytoplasmic, but nuclear and membrane localization has also been seen.

Applications

1. The *nm23* gene product was believed initially to play a role in suppressing tumor metastasis. This may be too simplistic a view, with both metastasis suppression and disease progression being linked to elevated gene expression in different tumors. Isotype-specific studies on breast neoplasms have indicated that it is nm23 HI and not nm23 H2 that correlates with metastases.
2. Somatic allelic deletions of nm23 HI have been reported in some human neoplasms, such as breast, kidney, colon, and lung cancer, in some cases associated with an increased incidence of metastases. The loss of nm23 function appears to correlate with phenotypic markers of metastatic potential in some human tumors.
3. In esophageal carcinoma, failure to express p53 and nm23 may be related to an unfavorable prognosis. Similarly, there is reduced staining of nm23 H1 in laryngeal squamous cell carcinoma compared with laryngeal polyps. In contrast, progression of ovarian carcinoma is accompanied by overexpression of nm23 protein.
4. In pituitary adenoma, strong expression of nm23 H2 is associated with noninvasive adenomas and may restrain tumor aggression.
5. Expression in uveal melanoma appears to be inversely proportional to the depth of scleral invasion.
6. Expression of nm23 protein is significantly decreased in complete hydatidiform moles that progress to gestational trophoblastic.
7. Similar studies have shown nm23 to be a significant factor for predicting a favorable prognosis in non-small-cell carcinoma of the lung and laryngeal squamous cell carcinoma.

Comments

Polyclonal antiserum to nm23 produces strong cytoplasmic staining after heat-induced epitope retrieval (HIER).

Selected references

Graham AN, Maxwell P, Mulholland K, et al. Increased nm23 immunoreactivity is associated with selective inhibition of systemic tumour cell dissemination. *J Clin Pathol* 2002;55:184–9.

Urano T, Furukawa K, Shiku H. Expression of *nm23/* NDP kinase proteins on the cell surface. *Oncogene* 1993;8:1371–6.

NTRK

Background

The t*ropomyosin* or tyrosine receptor kinases (TRK) are a receptor family composed of three transmembrane proteins: TRKA, TRKB, and TRKC. These proteins are in turn encoded by three n*eurotrophic* t*ropomyosin*/*tyrosine receptor kinase (NTRK)* genes: *NTRK1, NTRK2,* and *NTRK3*. Fusions of these proto-oncogenes are noted in several cancers and their significance been accentuated by the development of very specific, selective inhibitors of these *NTRK* gene fusions.

There are three *NTRK* genes that encode for three NTRK proteins: A, B, and C. There are monoclonal antibodies available to all three NTRK proteins (pan-NTRK) and a monoclonal antibody to NTRK-A.

There are three mechanisms of *NTRK* activation:

i) Somatic mutations are seen in colorectal cancer, lung cancer, melanoma, and acute myeloid leukemia.
ii) Activating splice variants and in-frame deletion mutations of *NTRK1* have been identified in neuroblastoma and acute myeloid leukemia, respectively.
iii) *NTRK* gene fusions are the principal abnormality involving the *NTRK1–3* genes. The mechanism of *NTRK* gene fusion is very consistent: the 3′ region (including the kinase domain) of the *NTRK* genes is fused with a 5′ sequence of a fusion partner gene resulting from an intrachromosomal or interchromosomal rearrangement. This results in a chimeric oncoprotein typified by ligand-dependent constitutive activation of TRK. A monoclonal pan-TRK antibody targeted to an amino acid sequence 880 at the C-terminus end of TRK A, B and C is available.

There is also an anti-TRKA monoclonal antibody that detects residues surrounding tyrosine 791 of TRKA.

Applications

1. Tumors with >90% fusions

Salivary gland mammary analogue secretory carcinoma
Breast secretory carcinoma
Infantile fibrosarcoma
Congenital mesoblastic nephroma
Lipofibromatosis-like neural tumor

2. Tumors with 5–25% fusions

Thyroid papillary carcinoma
Gastrointestinal stromal tumor
Spitzoid melanoma

3. Tumors with 1–5% fusions

High- and low-grade gliomas, lung squamous and adenocarcinomas, breast ductal cancer, acute myeloid leukemia, acute lymphoblastic leukemia.

Interpretation of staining

Several patterns of staining are encountered depending on staining localization: cytoplasmic, membrane, nuclear, and perinuclear.

Cytoplasmic staining: it is thought that >50% of tumor cells must show cytoplasmic decoration for the case to be regarded as NTRK positive; ETV6-NTRK3

Cytoplasmic membrane staining: TPM3/4-NTRK1/3 fusions

Nuclear staining: ETV6-NTRK3 and EML4-NTRK3 fusions and any nuclear staining is taken as evidence of a positive stain

Perinuclear staining: LMNA-NTRK1 fusion

Selected references

Chetty R. Neurotrophic tropomyosin or tyrosine receptor kinase (NTRK) genes. *J Clin Pathol* 2019;72:187–90.

Cocco E, Scaltriti M, Drilon A. NTRK fusion-positive cancers and TRK inhibitor therapy. *Nat Rev Clin Oncol* 2018;15:731–47.

Hechtman JF, Benayed R, Hyman DM, et al. Pan-Trk immunohistochemistry is an efficient and reliable screen for the detection of *NTRK* fusions. *Am J Surg Pathol* 2017;41:1547–51.

Rudzinski ER, Lockwood CM, Stohr BA, et al. Pan-Trk immunohistochemistry identifies NTRK rearrangements in pediatric mesenchymal tumors. *Am J Surg Pathol* 2018;42:927–35.

Weier HU, Rhein AP, Shadravan F, et al. Rapid physical mapping of the human trk protooncogene (NTRK1) to human chromosome 1q21-q22 by P1 clone selection, fluorescence in situ hybridization (FISH), and computer-assisted microscopy. *Genomics* 1995;26:390–3.

OCT2 (POU2F2)

Background

The POU2F2 protein, better known as OCT2, is a homeobox-containing transcription factor of the POU family of transcription factors. OCT2 derives its name from its ability to bind eight-nucleotide (octamer) recognition sites in the immunoglobulin genes, thus regulating their expression. It also regulates other genes such as CD20. While OCT2 typically has a positive effect on gene expression of B cells, it has a negative effect on gene expression in neuronal cells, the other major tissue type in which it is expressed. OCT2 is required for B-cell maturation and is associated with the BOB1 transcriptional coactivator. OCT2 has a further role in the control of brain development. In lymphoid tissues, the strong expression of OCT2 is observed in germinal center cells, plasma cells, and a subset of monocytoid B cells and marginal zone B cells. Expression in other B cells is weak. Further, OCT expression is also seen in T cells, including thymic medullary T cells, and in macrophages, but is weak.

Applications

Although OCT2 is an important transcription factor for B cells, its use to characterize B-cell neoplasia is restricted to use in specific contexts since it is not entirely lineage specific.

The most common use of OCT2 immunohistochemistry in diagnostic hematopathology is the distinction of classic Hodgkin lymphoma from large B-cell non-Hodgkin lymphoma, including gray zone lymphoma, and nodular lymphocyte-predominant Hodgkin lymphoma (NLPHL). OCT2 shows typically high expression in NLPHL, while the neoplastic cells of classical Hodgkin lymphoma either fail to express OCT2 or are only very weakly positive. In the rare CHL cases showing OCT2 expression, BOB1 (*see separate chapter in this volume*) is invariably negative. A third transcription factor, PU.1, is also absent in virtually all cases of CHL, although it is less commonly used in routine practice.

The singularly high level of OCT2 expression in the lymphocyte predominant (LP) Hodgkin cells of NLPHL can help distinguish it from T-cell/histiocyte-rich large B-cell lymphoma, with which it may be confused. This concerns especially the T-cell-rich variant of NLPHL.

OCT2 immunohistochemistry can also be helpful for the diagnosis of lymphomas with a plasmablastic immunophenotype. OCT2, in the proper context, serves as a B-cell marker in these lymphomas as B-cell surface markers are not expressed. These lymphomas include plasmablastic lymphoma, primary effusion lymphoma, and ALK-positive large B-cell lymphoma. Importantly, because of the occasional reports that OCT2 expression is not entirely lineage specific, one should try to find additional evidence of the B-lymphoid lineage in such cases, e.g., demonstration of cytoplasmic light chain restriction by immunohistochemistry or flow cytometry, or detection of a clonal immunoglobulin gene rearrangement by polymerase chain reaction.

Selected references

Gibson SE, Dong HY, Advani AS, Hsi ED. Expression of the B cell-associated transcription factors PAX5, OCT-2, and BOB.1 in acute myeloid leukemia: Associations with B-cell antigen expression and myelomonocytic maturation. *Am J Clin Pathol* 2006;126:916–24.

Marafioti T, Ascani S, Pulford K, et al. Expression of B-lymphocyte-associated transcription factors in human T-cell neoplasms. *Am J Pathol* 2003;162:861–71.

Ponzoni M, Arrigoni G, Doglioni C. New transcription factors in diagnostic hematopathology. *Adv Anat Pathol* 2007;14:25–35.

OCT4

Background

OCT4, also known as OCT3 or POU5F1, is a transcription factor that is required for the maintenance of pluripotency of primordial germ cells and embryonic stem cells. OCT4 is downregulated when embryonic stem cells are triggered for differentiation. The understanding of the role of OCT4 and its target genes and dimerization ability has provided insights into the understanding of early steps regulating mammalian embryogenesis. Additionally, OCT4 may also play a role in maintaining viability of the mammalian germline, thus functioning as a" stem cell survival" factor. OCT4 is associated with prognosis in esophageal squamous cell carcinoma and non-small-cell lung cancers.

Applications

1. OCT4 in the differential diagnosis of intratubular germ cell neoplasia unclassified (IGCNU):

    OCT4 expression is seen only in early stages of differentiation with progressive reduction of its immunohistochemical expression in normal spermatogenic cells in the second and third trimesters of fetal development. OCT4 has therefore become an extremely useful tool in detecting IGCNU with strong nuclear staining seen in 90–100% of atypical cells. The sensitivity of OCT4 in detecting IGCNU is similar to that of PLAP (placental like alkaline phosphatase) with the added advantage of minimal background and greater intensity.

2. OCT 4 in the differential diagnosis of germ cell tumors (GCT):

    On the basis of the nuclear reactivity for OCT4, GCTs may be divided into two groups: OCT4-positive group (embryonal carcinoma and seminoma) and OCT4-negative group comprising yolk sac tumor, spermatocytic seminoma, and choriocarcinoma. In the OCT4-positive group, embryonal carcinoma and seminoma can be differentiated by additional staining with CD30 stain (positive in embryonal carcinoma). CD30 positivity is seen in 93–100% of embryonal carcinomas, while seminoma is uniformly positive for OCT4 and trophoblastic cells that may be present are negative. OCT 4 is virtually 100% sensitive for embryonal carcinoma and seminoma, while the majority of other neoplasms of non-testicular origin are negative.

3. Rare cases of non-small-cell carcinoma of the lung, clear cell carcinoma of the kidney, and large B-cell lymphomas have been reported to be positive. Rare post-chemotherapy embryonal carcinomas can also be negative.

Interpretation

Nuclear staining.

Selected references

Cheng L, Sung MT, Cossu-Rocca P, et al. OCT4: Biological functions and clinical applications as a marker of germ cell neoplasia. *J Pathol* 2007;211:1–9.

de Jong J, Stoop H, Dohle GR, et al. Diagnostic value of OCT3/4 for pre-invasive and invasive testicular germ cell tumours. *J Pathol* 2005;206:242–9.

Jones TD, Ulbright TM, Eble JN, Baldridge LA, Cheng L. OCT4 staining in testicular tumors: A sensitive and specific marker for seminoma and embryonal carcinoma. *Am J Surg Pathol* 2004;28:935–40.

Jones TD, Ulbright TM, Eble JN, Cheng L. OCT4: A sensitive and specific biomarker for intratubular germ cell neoplasia of the testis. *Clin Cancer Res* 2004;10:8544–7.

Looijenga LH, Stoop H, de Leeuw HP, et al. POU5F1 (OCT3/4) identifies cells with pluripotent potential in human germ cell tumors. *Cancer Res* 2003;63:2244–50.

Sung MT, Jones TD, Beck SD, Foster RS, Cheng L. OCT4 is superior to CD30 in the diagnosis of metastatic embryonal carcinomas after chemotherapy. *Hum Pathol* 2006;37:662–7.

OLIG2 (oligodendrocyte transcription factor 2)

OLIG2 (oligodendrocyte transcription factor 2) is a member of the basic helix–loop–helix transcription factor family encoded by the gene *OLIG2*, with expression largely restricted to the central nervous system. *OLIG1/2* genes encode transcription factors that play a role as regulators of neuroectodermal progenitor cells and oligodendrocyte development. Initial studies by in situ hybridization demonstrated that OLIG2 was upregulated in oligodendroglial neoplasms and not in other primary brain tumors, suggesting this protein as a potential specific oligodendroglial marker while at the same time establishing the definite lineage of oligodendrogliomas as derived from oligodendroglial progenitors. Subsequent work, however, showed that OLIG2 expression is seen in all diffuse gliomas.

Applications

1. OLIG2 can be used as a general marker for gliomas, as it is expressed in tumor nuclei in all glioma subtypes. OLIG2 cannot be used to separate oligodendrogliomas from astrocytomas. A smaller percentage of ependymomas in adults show OLIG2 expression (10–30%) and pediatric ependymomas usually show minimal or no OLIG2 expression.
2. OLIG2 can be utilized in the differential diagnosis of glioma versus metastatic tumors to the brain. Metastatic tumors to the brain and lymphomas are OLIG2 negative.
3. Among other intracranial tumors, OLIG2 is not expressed by meningioma and variable expression has been reported in embryonal and neuronal tumors.
4. OLIG2 has been shown to be expressed in rhabdomyosarcoma with PAX3/7-FOXO1 fusion.

Selected references

Kaleta M, Wakulińska A, Karkucińska-Więckowska A, et al. OLIG2 is a novel immunohistochemical marker associated with the presence of PAX3/7-FOXO1 translocation in rhabdomyosarcomas. *Diagn Pathol* 2019;14: 103.

Ligon KL, Alberta JA, Kho AT, et al. The oligodendroglial lineage marker OLIG2 is universally expressed in diffuse gliomas. *J Neuropathol Exp Neurol* 2004;63:499–509.

Marie Y, Sanson M, Mokhtari K, et al. OLIG2 as a specific marker of oligodendroglial tumour cells. *Lancet* 2001;358:2980–300.

Popova SN, Bergqvist M, Dimberg A, et al. Subtyping of gliomas of various WHO grades by the application of immunohistochemistry. *Histopathology* 2014; 64: 365–79.

Yokoo H, Nobusawa S, Takebayashi H, et al. Anti-human Olig2 antibody as a useful immunohistochemical marker of normal oligodendrocytes and gliomas. *Am J Pathol* 2004;164:1717–25.

NOTES

Osteopontin

Background

Osteopontin (OPN, also designated bone sialoprotein 1, urinary stone protein, spp-1, eta-1, nephropontin, and uropontin) is an extracellular matrix cell adhesion phosphoglycoprotein. OPN is produced predominantly by osteoblasts but is also synthesized by brain and kidney cells. OPN is deposited into unmineralized matrix at the cement lines before calcification and between collagen fibrils of fully matured tissue. OPNs isolated from or secreted by various tissues have molecular weights between 44 and 75 kD due to post-translational modifications. OPN exists in multiple forms, such as glycosylated, phosphorylated, and cleaved mature forms of approximately 66–68 kD molecular weight protein, suggestive of diverse functions in various tissues.

OPN functions as a substrate for transglutaminase and is involved in cell adhesion. OPN (K-20) is an affinity-purified goat polyclonal antibody raised against a peptide mapping near the carboxy terminus of osteopontin of human origin.

Whilst OPN was originally extracted from bone extracellular matrix stroma, it has also been detected in normal epithelia of various organs with luminal epithelial surfaces.

Applications

1. It may have a role in the genesis of some cancers, such as hepatocellular carcinoma and squamous cell carcinoma of the lung.
2. OPN has been detected in breast, endometrial, and renal adenocarcinomas, where it has been postulated to function in adhesive interaction of cancer cells with the extracellular matrix, influencing biological behavior.
3. Lung, gastrointestinal, prostate, bladder, and other human carcinomas do not express OPN.

Selected references

Brown LF, Papadopoulos-Sergiou A, Berse B, et al. Osteopontin expression and distribution in human carcinomas. *Am J Pathol* 1994;145:610–23.

Butler WT. The nature and significance of osteopontin. *Connect Tiss Res* 1989;23:123–36.

Butler WT. Structural and functional domains of osteopontin. *Ann New York Acad Sci* 1995;760:6–11.

Denhardt T, Guo X. Osteopontin: A protein with diverse functions. *FASEB J* 1993;7:475–82.

p16

Background

p16 is a cyclin-dependent kinase-4 inhibitor that is expressed in a limited range of normal tissues and tumors. Infection with high-risk human papillomavirus (HPV) causes inactivation of the retinoblastoma (*RB*) gene by the HPV E7 protein. Normally Rb inhibits transcription of p16, resulting in accumulation of p16 protein.

The major diagnostic applications of p16 immunohistochemistry have been in pathology of the gynecologic tract and more recently in head and neck pathology. p16 overexpression is usually both cytoplasmic and nuclear, although sometimes only cytoplasmic staining is present.

Applications

1. Diffuse nuclear, or nuclear and cytoplasmic, p16 positivity (so-called "block positivity") in the lower one-third or full thickness of the cervical epithelium can be regarded as a surrogate marker of the presence of high-risk HPV infection. In normal cervical squamous epithelium p16 expression is absent or focally positive. In reactive changes and metaplastic lesions, p16 is generally negative or shows focal/weak positivity, whereas in low-grade squamous intraepithelial lesions (LSIL; CIN1) it can be negative or it can be expressed, usually confined to the lower third of the epithelium. Hence, p16 immunochemistry (IHC) should not be used either to establish when the diagnosis of LSIL is obvious morphologically or to exclude the diagnosis of LSIL (CIN1). Neither should p16 IHC be used to predict which cases might progress to high-grade squamous intraepithelial lesions (HSIL). In HSIL (CIN2/3), p16 is expressed strongly and diffusely and can be used to distinguish high-grade CIN from atrophy, immature squamous metaplasia, and transitional metaplasia. So, p16 is best used to establish the diagnosis of HSIL (particularly CIN II) and exclude benign/reactive mimics of HSIL (CIN II and CIN III).

2. Normal endocervical glands are p16 negative or weakly positive, in contrast to most neoplastic glandular lesions, which exhibit p16 positivity as a result of association with high-risk HPV infection. p16 is useful in distinguishing endocervical adenocarcinoma in situ (AIS) from microglandular hyperplasia, tuboendometrial metaplasia, and endometriosis. The patchy p16 positivity of endometriosis and tuboendometrial metaplasia differs from the diffuse positivity seen in AIS. The exceptions are endocervical adenocarcinomas that are not HPV driven, such as minimal deviation, adenoma malignum gastric type, and mesonephric types. However, 30% of adenoma malignum cases can express p16 through a mechanism that does not involve HPV infection.

3. On small biopsies, distinguishing between tumors of endocervical and endometrial origin can be challenging. In this situation p16 is a useful marker, which will be diffusely positive in HPV-related endocervical adenocarcinoma and negative or focally positive in endometrial adenocarcinoma. Of note, the benign squamoid elements or areas of tubal metaplasia in the endometrioid adenocarcinomas are usually p16 positive. One caveat in using and interpreting p16 in this scenario is that high-grade endometrial adenocarcinomas such as serous and clear cell types often show diffuse strong positivity for p16 and this overexpression is HPV independent. Since cervical small cell carcinoma is also driven by high-risk HPV infection, these tumors will be p16 positive.

4. In uterine smooth muscle tumors, gene expression studies have shown p16 expression in uterine leiomyosarcomas. A few studies have shown p16 staining to be diffuse and stronger in leiomyosarcomas when compared with leiomyomas, with no difference in staining pattern between smooth muscle tumors of uncertain malignant potential (STUMPs) and leiomyomas.

5. In the vulva, p16 may be used to distinguish HPV-associated vulvar intraepithelial neoplasia (VIN) (p16+, usual type VIN) from differentiated VIN that is not associated with HPV infection and is p16 negative.

6. In the ovary, serous carcinomas appear to express p16 more commonly than other subtypes, and p16 is usually negative in benign and borderline tumors.

7. Cervical metastases to the ovary are known to mimic primary mucinous or endometrioid ovarian carcinomas, and in this instance p16 expression is suggestive of a metastasis from a cervical adenocarcinoma.

8. p16 IHC is widely used in oropharyngeal squamous cell carcinomas (SCCs) as a surrogate marker of HPV positivity. The accepted criteria is 70% of tumor cells showing nuclear and cytoplasmic positivity for p16. p16-positive SCCs of the oropharynx have a better outcome and response to radiation therapy even at an advanced stage when compared with HPV-negative oropharyngeal SCCs. So, pathologists should perform HPV testing on all newly diagnosed oropharyngeal SCCs, and p16 IHC can be performed either on the primary site or on the metastatic tumor.

9. p16 loss has been proposed as a potential indicator of aggressive behavior in pleural malignant mesotheliomas (particularly when used along with BAP1 IHC).

10. p16 overexpression is seen in several malignancies and less commonly in benign differential diagnostic consideration. In examples such as atypical lipomatous tumors, leiomyosarcoma, and malignant peripheral nerve sheath tumors, the availability of more robust and specific markers limits the utility of p16 in such scenarios for establishing malignancy.

Comments

p16 usually shows nuclear and cytoplasmic positivity. Focal, discontinuous, or patchy p16 positivity or cytoplasmic-only p16 positivity is considered negative.

p16 IHC should be performed on formalin-fixed tissue and not on alcohol-fixed cytology smears.

Selected references

Ansari-Lari MA, Staebler A, Zaino RJ, et al. Distinction of endocervical and endometrial adenocarcinomas: Immunohistochemical p16 expression correlated with human papillomavirus (HPV) DNA detection. *Am J Surg Pathol* 2004;28:160–7.

Armes JE, Lourie R, De Silva M, et al. Abnormalities of the RB1 pathway in ovarian serous papillary carcinoma as determined by overexpression of the p16INK4A protein. *Int J Gynecol Pathol* 2005;24:363–8.

Bodner-Adler B, Bodner K, Czerwenka K, et al. Expression of p16 protein in patients with uterine smooth muscle tumors: An immunohistochemical analysis. *Gynecol Oncol* 2005;96:62–6.

Dray M, Russell P, Dalrymple C, et al. p16INK4a as a complementary marker of high-grade intraepithelial lesions of the uterine cervix: I: Experience with squamous lesions in 189 consecutive cervical biopsies. *Pathology* 2005;37:112–24.

Kalof AN, Evans MF, Simmons-Arnold L, Beatty BG, Cooper K. p16INK4A immunoexpression and HPV in situ hybridization signal patterns: Potential markers of high-grade cervical intraepithelial neoplasia. *Am J Surg Pathol* 2005;29:674–9.

Klaes R, Friedrich T, Spitkovsky D, et al. Overexpression of p16INK4A as a specific marker for dysplastic and neoplastic epithelial cells of the cervix uteri. *Int J Cancer* 2001;92:276–84.

Qiao X, Bhuiya TA, Spitzer M. Differentiating high-grade cervical intraepithelial lesion from atrophy in postmenopausal women using Ki-67, cyclin E, and p16 immunohistochemical analysis. *J Lower Genital Tract Dis* 2005;9:100–7.

Sano T, Oyama T, Kashiwabara K, et al. Expression status of p16 protein is associated with human papillomavirus oncogenic potential in cervical and genital lesions. *Am J Pathol* 1998; 153:1741–8.

p27kip1

Background

The p27kip1 (p27) gene encodes an inhibitor of cyclin-dependent kinase (CDK) activity. Two families of proteins that generally inhibit cell cycle progression regulate the activity of cyclin-dependent kinase complexes. These are the INK4 group of p16, p15, p18, and p19, which may have suppressor functions and whose activities are dependent on a normal retinoblastoma protein and show maximal expression during S-phase, and the group of CDK inhibitors, which include p21/WAF1/CIP1, p27kip1, and p57/kip2. Overexpression of the latter group inhibits kinase activities of several cyclins and causes cell cycle arrest. The role of kip protein in regulating cell cycle progression in normal and neoplastic cells has not been elucidated, although p27-deficient mice develop multiple organ hyperplasia, suggesting that this CDK inhibitor has antiproliferative activity in vivo.

Applications

1. Evaluation of p27 protein has the potential of predicting the biological behavior of various neoplasms and can be employed to study cell cycle regulation during tumor progression. Loss of or low immunoexpression of p57 is associated with poor prognosis for lymph node metastasis in patients with astrocytoma, cervical carcinoma, rectal carcinoma, papillary thyroid carcinoma, renal cell carcinoma, and gastric carcinoma.
2. The results in breast carcinoma have been conflicting. Decreased immunoexpression is described as being associated with lymph node metastasis in men, and high levels in tumors with nodal metastasis in women.
3. Paradoxical overexpression of p27 has been described in endometrioid adenocarcinoma of the uterus with lymph node metastasis, myometrial invasion, and advanced-stage disease.

Comments

The antigen is located in the nucleus.

Selected references

Lloyd RV, Jin L, Qian X, Kulig E. Aberrant p27[kip1] expression in endocrine and other tumors. *Am J Pathol* 1997;150:401–7.
Toyoshima H, Hunter T. p27, a novel inhibitor of G1 cyclin-Cdk protein kinase activity is related to p21. *Cell* 1994;78:67–74.
Hengst L, Reed SI. Translational control of p27[kip1] accumulation during the cell cycle. *Science* 1996;271:1861–4.

p40

Background

DeltaNp63 (p40) is a truncated p63 variant (a member of the *p53* gene family), which was originally found to label keratinocytes as well as kidney/adrenal, spleen, and thymus but not heart, testis, brain, or liver. DeltaNp63 was also noted to be an inhibitor of p53.

Applications

1. Antibody p40 was noted to label normal thymic cortical and medullary epithelial cells and thymomas, normal placentas, hydatidiform moles, invasive moles, choriocarcinoma, and epithelial trophoblastic tumors but not placental site trophoblastic tumors.
2. It is a specific marker for squamous differentiation. In lung cancer, p40 is a useful immunostain to differentiate squamous cell carcinoma from adenocarcinoma as well as from small cell carcinoma.

Selected references

Alomari AK, Glusac EJ, McNiff JM. p40 is a more specific marker than p63 for cutaneous poorly differentiated squamous cell carcinoma. *J Cutan Pathol* 2014;41:839–45.

Geddert H, Kiel S, Heep HJ, et al. The role of p63 and deltaNp63 (p40) protein expression and gene amplification in esophageal carcinogenesis. *Hum Pathol* 2003;34:850–6.

Righi L, Graziano P, Fornari A, et al. Immunohistochemical subtyping of nonsmall cell lung cancer not otherwise specified in fine-needle aspiration cytology: A retrospective study of 103 cases with surgical correlation. *Cancer* 2011;117:3416–23.

Tilson MP, Bishop JA. Utility of p40 in the differential diagnosis of small round blue cell tumors of the sinonasal tract. *Head Neck Pathol* 2014;8:141–5.

Zhang HJ, Xue WC, Siu MK, et al. P63 expression in gestational trophoblastic disease: Correlation with proliferation and apoptotic dynamics. *Int J Gynecol Pathol* 2009;28:172–8.

p53

Background

In the current constellation of oncogenes and recessive tumor suppressor genes, the *p53* molecule represents one of the most common genetic changes associated with human cancer, being implicated in a wide range of malignancies. The *p53* gene displays several unusual features, the most important of which is the ability to act as either a dominant oncogene or a recessive tumor suppressor gene. A combination of genetic events that affect both alleles of the gene results in the loss of expression of wild-type (WT) *p53*. This may occur as a complete loss of one allele of the gene as a result of a large chromosomal deletion combined with a point missense mutation on the other allele. Mutation leads to the loss of DNA binding and transcriptional regulatory activities of the p53 phosphoprotein with a corresponding loss of its growth suppressive activity and its role as "the guardian of the genome." The mutated protein has abnormal conformation, impaired DNA binding, and a prolonged or stabilized half-life, the last of which results in immunohistochemically stainable levels within nuclei in nearly all tumors showing *p53* gene mutation. While a loss of transformation suppression activity and a gain of transforming potential often accompany mutation of *p53*, not all p53 mutants are equal in terms of their biological activity. Mutations at different hotspots manifest different and distinct phenotypes, and there is geographic variation in the sites of mutations, thought to reflect the effects of different environmental and regional carcinogens and cofactors.

Binding of WT p53 to a variety of viral proteins such as protein E6, a product of the human papillomavirus, simian virus 40T antigen, and the Epstein–Barr nuclear antigen, as well as to cellular proteins such as heat shock protein 70 and MDM-2 replication protein, may result in an inactivated complex and a loss of transformation suppression activity.

p53 immunohistochemistry (IHC) is a surrogate for molecular testing of p53 and is widely utilized in clinical practice in the workup of tumors to aid in differential diagnosis or as a prognostic marker.

Applications

Gynecologic pathology

a. Ovary: IHC for p53 is used widely to confirm/favor the diagnosis of high-grade serous carcinoma over endometrioid adenocarcinoma. Although IHC can be challenging to use in separating G3 endometrioid carcinoma from serous carcinoma, strong diffuse block type positivity with mutant type p53 positivity favors serous carcinoma diagnosis. Additionally, unlike high-grade ovarian serous carcinomas, low-grade serous carcinomas typically show wild-type expression and can be useful in challenging cases.

b. Vulva: p53 mutant type IHC staining pattern (basal or parabasal staining or complete absence of staining) can be used to support the diagnosis of differentiated vulvar epithelial neoplasia (VIN) (non-HPV pathway). One limitation is that p53 positivity can be seen in reactive conditions in basal keratinocytes. A more reliable use is in those cases where there is loss of p53 IHC. This can be of potential use in evaluating margin involvement as well.

c. Endometrial carcinoma: Serous carcinomas show mutant p53 staining pattern, which, in the appropriate morphologic context, can be used to support the diagnosis of serous carcinoma (unlike endometrioid carcinomas and the majority of clear cell carcinomas, which are p53 wild type). *See Comments section for discussion.* p53 IHC along with mismatch repair (MMR) and polymerase epsilon (POLE) testing allows a molecular classification of endometrial carcinoma. Endometrial carcinoma with p53 abnormalities has the worst prognosis compared with *POLE* mutated, MMR-D, and p53 WT tumors. Subclonal p53 staining has also been described and is often associated with endometrial carcinoma with MMR deficiency and POLE mutation.

d. Fallopian tube lesions: p53 along with Ki-67 is useful in classifying cases of serous tubal intraepithelial carcinoma (STIC) in which the morphology is equivocal. A mutant pattern of p53 is usually associated with high Ki-67 and helps support the diagnosis of STIC.

Neuropathology

p53 overexpression supports the diagnosis of astrocytoma in the setting of IDH-mutant glioma. Usually, oligodendrogliomas show absent or weak p53 expression.

Comments

Interpretation of p53 IHC: WT staining is usually a faint blush of nuclear staining. Patterns of mutant type staining are as follows: 1. Diffuse nuclear positivity (80–100%% tumor nuclei), 2. complete absence of staining ("null type"), 3. cytoplasmic positivity (a rare pattern).

In vulvar specimens, WT pattern includes variable intensity of positivity in basal and parabasal nuclei or a more recently described mid-epithelial staining (with basal sparing). Mutant staining patterns include strong basal nuclear expression, diffuse basal/parabasal staining, total absence of staining, and diffuse cytoplasmic staining.

It is important to evaluate for internal control, usually in the form of faint staining (reflecting WT positivity), in stromal cells or endothelial cells. Mutant type p53 positivity usually results in diffuse strong nuclear staining in at least 80% of tumor cells, or in the case of loss of function mutation, in complete absence of staining. Cytoplasmic p53 staining has been described as being caused by a loss of function mutation disrupting the nuclear localization domain and rarely (5% in ovarian serous carcinoma) a WT staining caused by a truncating mutation.

Reporting: p53 results should be reported as "wild-type" or "mutation/aberrant type."

Selected references

Batsakis JG, El-Naggar AK. p53: 15 years after discovery. *Adv Anat Pathol* 1995;2:71–88.

Casey L, Kobel M, Ganesan R, et al. A comparison of p53 and WT1 immunohistochemical expression patterns in tubo-ovarian high-grade serous carcinoma before and after neoadjuvant chemotherapy. *Histopathology* 2017;71(5):736–42.

Chang F, Syrjanen S, Tervahauta A, Syrjanen K. Tumorigenesis associated with the p53 tumour suppressor gene. *Br J Cancer* 1993;68:653–61.

Kobel M, Ronnett BM, Singh N, Soslow RA, Gilks CB, McCluggage WG. Interpretation of P53 immunohistochemistry in endometrial carcinomas: Toward increased reproducibility. *Int J Gynecol Pathol* 2019;38 Suppl 1:S123–S131.

Singh N, Leen SL, Han G, et al. Expanding the morphologic spectrum of differentiated VIN (dVIN) through detailed mapping of cases with p53 loss. *Am J Surg Pathol* 2015;39(1):52–60.

Singh N, et al. p53 IHC is an accurate surrogate for TP53 mutational analysis in endometrial carcinoma biopsies. *J Pathol* 2020;250:336–345.

Talhouk A, McConechy MK, Leung S, et al. Confirmation of ProMisE: A simple, genomics-based clinical classifier for endometrial cancer. *Cancer* 2017;123(5):802–13.

Visvanathan K, Vang R, Shaw P, et al. Diagnosis of serous tubal intraepithelial carcinoma based on morphologic and immunohistochemical features: A reproducibility study. *Am J Surg Pathol* 2011;35(12):1766–75.

p63

Background

The *p63* gene (chromosome 3q27-19) is part of the p53 tumor suppressor family and has structural similarity to both p53 and p73. During embryogenesis, it is responsible for epithelial development. Germline mutations lead to cleft lip and palate syndrome, ectrodactyly, ectodermal dysplasia, and limb-mammary syndrome – a group of disorders resulting in variable ectodermal abnormalities.

p63 expression is nuclear in location and is seen in normal squamous epithelium, including that of skin, esophagus, uterine ectocervix, tonsil, and bladder, or other sites that exhibit squamous metaplasia.

p63 is expressed in basal epithelial and/or myoepithelial cells of several organs, including breast, skin, uterine cervix, urogenital tract, and prostate.

p63 is also expressed in thymic epithelial cells and cytotrophoblastic cells.

Applications

1. Useful for identification of squamous carcinomas, urothelial carcinoma, a proportion of anaplastic large cell lymphoma, mucoepidermoid carcinoma, adenoid cystic carcinoma, metaplastic carcinoma of the breast, sarcomatoid carcinoma, and giant cell tumor of bone.
2. Key applications in daily practice include identification of squamous differentiation, baso-myoepithelial cells in the breast (ductal carcinoma in situ [DCIS] vs invasive carcinoma), and prostate (atypical glands vs invasive carcinoma).
3. Cytoplasmic p63 staining has been reported in tumors with skeletal muscle differentiation.

Selected references

Di Como CJ, Urist MJ, Babayan I, et al. p63 expression profiles in human normal and tumor tissues. *Clin Cancer Res* 2002;8:494–501.

Martin SE, Temm CJ, Goheen MP, et al. Cytoplasmic p63 immunohistochemistry is a useful marker for muscle differentiation: An immunohistochemical and immunoelectron microscopic study. *Mod Pathol* 2011;24:1320–6.

Weinstein MH, Signoretti S, Loda M. Diagnostic utility of immunohistochemical staining for p63, a sensitive marker of prostatic basal cells. *Mod Pathol* 2002;15(12):1302–8.

Pancreatic hormones (insulin, somatostatin, vasoactive intestinal polypeptide, gastrin, glucagon, pancreatic polypeptide)

Pancreatic endocrine tumors have been associated with several distinct clinical syndromes, such as hypoglycemia, glucagonoma syndrome, Zollinger–Ellison syndrome, and WDHA (watery diarrhea, hypokalemia, and achlorhydria) syndrome. Routine histological examination usually fails to predict the behavior and endocrine manifestations of these neoplasms. Immunohistochemistry permits the specific demonstration of various pancreatic hormones in tissue sections.

Background

The antigens used as immunogens to raise rabbit antibodies against the pancreatic hormones were as follows: insulin – porcine pancreatic insulin; somatostatin – synthetic peptide somatostatin 14; vasoactive intestinal polypeptide (VIP) – natural porcine VIP conjugated to glutaraldehyde as carrier protein; gastrin – synthetic human gastrin-17 non-sulfated form conjugated to bovine serum albumin; glucagon – porcine glucagon.

Although there are at least eight different cell types identified in the pancreatic islets, only the resident four major cell types (A, B, D, and PP cells) and G and VIP cells (in neoplastic conditions) will be considered here. In the normal adult islet, insulin-containing B cells account for 60–80% of endocrine cells and occupy the central portion of the islets. Glucagon-containing A cells constitute 20–30% and somatostatin-containing D cells 5–11%. A and D cells are mostly present in the periphery of the islets and are also scattered within the islets along capillaries. Physiologically, glucagon increases hepatic glucose production and opposes hepatic glucose storage; insulin increases peripheral glucose uptake and opposes glucagon-mediated hepatic glucose production. Hence, the delicate balance of these two hormones maintains blood glucose homeostasis. Somatostatin has inhibitory actions on both A and B cells through a "paracrine" effect, thereby regulating the balance of A and B cell functions. PP cells are the least numerous and are present

both within and outside the islets. The function of pancreatic polypeptide is not fully understood. PP cells have a variable distribution in the pancreas, with PP-cell-rich islets being occasionally present in the posterior lobe of the pancreatic head. Hence, caution should be exercised when evaluating hyperplastic changes of PP cells.

Although the presence of gastrin in D cells has been disputed, recent studies indicate that gastrin is not present in normal adult islets. VIP has been localized in human islets but the exact cellular origin is not fully understood. In the rat, diabetes mellitus induced by streptozotocin resulted in a reduction of the number of insulin-positive cells in the islet of Langerhans, while VIP and neuropeptide-Y increased significantly after the onset of diabetes. Both these hormones evoked large and significant increases in insulin release from pancreatic tissue fragments of normal rats.

In the gastro-duodenal segment, gastrin has been immunolocalized to the G cells of the gastric antrum, whilst somatostatin has been found in endocrine cells and nerves of the intestinal wall digestive mucosa.

Applications

1. With the availability of antibodies to the secretory products, specific designation of these neoplasms has led to terms such as insulinoma, glucagonoma, gastrinoma, somatostatinoma, and VIPoma.
2. The common clinical syndromes and their causative hormones are as follows: hypoglycemia (insulin), Zollinger–Ellison syndrome (gastrin), glucagonoma syndrome (glucagon), WDHA syndrome (Verner–Morrison syndrome) (vasoactive intestinal pancreatic polypeptide), and somatostatinoma syndrome (somatostatin). Apart from the first two syndromes, which are relatively frequent, the remaining three are either infrequent or rare. Occasionally, pancreatic endocrine tumors fail to demonstrate immunoreaction in the presence of clinical syndromes. Explanations for

this aberrant phenomenon include abnormal peptides (although biologically active), which may not react with specific anti-hormone antibodies, fixation artifact, or alternatively, rapid turnover in tumor cells resulting in only minute amounts being stored.

3. Tumors from some patients with WDHA syndrome have been found to secrete PP. PP also appears to be the most commonly found in hormone-silent/nonfunctioning tumors. Whilst the physiologic function of PP is not yet fully understood, PP cells are nevertheless a component often demonstrated in multihormonal tumors. The frequency of multihormone production by islet cell tumors has been stated to be as high as 50%. These tumors usually cause only one clinical syndrome, and a combination of syndromes is extremely rare. In fact, the predominant cell type in a tumor does not necessarily cause the corresponding syndrome. Any combination of cell types is possible in pancreatic endocrine tumors, the most striking example being the high frequency of PP cells in tumors secreting VIP and causing the WDHA syndrome. The most likely explanation for the common presence of several cell types in pancreatic endocrine tumors is that they derive from a multipotential stem cell that may differentiate in various directions.

4. Antibodies to pancreatic hormones may also be applied to the diagnosis of islet cell hyperplasia seen in the nonneoplastic pancreas of patients with islet cell tumors and primary G-cell hyperplasia (gastrin producing) in the antrum of the stomach. The latter is clinically indistinguishable from Zollinger–Ellison's syndrome due to gastrinoma.

5. Duodenal (periampullary) somatostatin-rich carcinoid tumors (psammomatous somatostatinoma) need to be distinguished from adenocarcinoma, because the prognosis is better in the former even though lymph node metastases may occur with carcinoids. Other neuroendocrine tumors of the duodenum that require immunohistochemistry for their recognition include gastrinomas (most common), gangliocytic paraganglioma, serotonin-/calcitonin-/pancreatic polypeptide-producing tumors, and poorly differentiated neuroendocrine carcinomas. A characteristic feature of multiple endocrine neoplasia (MEN)-associated gastrinomas is their frequent multicentricity.

6. Gastrointestinal carcinoid tumors have also benefited from the development of immunohistochemical technology: gastrin, VIP, PP, and glucagon have been demonstrated (apart from serotonin in cases of carcinoid syndrome). In children, WDHA syndromes have been reported in association with VIP-secreting ganglioneuromas and ganglioneuroblastomas.

7. Increased neuroproliferation in the appendix is associated with an increase in VIP, substance P, and growth-associated protein-43 in adults with acute right lower quadrant abdominal pain.

Selected references

Bouchard S, Russo P, Radu AP, Adzick NS. Expression of neuropeptides in normal and abnormal appendices. *J Pediatr Surg* 2001;36:1222–6.

Parathyroid hormone

Background

The parathormone gene, closely linked to that of β-globin, is located on the short arm of chromosome 11 in humans (as are the genes for calcitonin and insulin). The initial form in which parathormone is synthesized within the cell is a single-chain polypeptide of 115 amino acid residues, preproparathyroid hormone. This is cleaved within the cell to form a proparathyroid hormone, from which a further 6 amino acids are split, leaving the 84–amino acid chain of parathormone. The rate of parathormone secretion is directly responsive to the level of calcium in the serum, and indeed the cytoplasm, of parathyroid cells, as has been shown by studies both in vivo and in vitro. Recent in vitro studies of osteoclast turnover suggest that both PTH and PTH-related protein exert both pro- and anti-apoptotic effects in mesenchymal cells.

Applications

Surgical pathologists are familiar with the ability of parathyroid proliferations to assume a variety of histological guises, posing difficulty in categorizing any given lesion as hyperplastic, adenomatous, or carcinomatous in nature. This is usually resolved with the macroscopic appearance of the remaining parathyroid glands as assessed by the surgeon. The role of the surgical pathologist is to identify the lesion as parathyroid in nature and to assess whether it is normocellular or hypercellular. Although this is easily accomplished in the majority of instances, rare examples of parathyroid hyperplasia/adenoma showing a follicular/trabecular arrangement may cause concern over the alternative diagnosis of a thyroid adenoma. This becomes more pertinent when the parathyroid lesion abuts into the thyroid gland or lies within the thyroid capsule. Immunodetection for thyroglobulin and parathyroid hormone (PTH) is especially useful to resolve the problem. Nevertheless, caution should be exercised, since parathyroid cells often discharge their hormonal product almost as soon as it is packaged in the cytoplasm, resulting in false-negative PTH immunostaining although the cells are biologically synthetic.

PTH antibody is also useful to distinguish cell parathyroid hyperplasia/neoplasms from thyroid and metastatic neoplasms, although the pathologist is typically aware of the preoperative hypercalcemic status. Occasionally, when the surgeon does not supply this information, PTH immunohistochemistry is essential. Even more problematic are situations in which clear cell parathyroid carcinomas are nonsecretory, without an abnormality in mineral metabolism. In such situations, metastatic renal cell carcinoma or metastatic clear cell carcinoma of the lung is evident, warranting PTH immunohistochemistry to arrive at the correct diagnosis. The other instance in which PTH antibodies are useful is in the consideration of parathyroid carcinomas located primarily in the anterior mediastinum (intrathymically). In this situation, distinction from primary thymic metastatic carcinomas, non-Hodgkin's lymphoma, and germ cell tumors is necessary.

Selected references

Aldinger KA, Hickey RC, Ibanez ML, Samaan NA. Parathyroid carcinoma: A clinical study of seven cases of functioning and two cases of nonfunctioning parathyroid cancer. *Cancer* 1982;49:388–97.

Brown EM. PTH secretion in vivo and in vitro: Regulation by calcium and other secretagogues. *Mineral Electrolyte Metal* 1982;8:130–50.

Chen HL, Demiralp B, Schneider A, et al. Parathyroid hormone and parathyroid hormone-related protein exert both pro- and anti-apoptotic effects in mesenchymal cells. *J Biol Chem* 2002;277:19374–81.

Parathyroid hormone-related protein (PTHrP)

Background

Humoral hypercalcemia of malignancy (HHM) is a syndrome characterized by low levels of parathyroid hormone (PTH), few/absent bone metastases, and hypophosphatemia. Parathyroid hormone-related protein (PTHrP) has been isolated from tumors with HHM and shown to be responsible for the PTH-like effects and disruption of calcium homeostasis. The amino acid sequence of PTHrP bears homology to PTH from amino acid 1 to 13 but is unique thereafter. Although functioning via the PTH receptor, PTHrP is the product of a separate gene located on the short arm of chromosome 12. Antibody to PTHrP (Ab-1) reacts with amino acid residues 38–64 of human PTHrP and shows no cross-reactivity with human PTH.

In addition to being produced by malignant tumors, PTHrP is found in normal keratinocytes, lactating mammary tissue, placenta, parathyroid glands, the central nervous system, and a number of other sites, suggesting that it may have a widespread physiologic role. PTHrP is thought to act in an autocrine and paracrine manner in various tissues to modulate other functions in addition to regulating calcium mobilization.

Through studies of osteoblast turnover in vitro it was suggested that PTHrP and the PTH-1 receptor might play an important role in exerting both pro- and anti-apoptotic effects in mesenchymal cells.

Immunostaining for PTHrP suggests that production of the peptide by stromal cells and giant cells may be involved in the formation of osteoclast-like cells in giant cell tumor of tendon sheath by acting in an autocrine/paracrine fashion.

Applications

Most squamous cell carcinomas from a variety of sites synthesize PTHrP irrespective of the calcium status of the patient. Using a polyclonal antibody to PTHrP (1–130), 93% of 40 invasive squamous cell carcinomas were found to be immunopositive. Interestingly, the strongest immunoreactivity for PTHrP in the squamous carcinomas was in areas of invasion and with desmoplasia. Adenocarcinomas (a smaller percentage than squamous cancers) of breast, lung, and kidney, hepatocellular carcinoma, mesothelioma, neuroendocrine tumors, and T-cell leukemias are other neoplasms that may express PTHrP. The presence of PTHrP and its receptor has been demonstrated in normal breast epithelium and breast carcinomas, suggesting that most breast tumors are able to respond to PTHrP.

Cholangiocarcinomas may be immunopositive for PTHrP (and chromogranin A), whilst all hepatocellular carcinomas were negative. Mixed primary liver tumors contained PTHrP immunoreactivity only in areas of cholangiocellular differentiation. Moreover, all metastatic adenocarcinomas (especially from the gastrointestinal tract) were negative except for 2/5 metastatic breast carcinomas.

Using polyclonal antibodies against synthetic PTHrP peptides, immunopositivity was demonstrated in primary parathyroid adenomata and hyperplastic glands from patients with chronic renal failure, whilst primary hyperplastic glands were negative.

Comments

The frequency of expression of PTHrP is so great and widespread that it may be useful as a tumor marker in the histological diagnosis of certain cancers, e.g., squamous cell carcinoma of the lung. The protein has been shown to be a potential marker of pancreatic adenocarcinoma, and the coexpression of PTHrP and PTH/PTHrP receptor in chondrosarcomas may be of value in differentiating between benign and malignant cartilaginous lesions. Furthermore, the role of PTHrP in distinguishing between primary hepatocellular carcinoma and cholangiocarcinoma in the liver appears to be fairly reliable. Reactive bile ductules or squamous epithelium of epidermis are recommended control tissue. PTHrP has also been demonstrated in uterine tumors resembling ovarian sex cord tumors, multiple myeloma, endometrium, and salivary glands.

Selected references

Bouvet M, Nardin SR, Burton DW, et al. Parathyroid hormone-related protein as a novel tumor marker in pancreatic adenocarcinoma. *Pancreas* 2002;24:284–90.

Burtis WJ, Brady TG, Orloff JJ, et al. Immunochemical characterization of circulating parathyroid hormone-related protein in patients with humoral hypercalcemia of cancer. *N Engl J Med* 1990;322:1106–12.

PAX-2 (paired box gene 2)

Background

PAX2 is a transcriptional protein that, together with PAX8, plays a role in the development of the urogenital system and it is expressed in Wolffian and Mullerian ducts during early embryologic stages.

Applications

1. PAX2 is expressed in a spectrum of urologic neoplasms, including renal cell carcinomas, papillary renal cell carcinomas, chromophobe, and oncocytoma, but not in urothelial renal carcinomas. In addition, it has been shown to be expressed in Wilms tumor and nephrogenic adenomas.

2. PAX2 is a diagnostically useful marker for both primary and metastatic renal neoplasms, especially in small core needle biopsies.

3. PAX2 is also normally expressed in epithelium of rete testis to ejaculatory duct, and neoplasms arising from these cells (carcinoma rete testis, Wolffian adnexal tumor of the seminal vesicle and endometrioid carcinoma of the seminal vesicle) will express PAX2. In contrast, it is not expressed in prostatic adenocarcinomas.

4. PAX2 has been reported in some normal Mullerian tissues, including endometrium, fallopian tube mucosa, endocervix, and foci of endosalpingiosis and endometriosis. In addition, it is present in mesonephric remnants and mesonephric hyperplasia.

5. In Mullerian epithelial neoplasms, PAX2 expression is seen in approximately 55% of serous tumors from ovary, uterus, and peritoneum; 25% of endometrioid adenocarcinomas; 19% of clear cell tumors, 10% of undifferentiated tumors;

and 10% of mucinous tumors. When compared with PAX8, although both stain the same tumors, PAX2 staining is usually less intense and in fewer cells, indicating that PAX2 sensitivity for epithelial tumors is lower than that of PAX8.

6. In the uterine cervix, PAX2 is not expressed in minimal deviation adenocarcinoma, and it is useful to distinguish this entity from mesonephric hyperplasia and lobular endocervical hyperplasia, both of which will be positive for PAX2. In addition, endocervical adenocarcinoma in situ is negative for PAX2, in contrast to endocervical tubal metaplasia or cervical endometriosis. A strong, diffuse nuclear PAX2 expression in cervical glandular epithelium suggests a benign diagnosis.

Selected references

Daniel L, Lechevallier E, Giorgi R, et al. Pax-2 expression in adult renal tumors. *Hum Pathol* 2001; 32:282–7.

Dressler GR, Douglass EC. Pax-2 is a DNA-binding protein expressed in embryonic kidney and Wilms tumor. *Proc Natl Acad Sci USA* 1992;89:1179–83.

Ordonez NG. Value of Pax2 immunostaining in tumor diagnosis: A review and update. *Adv Anat Pathol* 2012:19:401–9.

Ozcan A, Liles N, Coffey D, et al. PAX2 and PAX8 expression in primary and metastatic mullerian epithelial tumors: A comprehensive comparison. *Am J Surg Pathol* 2011;35:1837–47.

Rabban JT, Mcalhany S, Lerwill MF, et al. Pax2 distinguishes benign mesonephric and mullerian glandular lesions of the cervix from endocervical adenocarcinoma, including minimal deviation adenocarcinoma. *Am J Surg Pathol* 2010;34:137–46.

PAX-5

Background

PAX-5, also known as B-cell-specific activator protein (BSAP), is a nuclear transcription factor thought to play a critical role in the commitment of the common lymphoid progenitor to the B-cell lineage. *Pax* genes constitute a family of nine transcription factors that have important roles in regulating cell proliferation, migration, and differentiation during embryonic development and organogenesis. PAX-5 expression is thought to trigger B-cell development by transcriptionally activating target genes such as CD19, which in turn drive B-cell differentiation. PAX-5 is expressed in all B-cell differentiation, including the entire range of immature B-cell stages in the bone marrow and the full range of mature B cells in peripheral lymphoid tissues, the blood, and bone marrow. As B cells terminally differentiate into plasma cells, PAX-5 is normally downregulated by the coordinate activity of several proteins involved in plasmacytic differentiation, primarily BLIMP and APRIL. The ubiquitous expression of PAX-5 in immature and mature B cells makes it an excellent marker for the entire range of B-cell differentiation prior to the plasma cell stage.

Applications

1. In normal bone marrow, PAX-5 is uniformly and strongly expressed in all immature and mature B cells but not in plasma cells. Similarly, in peripheral lymphoid tissue, PAX-5 is uniformly expressed in B-cell follicles, including both primary and secondary follicles. It tends to be somewhat more highly expressed in naïve/mantle zone–type B cells compared with germinal center B cells. PAX-5 expression can be seen in marginal zone B cells and in virtually all mature B-cell non-Hodgkin lymphomas.

2. PAX-5 is uniformly expressed in the neoplastic cells of nodular lymphocyte-predominant Hodgkin lymphoma (lymphocyte predominant [LP] cells), although typically at a lower level than normal germinal center-derived B cells. Roughly 90% of classical Hodgkin lymphomas are thought to show PAX-5 expression in the Hodgkin/Reed–Sternberg (HRS) cells, always at low level and sometimes on only a small portion of the HRS cells. Rare cases of classical Hodgkin lymphomas are thought to include PAX-5-negative HRS cells, although in such cases exclusion of anaplastic large cell lymphoma of T lineage would be required.

3. While **normal** plasma cells lack PAX-5 expression, the neoplastic plasma cells in several B-lymphoid malignancies will show PAX-5 expression. In B-cell lymphomas with significant plasmacytic differentiation, most notably lymphoplasmacytic lymphoma (LPL) and marginal zone lymphoma (MZL), both the neoplastic B cells and plasma cells typically express PAX-5. In contrast, true plasma cell neoplasms, including plasma cell myeloma and extramedullary plasmacytoma, lack PAX-5 expression in the large majority of cases. The one exception is plasma cell neoplasms containing t(11;14), which frequently do aberrantly retain PAX-5 expression.

4. Importantly, rare nonhematopoietic neoplasms are known to express PAX-5. The most important such neoplasm is Merkel cell carcinoma (MCC).

   Other neoplasms known to express PAX-5 include neuroendocrine tumors of the lung, especially small cell carcinoma (80%), atypical carcinoids (70%), and large cell neuroendocrine carcinomas (75%).

Selected references

O'Brien P, Morin P Jr, Ouellette RJ, et al. The Pax-5 gene: A pluripotent regulator of B-cell differentiation and cancer disease. *Cancer Res* 2011;71:7345–50.

Baker SJ, Reddy EP. B cell differentiation: Role of E2A and Pax5/BSAP transcription factors. *Oncogene* 1995 11:413–26.

Desouki MM, Post GR, Cherry D, et al. PAX-5: A valuable immunohistochemical marker in the differential diagnosis of lymphoid neoplasms. *Clin Med Res* 2010;8:84–8.

Morgenstern DA, Hasan F, Gibson S, et al. PAX5 expression in nonhematopoietic tissues: Reappraisal of previous studies. *Am J Clin Pathol* 2010;133:407–15.

PAX-8

Background

PAX-8 is a member of the paired box (PAX) gene family of transcription factors that is expressed in the epithelium of the thyroid gland, kidney, and Mullerian tract. PAX-8 positivity is seen as nuclear positivity by immunohistochemistry. In the normal female genital tract, PAX-8 is expressed in normal epithelial cells of the endocervix, endometrium, nonciliated cells of the fallopian tube, and ovarian inclusion cyst lining cells. In the normal kidney, PAX-8 is expressed in epithelium of proximal and distal tubules, loops of Henle, collecting ducts, and parietal cells of Bowman's capsule. In the normal thyroid gland, PAX-8 is expressed in follicular cells and focally in C cells. PAX-8 is also seen expressed in thymic epithelial cells and the parathyroid gland.

Applications

1. Gynecologic tumors:
   a. Ovary: PAX-8 is expressed in the vast majority of serous, endometrioid, and clear cell carcinomas of the ovary. Serous carcinomas (99%) are more frequently positive for PAX-8 as compared with nonserous carcinomas. Mucinous carcinomas of ovary show much more variable positivity, ranging from being negative to showing heterogeneous or weak positivity. Primary mucinous tumors of the ovary are an exception, with variable staining, and 50% of these tumors can be PAX-8 negative.
   b. Endometrial tumors: Endometrioid, clear cell, and serous carcinomas are PAX-8 positive. Typically, undifferentiated carcinomas of the endometrium are PAX-8 negative (80% or more cases).
   c. Cervix: Benign and malignant cervical epithelial tumors are positive for PAX-8, although the benign and precursor lesions (adenocarcinoma in situ) can show strong positivity compared with invasive adenocarcinomas.

2. PAX-8 is a very useful marker to confirm the diagnosis of primary thyroid carcinomas and is seen in 90% of follicular adenomas and follicular and papillary carcinomas. While it is also expressed in the majority of anaplastic thyroid carcinoma, the extent of positivity can be highly variable, but when positive, it can help support the diagnosis of anaplastic thyroid carcinoma over metastatic carcinoma (except from the kidney and gynecologic tract) or other sarcoma. Medullary carcinomas can be focally positive or negative.

3. Additionally, PAX-8 expression is seen consistently in benign and malignant thymic neoplasms.

4. In renal tumors, PAX-8 is expressed in renal cell carcinoma (clear cell, papillary chromophobe, and Xp11.2 translocation types), Wilms tumor, and nephrogenic adenoma. Less common variants such as collecting duct and medullary carcinoma also are frequently PAX8 positive. This makes it a valuable biomarker in the workup of metastatic carcinoma where metastatic renal cell carcinoma is a differential diagnostic consideration. Conventional urothelial carcinomas of the urinary bladder are PAX-8 negative. A subset of renal pelvic urothelial carcinoma and clear cell adenocarcinoma of the urinary bladder can express PAX-8.

5. Serous carcinoma versus mesothelial proliferations: 99% or more of serous carcinomas express PAX-8 and the vast majority of malignant mesotheliomas are negative for PAX-8, although a small percentage will show weak expression. Well-differentiated papillary mesothelioma in particular can show PAX-8 expression in 30–60% of cases. Additionally, PAX-8 expression has been seen in both benign mesothelial cells and benign mesothelial lesions such as peritoneal inclusion cysts. However, diffuse strong positivity (as is typically seen in serous carcinomas) will be most unusual.

6. PAX-8 can show strong expression in mammary carcinoma and carcinomas of the lung, and also, rarely, in urothelial carcinoma, adenocarcinoma of the esophagus and pancreas, and cholangiocarcinoma.

7. Hemangioblastoma in the central nervous system can be PAX-8 positive. Since clear cell renal cell carcinoma is PAX-8 positive and often a differential diagnostic consideration of hemangioblastoma, this is another pitfall.

8. Among small round cell tumors, PAX-8 can be seen expressed in Ewing sarcoma and occasionally in synovial sarcoma.

9. PAX8 can be used to establish the origin of a low-grade neuroendocrine tumor. However, pancreatic neuroendocrine tumors and duodenal and rectal low-grade neuroendocrine tumors can show PAX-8 expression.

Selected references

Laury AR, Perets R, Piao H, et al. A comprehensive analysis of PAX8 expression in human epithelial tumors. *Am J Surg Pathol* 2011;35:816–26.

Liang L, Zheng W, Liu J, et al. Assessment of the utility of PAX8 immunohistochemical stain in diagnosing endocervical glandular lesions. *Arch Pathol Lab Med* 2016;140:148–52.

PDX1

Background

Pancreatic duodenal homeobox 1 (PDX1) (also known as insulin promoter factor 1 or IPF1) is a transcription factor located on chromosome 13q12.1 involved in pancreatic development and β-cell maturation. Mutations in IPF-1 have been implicated in cases of pancreatic agenesis and in mature onset of diabetes of the young, type 4.

Applications

1. Expression is normally noted in the nucleus of islet cells, centroacinar cells, and nonneoplastic ductal epithelium of the pancreas, and is normally negative in nonneoplastic acinar cells.
2. Positive staining tends to be present in well-differentiated neuroendocrine tumors of the gastrointestinal tract, although site-specificity has not been seen. In the select setting of gastrinomas, it can be useful in distinguishing pancreatic from duodenal tumors, as positive staining is noted only in those tumors arising from the pancreas.
3. Pancreatic ductal carcinomas, intraductal papillary mucinous neoplasms, and pancreatic precursor lesions (PAN-Ins) may show staining.
4. Acinar cell carcinomas also tend to show expression, despite the fact that nonneoplastic acinar cells do not express PDX1.
5. Outside the pancreas, expression has also been noted in pseudopyloric glands and intestinal metaplasia of the stomach, as well as a subset of cases of hilar cholangiocarcinoma.

Selected references

Park JY, Hong SM, Klimstra DS, et al. Pdx1 expression in pancreatic precursor lesions and neoplasms. *Appl Immunohistochem Mol Morphol* 2011;19(5):444–9.

Sakai H, Eishi Y, Li X-L, et al. PDX1 homeobox protein expression in pseudopyloric glands and gastric carcinomas. *Gut* 2004;53(3):323–30.

Srivastava A, Hornick .L. Immunohistochemical staining for CDX-2, PDX-1, NESP-55, and TTF-1 can help distinguish gastrointestinal carcinoid tumors from pancreatic endocrine and pulmonary carcinoid tumors. *Am J Surg Pathol* 2009;33(4):626–32.

P-glycoprotein (P-170), multidrug resistance (MDR)

Background

P-glycoprotein (P-170) is a transmembrane protein of 170 kD molecular weight. It has been associated with both intrinsic and acquired resistance to certain chemotherapeutic agents, particularly anthracyclines and vinca alkaloids. It is an energy-dependent pump, which functions in drug efflux, reducing intracellular accumulation of chemotherapeutic agents and thus conferring the so-called multidrug resistance (MDR) phenomenon on cells expressing increased levels of this protein. One of the most perplexing problems encountered in chemotherapy is the resistance of certain tumors to all chemotherapeutic regimens, while other tumors, which are initially chemosensitive to a particular agent, show resistance to treatment over time and with disease progression. Furthermore, tumor cells that are resistant to one drug often show cross-resistance to a wide variety of other, structurally unrelated drugs. For example, tumor cells resistant to adriamycin can show cross-resistance to diverse drugs to which they have never been exposed, including vinca alkaloids and mitomycin C, but not to other drugs such as alkylating agents. This is known as the MDR phenomenon. A family of so-called *MDR* genes encodes the P-glycoprotein, apparently with only the protein encoded by the MDR 1 gene inducing the MDR phenotype.

There is extensive evidence from in vitro studies, especially with nonhuman cell lines, that overexpression of P-glycoprotein results in reduced accumulation of drug within the cell. Recently, mice have been generated with knockout of MDR 1, and these animals show abnormalities of transport at the blood–brain barrier and are more sensitive to drugs.

Applications

Molecular and immunohistochemical studies of P-glycoprotein reveal that it is overexpressed in a number of intrinsically resistant tumors, such as carcinomas of the liver, pancreas, colon, adrenal cortex, and kidney, and appears to vary according to the differentiation of the cells. Interestingly, in these cases, high levels of the protein have also been demonstrated in the normal tissues from which the tumors are derived. The physiologic function of P-glycoprotein can be deduced from its normal tissue distribution in that high levels of expression are seen in endothelial cells of the blood–brain barrier and in renal proximal tubules, both cell types having the primary function of moving toxic molecules across cell membranes.

P-glycoprotein expression has been found significantly more frequently in soft tissue sarcomas, neuroblastomas, and hepatoblastomas and generally in disseminated tumors but not in malignant brain tumors and nephroblastoma. Tumors responsive to chemotherapy generally show low levels of P-glycoprotein expression, and solid tumors that are most responsive to systemic chemotherapy, such as seminomas and embryonal carcinomas, rarely display detectable levels of the protein. Tumors from patients previously treated with chemotherapy show frequent elevation of P-glycoprotein, suggesting that the MDR phenotype is induced by exposure to chemotherapy. The detection of elevated levels of P-glycoprotein expression has the potential to identify tumors likely to be resistant to conventional chemotherapy and may provide a rationale for the use of alternative treatments for such patients. Immunohistological evaluation appears to be the method of choice for the assessment of P-glycoprotein, largely because it allows morphological correlation and discrimination from P-glycoprotein in nontumor cells. However, the published results are conflicting, with immunoexpression of P-glycoprotein and other multidrug resistance–related proteins not changing significantly after chemotherapy. It was shown that there was no significant correlation between P-glycoprotein expression in tumor cells and clinical course, stage, and grade of nephroblastoma. However, positivity in tumor capillary endothelial cells correlated significantly with unfavorable outcome, suggesting that chemoresistance depended on an active blood–tumor barrier.

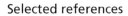

P

Selected references

Cordon-Cardo C, O'Brien JP, Boccia J, et al. Expression of the multidrug resistance gene product (P-glycoprotein) in human normal and tumor tissues. *J Histochem Cytochem* 1990;38:1277–87.

Lopes JM, Bruland OS, Bjekehagen B, et al. Synovial sarcoma: Immunohistochemical expression of P-glycoprotein and glutathione S transferase-pi and clinical drug resistance. *Pathol Res Pract* 1997;193:21–36.

Scheffer GL, Pijnenborg AC, Smit EF, et al. Multidrug resistance related molecules in human and murine lung. *J Clin Pathol* 2002;55:332–9.

Phosphohistone H3 (pHH3)

Background

Histone H3, a core histone protein, and other histone proteins form the major protein constituents of eukaryotic chromatin. In mammalian cells, phosphorylation of the serine 10 residue of histone H3, a rare event during interphase, reaches a maximum for chromatin condensation during mitosis. No phosphorylation of the histone H3 has been noted during apoptosis or karyorrhexis. Additionally, in comparison to the Ki-67 immunostain, which stains cells in all phases of the cell cycle (except G0), studies have shown that the antibody directed against the pHH3 is a more sensitive and effective marker for identifying mitotic activity.

Applications

Studies have shown that the pHH3 immunostain helps focus attention on the most mitotically active areas of a tumor, allows easy and objective differentiation of mitotic from apoptotic nuclei, and consequently reduces intra- and interobserver variability. Its role in facilitating the rapid reliable grading of meningiomas, astrocytomas, melanomas, and well-differentiated neuroendocrine tumors of the pancreas has been well studied.

Selected references

Juan G, Traganos F, James WM, et al. Histone H3 phosphorylation and expression of cyclins A and B1 measured in individual cells during their progression through G2 and mitosis. *Cytometry* 1998;32:71–7.

Ribalta T, McCutcheon IE, Aldape KD, et al. The mitosis-specific antibody anti-phosphohistone-H3 (PHH3) facilitates rapid reliable grading of meningiomas according to WHO 2000 criteria. *Am J Surg Pathol* 2004;28:1532–6.

Shibata K, Ajiro K. Cell cycle-dependent suppressive effect of histone H1 on mitosis-specific H3 phosphorylation. *J Biol Chem* 1993;268:18431–34.

Tetzlaff MT, Curry JL, Ivan D, et al. Immunodetection of phosphohistone H3 as a surrogate of mitotic figure count and clinical outcome in cutaneous melanoma. *Mod Pathol* 2013;26:1153–60.

Voss SM, Riley MP, Lokhandwala PM, et al. Mitotic count by phosphohistone H3 immunohistochemical staining predicts survival and improves interobserver reproducibility in well-differentiated neuroendocrine tumors of the pancreas. *Am J Surg Pathol* 2015;39:13–24.

Pituitary hormones (ACTH, FSH, hGH, LH, PRL, TSH)

Background

In all instances antibodies against the pituitary hormones were raised using purified extract from human pituitary glands as immunogen. The adenohypophysis comprises approximately 75% of the normal pituitary gland. It consists of the pars distalis, pars intermedia, and pars tuberalis. The pars distalis is roughly divided into a midline zone (periodic acid–Schiff [PAS]-positive mucosubstance containing adrenocorticotropic hormone [ACTH] [15–20%], follicle stimulating hormone/luteinizing hormone [FSH/LH] [10%], and thyroid stimulating hormone [TSH] [5%] cells) and two lateral portions that stain positively with acidic dyes (PBX 15–20% and growth hormone [GH] 50%). It should be noted that cells are not strictly limited in their geographic distribution. Trichrome stains such as the PAS–orange G method serve to highlight the PAS-positive basophils and the orange G–positive acidophils. Since this reactivity correlates only crudely with hormonal function, it is necessary to resort to immunohistochemical characterization for proper identification. The cells are arranged in cords and are encircled by well-formed basement membrane. These cells lie in the immediate proximity of a capillary to facilitate the secretory process.

Applications

The major role of antibodies to pituitary hormones is that they serve as the primary basis of adenoma classification. In adults, adenomas may present with hyperfunction (amenorrhea-galactorrhea, Cushing's disease, Nelson's syndrome, and acromegaly or gigantism), hypofunction (insufficiency of gonadal, thyroidal, or adrenal function) or with compressive signs (visual disturbance, headache, or raised intracranial pressure). Aggression of pituitary adenomas is based on the radiological assessment: Grade I, microadenomas (<10 mm); grade 2, intrasellar adenoma; grade 3, diffuse adenomas with erosion of sellar floor; and grade 4, invasive adenomas with widespread sellar erosion and destruction.

The conventional tinctorial classification of adenomas, based on affinity of tumor cells for acid or basic dyes, correlated crudely with the functional characteristics. Acidophil adenomas were presumed to produce growth hormone, whilst basophilic adenomas were considered synonymous with ACTH secretion and Cushing's disease. Chromophobe adenomas, in contrast, were considered nonfunctioning, with symptoms being attributed to local destructive or compressive effects.

Comments

Histopathology laboratories servicing neurosurgical units need to provide a comprehensive functional characterization of pituitary adenomas. The use of the normal pituitary gland will suffice as a positive control for the six hormones.

Selected references

Earle KM, Dillard SH Jr. Pathology of adenomas of the pituitary gland. *Excerpta Medica International Congress Series* No. 303, 1973, pp. 3–16.

Hardy J, Vezina JL. Transsphenoidal neurosurgery of intracranial neoplasm. *Adv Neurol* 1976;15:261–5.

Robert F. Electron microscopy of human pituitary tumors. In: Tindall GT, Collins WF. eds. *Clinical management of pituitary disorders*. New York: Raven Press, 1979, pp. 113–31.

NOTES

Placental alkaline phosphatase (PLAP)

Background

The alkaline phosphatases (APs) are a heterogenous group of glycoproteins, which are usually confined to the cell surface. The isoenzymes differ in terms of their biochemical properties, anatomical sites of production, and reactivity with different antibodies. APs probably have a role in cellular transport, regulation of metabolism, gene transcription, and cellular differentiation. At least three genes encode the human AP isoenzymes, one for tissue-nonspecific AP present in the liver, bone, and kidney, one for the synthesis of intestinal AP, and one or more genes for the placental isoenzyme (PLAP). The different isoenzymes differ in molecular weight and amino acid composition and have different properties. The tissue-nonspecific and intestinal variants are heat sensitive, whereas the PLAP isoenzymes are heat resistant. PLAP occurs only in higher primates and displays a high degree of genetic polymorphism. It is a dimer of 65 kD subunits and is synthesized during the G phase of the cell cycle. The enzyme is produced by trophoblasts and is responsible for the hyperphosphatemia observed during pregnancy. Biochemically, immunologically, and electrophoretically, PLAP can be separated into three distinct subtypes. The phase 1 isoenzyme corresponds to that produced by 6–8-week trophoblasts, the second is a mixture of the early phase and term placental isoenzymes, and phase 3 corresponds to the 13 weeks to term gestation AP isoenzymes. PLAP-like reactivity has been reported in the serum of about 5% of patients with tumors that included carcinoma of the lung, ovary, breast, colon, and endometrium, as well as malignant lymphoma and multiple myeloma. Raised levels of serum PLAP were found in 25% of patients with seminoma. Several isoenzymes of AP have been specifically named. The Regan isoenzyme was named after a patient with lung cancer whose serum had the phase 3-type isoenzyme. It was also found in 4–14%

of patients with a variety of neoplasms including testicular germ cell tumors and carcinomas of the breast, ovary, lung, stomach, and pancreas as well as in the serum of patients with ulcerative colitis, familial polyposis, and cirrhosis of the liver. The Nagao isoenzyme was named after a patient with pleural carcinomatosis and bears some similarities to the phase 3 PLAP. The Nagao AP has been found in the serum and tumor cells of patients with adenocarcinoma of the bile ducts and pancreas. The Kashahara variant was detected in tumor extracts of hepatocellular carcinoma and possesses some of the properties of the placental isoenzyme. Other non-Regan isoenzymes have been described in patients with gastrointestinal cancer, benign gynecological disease and female genital cancer, testicular teratomas, and lung tumors.

Applications

1. Antibodies to PLAP are primarily used as a diagnostic discriminator of germ cell tumors in the context of separation from somatic carcinomas and mediastinal tumors. Membrane-based PLAP has been documented immunohistochemically in seminoma, embryonal carcinoma, gonadoblastoma, endodermal sinus tumor, and choriocarcinoma and metastatic deposits of seminoma, making this marker an important one for the identification of germ cell tumors. Spermatocytic seminoma and immature teratomas were negative.
2. Epithelial neoplasms of the ovary and intratubular neoplastic germ cells also label for PLAP. It has been suggested that PLAP immunostaining may help separate partial and complete hydatidiform moles and choriocarcinoma. Partial moles show weak human chorionic gonadotrophin (hCG) and strong PLAP, complete moles show strong expression of hCG and weak PLAP, and choriocarcinomas display strong expression of hCG and weak PLAP and hPL (human placental lactogen).

Selected references

Koshida K, Uchibayashi T, Yamamoto H, et al. A potential use of a monoclonal antibody to placental alkaline phosphatase (PLAP) to detect lymph node metastases of seminoma. *J Urol* 1996;155:337–41.

Losch A, Kainz C. Immunohistochemistry in the diagnosis of the gestational trophoblastic disease. *Acta Obstet Gynecol Scand* 1996;75:753–6.

Manivel JC, Jessurun J, Wick MR, et al. Placental alkaline phosphatase immunoreactivity in testicular germ cell neoplasms. *Am J Surg Pathol* 1987;11:21–9.

Wick MR, Swanson PE, Manivel JC. Placental-like alkaline phosphatase reactivity in human tumors: An immunohistochemical study of 520 cases. *Hum Pathol* 1987;18:946–54.

PMS2

Background

There are four main mismatch repair genes (*MLH1*, *MSH2, MSH6, and PMS2*). The products of these genes are necessary to identify and correct errors that occur during DNA replication at microsatellite loci, small repetitive sequences scattered throughout the genome. These areas are prone to DNA slippage, resulting in insertion and deletion loops. The mismatch repair proteins form heterodimers, with the MSH2–MSH6 complex recognizing the impaired bases, while MLH1 and PMS2 excise the mismatched nucleotides. Germline mutations in these genes are associated with Lynch syndrome (hereditary nonpolyposis colorectal carcinoma [HNPCC]), an autosomal dominant disorder characterized by early onset colorectal cancer and increased risk of cancer of the endometrium, stomach, ovary, skin, and other sites.

PMS2 (postmeiotic segregation increased 2) comprises 15 exons encoding a protein of 862 amino acids and is located on chromosome 7p22. It was first identified due to its homology with the yeast mismatch repair gene mutL homologue yPMS1 and is associated with multiple pseudogenes. Its function as a mismatch repair gene in humans was confirmed when knockout mice lacking both PMS2 alleles were shown to have microsatellite instability (MSI) in both germline and tumor DNA. Genetic testing has confirmed the presence of heterozygous truncating mutations in cohorts of HNPCC families lacking mutations in MLH1, MSH2, and MSH6. Germline mutations in PMS2 are rare, and patients with these mutations tend to show decreased penetrance in comparison with patients with MLH1 and MSH2 mutations.

Applications

In practice, the PMS2 immunohistochemical stain is most commonly used in a panel with MLH1, MSH2, and MSH6 to screen tumors for MSI and Lynch syndrome. It is important to remember that PMS2 mutations are usually associated with a truncated protein product and loss of function, and therefore, one must assess for the absence of staining in tumor nuclei. As the proliferating epithelium of the gastrointestinal tract should show strong nuclear staining, most slides should have ample tissue as an internal positive control. Although the four-stain panel is most commonly used, studies have shown that a panel consisting of MSH6 and PMS2 is as sensitive as the four-stain panel with the added benefit of decreased cost.

Loss of PMS2 may be seen in three distinct scenarios. The first, and most common, is in the setting of sporadic cancers with hypermethylation of the MLH1 promoter region, causing loss of expression of both MLH1 and PMS2 by immunohistochemistry. Loss of both markers can also be seen in the setting of a germline mutation of MLH1, while germline mutations of PMS2 usually result in loss of expression of PMS2 only. This is most likely related to the biochemical properties of the MLH1 protein, which has the ability to form a heterodimer with PMS1 in the absence of PMS2 (and may also explain the decreased penetrance seen in patients with PMS2 mutations).

Immunohistochemistry to predict MSI is used outside colorectal carcinoma with increasing frequency. Studies have confirmed its accuracy in detecting MSI in endometrial carcinomas and it can also be used to screen for Lynch syndrome in patients with sebaceous neoplasms.

Pneumocystis carinii

Background

The DAKO antibody (IgM, Kappa) reacts with an 82 kD parasite-specific component of human *Pneumocystis carinii*. No cross-reactivity was found with a number of parasites and fungi.

Applications

The AIDS epidemic brought about an increased need for specific markers that recognize *Pneumocystis carinii*. While the sensitivity of the immunohistochemical method appears to be greater than that of the Giemsa stain, it is only slightly better than the GMS stain, warranting the use of immunostaining in sputum, where identification of the pathogen is more difficult than in bronchoalveolar lavage. The other advantage of immunostaining is that both cyst wall and trophozoites are stained, whereas the silver stain only labels the cyst wall. However, the former staining pattern may appear amorphous or focally granular, which may be confused with nonspecific staining of mucin or intracellular/free particulate material.

Selected references

Amin MB, Mezger E, Zarbo RJ. Detection of *Pneumocystis carinii*: Comparative study of monoclonal antibody and silver staining. *Am J Clin Pathol* 1992;98:13–18.

Pregnancy-specific β-1-glycoprotein (SP1)

Background

Pregnancy-specific β-1-glycoprotein (SP1), human chorionic gonadotrophin (hCG), and placental alkaline phosphatase (PLAP) are three major proteins produced by the trophoblasts of the human placenta. Immunohistochemical studies suggest that SP1 and hCG are also present in the human amnion. Recent molecular cloning studies indicate that the human SP1s form a group of closely related placental proteins that, together with the carcinoembryonic antigen family members, comprise a subfamily within the immunoglobulin superfamily. The main source of SP1 is the syncytiotrophoblast, but it has been demonstrated that amniotic as well as chorionic membranes express low levels of SP1 genes, although only certain subpopulations of SP1 transcripts were expressed, with differences in species expression between amnion, chorion, and trophoblasts. The function of the SP1s is largely unknown. Recent information suggests that the SP1 family induce secretion of anti-inflammatory cytokines in mononuclear phagocytes, and the tetraspanin CD9 has been identified as a receptor of murine SP1.

Applications

1. The immunohistochemical applications of SP1 have been mainly in the study of placental elements and their corresponding tumors. Differing levels of expression of hCG, human placental lactogen (hPL), and SP1 were observed in the feto-maternal tissues throughout pregnancy. The presence of SP1, vimentin, cytokeratin, and PLAP, particularly the first three antigens, has been used to identify intermediate trophoblasts in the placental site nodule.
2. SP1 is not specific to placental cells. It is expressed in a variety of nonplacental tumors.
3. SP1 has been employed in the panel for the distinction of mesothelioma from adenocarcinoma, being positive in almost 60% of adenocarcinomas. However, SP1 is also expressed in mesotheliomas, albeit in lower frequency (6%). In lung carcinomas, SP1 was immunostained in 90% of non-small cell carcinomas and in 50% of small cell carcinomas with a significant negative correlation of both SP1 and CEA immunoexpression with grade of differentiation of adenocarcinoma.

Selected references

Plouzek CA, Leslie KK, Stephens JK, et al. Differential gene expression in the amnion, chorion, and trophoblast of the human placenta. *Placenta* 1993;14:277–85.

Sabet LM, Daya D, Stead R, et al. Significance and value of immunohistochemical localization of pregnancy specific proteins in feto-maternal tissue throughout pregnancy. *Mod Pathol* 1989;2:227–32.

Waterhouse R, Ha C, Dvcksler GS. Murine CD9 is the receptor for pregnancy-specific glycoprotein 17. *J Exp Med* 2002;195:277–82.

Wright C, Angus B, Napier J, et al. Prognostic factors in breast cancer: Immunohistochemical staining for SP1 and NCRC 11 related to survival, tumour epidermal growth factor receptor and oestrogen receptor status. *J Pathol* 1987;153:325–31.

NOTES

412

Progesterone receptor (PR)

Background

In selected target tissues, estrogens have been found to stimulate not only mitogenesis but also the synthesis of specific proteins. One of these estrogen-induced proteins is the progesterone receptor (PR). Progesterone and synthetic progestins activate the receptor, provoke its phosphorylation and DNA-binding ability, and induce its regulatory activities. Since the PR is an estrogen-inducible protein, its expression is indicative of an intact estrogen receptor pathway and may identify tumors that are hormonally responsive to estrogen, thereby improving the overall predictive value of steroid receptor assays in selected tumors such as breast carcinoma.

The PR displays the typical three-domain structure of the steroid-thyroid receptor family. The central domain contains two "zinc finger" structures responsible for the specific recognition of the cognate DNA sequences. The carboxyl-terminal domain contains the hormone and anti-hormone binding sites. The complete organization of the human PR gene has been determined. It spans over 90 kb and contains eight exons. The first exon encodes the N-terminal part of the receptor, the DNA binding domain is encoded by two exons, each corresponding to one zinc finger, and the steroid binding domain is encoded by five exons.

The signal responsible for the nuclear localization of the PR is a complex one. The receptor continuously shuttles between the nucleus and the cytoplasm. The receptor diffuses into the cytoplasm and is constantly and actively transported back into the nucleus, similarly to the phenomenon for estradiol and glucocorticosteroid receptors. Immunolocalization of PR is confined to the nucleus.

Applications

1. The value of estrogen receptor (ER) and PR assays in predicting response to hormonal treatment in advanced breast cancer patients has been well supported by both studies employing cytosol-based ligand-binding methods

and immunohistochemical assays, the prognostic utility being strongest in premenopausal women. Approximately 50% of breast cancers are ER+PR+, 20% ER+PR−, 5% ER−PR+, and 25% ER−PR−.

Those women whose cancers express both ER and PR show the greatest likelihood of responding to endocrine treatment. Using conventional biochemical assays, the response rate is about 77% for ER+PR+, 46% for ER−PR+, 27% for ER+PR−, and 11% for ER−PR− tumors. However, it is clinically recognized that a small proportion of women with tumors that are receptor negative will show a positive response to hormonal therapy, and as many as one-third of those with receptor-positive tumors may fail to respond to such treatment. The significance of breast carcinomas biochemically negative for ER but positive for PR is poorly understood. It has been proposed that these tumors, more common in younger women, contain ER, whose presence is masked in a biochemical binding assay by endogenous estrogen. Such tumors should be positive for ER by immunocytochemical assay, but this was not proven in one study, which found that ER−PR+ tended to have larger tumor size and higher histologic grade and S-phase fractions compared with ER+PR+ tumors. It was concluded that biochemically, ER−PR+ breast carcinomas are biologically different from ER+PR+ tumors.

There has been some suggestion that PR may be a more important predictor, as there are more responders among patients with ER−PR4+ compared with ER+PR− tumors. In some series, although this remains to be proven, the prognostic advantage of steroid receptor positivity was lost after 4–5 years of follow-up. As with the ER, there is increasing evidence that immunohistological assays provide more accurate prognostication than cytosol-based methods.

Selected references

Keshgegian AA. Biochemically estrogen receptor-negative, progesterone receptor-positive breast carcinoma: Immunocytochemical hormone receptors and prognostic factors. *Arch Pathol Lab Med* 1994;118:240–4.

Leong AS-Y, Milios J. Comparison of antibodies to estrogen and progesterone receptors and the influence of microwave antigen retrieval. *Appl Immunohistochem* 1993;1:282–8.

MacGrogan G, Soubeyran I, De Mascarei I, et al. Immunohistochemical detection of progesterone receptors in breast invasive ductal carcinomas: A correlative study of 942 cases. *Appl Immunohistochem* 1996;4:219–27.

Programmed death-1

Background

Programmed death 1 (PD-1) (CD279) is an inhibitory cell receptor that belongs to the CD28/CTLA-4 family of receptors and binds two ligands: PD-L1 (also known as B7-H1 or CD274) and PD-L2 (also known as B7-DC or CD273). While PD-1 expression is induced on activated T cells, B cells, and myeloid cells, the function of PD-1 has been best characterized in T cells, where it inhibits T-cell receptor (TCR) signaling. Upon engagement with PD-L1 or PD-L2, PD-1 suppresses the activation and function of T cells through the recruitment of SHP-2, which dephosphorylates and inactivates ZAP-70, an important integrator of TCR-mediated signaling. Interfering with the PD-1/PD-L1 pathway during the early stage of immune activation can result in improved T-cell responses and has been used as a treatment modality in advanced cancer patients.

Applications

1. PD-1 is normally expressed by germinal center–associated helper T cells (follicular helper T cells), a CD4-positive T-cell subset that typically resides in the germinal center and helps coordinate immunologic reactions in this location. Activated T cells outside lymph node germinal centers and in other tissues can also transiently express PD-1, but sustained non-germinal center PD-1 expression is associated with T-cell dysfunction. In reactive nodal lymphoid proliferations, immunohistochemical staining for PD-1 will highlight a small subset of T cells within the germinal centers, as would be expected for germinal center helper T cells, and only occasional interfollicular T cells. In reactive lymphoid proliferations in the skin, a small subset of the T cells may also express weak PD-1. The pattern of staining seen with PD-1 is typically both surface and cytoplasmic immunoreactivity.
2. PD-1 immunohistochemical staining has clinical applications in the diagnostic workup of both Hodgkin and non-Hodgkin lymphomas. Nodular lymphocyte-predominant Hodgkin lymphoma (NLPHL) is clinically and immunophenotypically distinct from classical Hodgkin lymphoma and is characterized by scattered large neoplastic B cells (so-called "popcorn" or LP cells) surrounded by small lymphocytes. Classically, the neoplastic cells are ringed by small T cells, which exhibit the immunophenotype of follicular helper T cells. These T-cell rosettes are considered to be a diagnostic feature of NLPHL (when present) and express strong PD-1 as well as CD57. PD-1+ T-cell rosettes are not entirely specific for NLPHL, as the Reed–Sternberg cells in classical Hodgkin lymphoma can reportedly also be surrounded by varying numbers of PD-1+ T cells.
3. Angioimmunoblastic T-cell lymphoma (AITL) is a peripheral T-cell lymphoma characterized by numerous high endothelial venules, expanded follicular dendritic cell meshworks, and a proliferation of neoplastic small–intermediate-sized T lymphocytes with clear/pale cytoplasm and distinct cell membranes. The neoplastic T cells are derived from follicular helper T cells and consequently express CD10, bcl-6, CXCL13, and PD-1. Uniform and/or strong expression of PD-1 is unusual in other T-cell lymphoproliferative disorders but has been reported in a subset of peripheral T-cell lymphoma, not otherwise specified (PTCL-NOS) that lacks the characteristic clinical and histologic features of AITL. PD-1 expression has also been reported in a small subset of ALK+ and ALK-negative anaplastic large cell lymphomas. Similarly, some authors have suggested a provisional category of "primary cutaneous follicular helper T-cell lymphoma" for cases with cutaneous involvement by a T-cell population with a TFH phenotype (including expression of PD-1), in which the patients lack significant adenopathy at the onset of disease or the clinical signs/symptoms suggestive of AITL. However, PD-1 expression is most commonly seen in AITL, is expressed by few B cells (unlike CD10 and bcl-6), and is a useful diagnostic feature.

4. Primary cutaneous CD4+ small/medium-sized pleomorphic T-cell lymphoma is a provisional diagnostic entity in the most recent 2008 World Health Organization classification. The atypical CD4+ T cells in this disorder characteristically express PD-1, bcl-6, and CXCL13, without CD10, and PD-1 usually highlights the greatest proportion of the cells of interest. Other primary cutaneous T-cell lymphoproliferative disorders/T-cell lymphomas are largely negative for PD-1. A small subset of mycosis fungoides cases is reportedly positive for PD-1; however, no significant PD-1 expression has been reported in cutaneous anaplastic large cell lymphoma, lymphomatoid papulosis, or aggressive CD8+ epidermotropic cytotoxic cutaneous T-cell lymphoma.

5. PD-1 immunoreactivity can be seen in chronic lymphocytic leukemia/small lymphocytic lymphoma (CLL/SLL); however, this immunophenotypic finding is not reliable enough for primary histopathologic diagnosis of CLL/SLL. PD-1 expression is generally not preset on neoplastic cells in other B-cell non-Hodgkin lymphomas. Similarly, the neoplastic B cells in cutaneous B-cell lymphomas rarely express PD-1. Of note, increased numbers of PD-1+ "tumor infiltrating" T cells have been described in primary cutaneous follicle center lymphomas, in follicular lymphoma, and in classical Hodgkin lymphoma, with varying prognostic implications.

6. PD-1 expression has also been investigated in several reactive lymphadenopathies. In HIV-associated lymphadenopathy, the number of PD-1+ cells within germinal centers is reportedly low with increased marginalization of the PD1+ cells beneath the mantle zones. Increased numbers of PD-1+ T cells are also seen within the paracortex of lymph nodes in patients with Castleman's disease.

Selected references

Carreras J, Lopez-Guillermo A, Roncador G, et al. High numbers of tumor-infiltrating programmed cell death 1-positive regulatory lymphocytes are associated with improved overall survival in follicular lymphoma. *J Clin Oncol* 2009; 27(9):1470–6.

Cetinozman F, Koens L, Jansen PM, et al. Programmed death-1 expression I cutaneous B cell lymphoma. *J Cutan Pathol* 2014; 41:14–21.

Dorfman DM, Brown JA, Shahsafaei A, et al. Programmed Death-1 (PD-1) is a marker of germinal center-associated T cells and angioimmunoblastic T cell lymphoma. *Am J Surg Pathol* 2006; 30(7):802–10.

Muenst S, Dirnhofer S, Tzankov A. Distribution of PD-1+ lymphocytes in reactive lymphadenopathies. *Pathobiology* 2010;77:24–27.

Muenst S, Hoeller S, Willi N, et al. Diagnostic and prognostic utility of PD-1 in B cell lymphomas. *Dis Markers* 2010; 29: 47–53.

Nam-Cha SH, Roncador G, Sanchez-Verde L, et al. PD-1, a follicular T-cell marker useful for recognizing nodular lymphocyte-predominant Hodgkin lymphoma. *Am J Surg Pathol* 2008;32(8):1252–7.

Proliferating cell nuclear antigen (PCNA)

Background

PCNA, formerly called cyclin (now recognized to be a much wider class of proteins associated with cell proliferation), represents a component of DNA polymerase-δ and is a 36 kD intranuclear proliferation-associated antigen. An antibody to this antigen was first described in the blood of selected patients with systemic lupus erythematosus. This polypeptide has since been found in both normal and transformed cells and is tightly associated with the sites of DNA replication. Its expression is highest during S-phase of the cell cycle, and there is generally a good correlation between expression of PCNA and the S-phase fraction determined by flow cytometry in a given tumor cell population. However, certain caveats apply to the use of anti-PCNA antibodies as a marker of cell proliferation. In malignant cell lines such as HeLa, PCNA levels increase during S-phase but are not zero during the other phases of the cell cycle. Indeed, in this cell line the levels of PCNA increase only by a factor of 2–3 during S-phase. There are also at least two forms of PCNA, one associated with the "replicon" structure and the other more loosely associated in the cell nucleus. Both proteins are retained by formalin fixation but only the former is retained by alcoholic fixatives such as methacarn. Furthermore, the antigen persists in cells that are no longer in the cycling phase and are in G_0. Generally, PCNA counts obtained with clone PC 10 have been higher that those obtained with Ki-67 or S-phase fraction measured by flow cytometry, despite PCNA being considered to be primarily an S-phase-associated protein. PCNA has a relatively long half-life of 20 hours and may be immunohistochemically detected in cells that have recently left the cell cycle and may be in G_0. Discrepancies have also been demonstrated between PCNA counts obtained with PC 10 and those of the S-phase fraction by thymidine and bromodeoxyuridine uptake in a variety of tumors and in the experimental situation. The PCNA index was found to be two to three times higher than values obtained with DNA polymerase-alpha. There is ample evidence that the antigen is very fixation dependent, and different antibody clones show vastly different sensitivities for the antigen.

Applications

PCNA immunostaining offers an alternative to the well-established but cumbersome methods of assessing tumor growth fractions, namely, tritiated thymidine or bromodeoxyuridine incorporation or flow cytometry, and has been enthusiastically employed in numerous publications, despite the limitations discussed earlier.

Selected references

Bravo R, Macdonald-Bravo H. Existence of two populations of cyclin/proliferating cell nuclear antigen during the cell cycle: Association with DNA replication sites. *J Cell Biol* 1987;105:1549–54.

Burford-Mason AP, MacKay AJ, Cummins M, et al. Detection of proliferating cell nuclear antigen in paraffin-embedded specimens is dependent on preembedding tissue handling and fixation. *Arch Pathol Lab Med* 1994;118:1007–13.

Prostate-specific antigen (PSA)

Background

Prostate-specific antigen (PSA) is a chymotrypsin-like, 33 kD single-chain glycoprotein with selective serine protease activity for cleaving specific peptides. The PSA gene is a member of the human kallikrein gene family and is located on the 13q region of chromosome 19. PSA is selectively produced by the epithelial cells of the acini and ducts of the prostatic gland and is secreted into the semen, where it is directly involved in the liquefaction of the seminal coagulum that is formed at ejaculation. The sequence of PSA shows extensive homology with γ-nerve growth factor (56%), epidermal growth factor-binding protein (53%), and OC-nerve growth factor (51%). This feature, together with its ability to digest insulin growth factor-binding protein-III (IGFBP-3) to release biologically active IGF-I, makes PSA a candidate growth factor or cytokine or modulator of cell growth. It has also recently been suggested that PSA is capable of being produced by cells bearing steroid hormone receptors under conditions of steroid hormone stimulation.

Applications

PSA is a useful biochemical marker, as any disruption of the normal architecture of the prostate allows diffusion of PSA into the stoma, where it gains access to the peripheral blood through the microvasculature. Elevated serum PSA levels are thus seen with prostatitis, infarcts, benign hyperplasia, and transiently after manipulation and biopsy. Most importantly, significant elevations are seen with prostatic adenocarcinoma, making it an important tool for diagnosis as well as monitoring response to treatment. Although cancers produce less PSA per cell than normal prostatic epithelium, the greater number of malignant cells and the disruption of stroma in the malignant gland account for the elevated serum PSA levels.

Immunostaining for PSA has proven to be an effective method of identifying cells of prostatic origin; however, the presence of PSA cannot be used to differentiate between benign and malignant. Antibodies to PSA show high sensitivity, although very occasional carcinomas have been reported to be negative for PSA. Correlations of PSA tissue reactivity with Gleason's grade of prostatic cancer have shown that high-grade tumors may be entirely negative by immunolabeling. There was an initial suggestion that the presence of PSA-negative cells in a prostatic carcinoma correlates with a more aggressive clinical course, but this has not been confirmed, and most tumors display very heterogeneous staining.

Selected references

Bostwick DG. Prostate-specific antigen: Current role in diagnostic pathology of prostatic cancer. *Am J Clin Pathol* 1994;102 (Suppl 1):S31–S37.

Prostatic acid phosphatase (PAP)

Background

Acid phosphatases hydrolyze phosphoric acid esters at acid pH. They are found in a variety of tissues, and differences in electrophoretic patterns or sensitivity to isoenzyme inhibitors allowed the distinction of isoforms of the enzyme to specific tissues. Normal prostatic tissue contains several isoforms but only two are secreted in the seminal fluid. Acid phosphatase activity is mainly localized to the lysosomes of prostatic epithelial cells and, ultrastructurally, is identified within microvilli of the apical cell membranes and in the secretory granules at the supranuclear or apical regions of benign cells. Although synthesized in rough endoplasmic reticulum, PAP is not demonstrable in this site, and because it is only recognized in lysosomes, it is assumed that antibodies recognize PAP only when packaged into granules. Basal cells are negative for PAP. Serum levels of the enzyme reflect the amount of enzyme released into the circulation and are dependent on the tumor mass and also the rate of synthesis and access to the intravascular space. Low levels of the enzyme have been suggested to represent low rates of synthesis by poorly differentiated tumors.

Applications

PAP immunostaining is a useful discriminator for prostatic tissue and its diagnostic specificity and sensitivity are increased when used in a panel in conjunction with prostate-specific antigen (PSA) and CD57 (Leu 7). Like PSA, immunoreactivity for PAP is more intense and homogeneous in benign prostatic tissue than in prostatic carcinoma. PAP is localized within prostatic acini and ducts, although the latter tend to show weaker and more heterogeneous staining.

Rare cases of squamous metaplasia of the prostatic epithelium show staining for PAP. There is weak positivity in seminal vesicle epithelium, and as with PSA, periurethral glands in both men and women are positive for the enzyme. Other nonprostatic tissues that may show PAP immunostaining are anal glands in men, neuroendocrine cells of the rectum, transitional epithelium and von Brun's nests of the bladder, renal tubular epithelium, pancreatic islet cells, hepatocytes, gastric parietal cells, and mammary ductal epithelium. Neutrophils show the strongest concentration of PAP among nonprostatic tissues. Neoplasms that show cross-reactivity are mainly those derived from the cloaca, such as urinary bladder, periurethral glands, and colon and neuroendocrine tumors.

Comments

In general, PAP is relatively specific for prostatic neoplasms. However, because of the cross-reactivity of both PAP and PSA with the tissues listed earlier, it is still best to use PAP in conjunction with PSA, particularly in the context of a tumor in the perineum whose differential diagnosis includes prostatic carcinoma, transitional carcinoma and adenocarcinoma of the bladder, and rectal carcinoma.

Selected references

Epstein JI. PSA and PAP as immunohistochemical markers in prostatic cancer. *Urol Clin North Am* 1993;20:757–70.

pS2

Background

pS2 is a 6660 Dalton, 60–amino acid secretory polypeptide protein that was isolated from the breast carcinoma cell line MCF-7. It belongs to a recently described family of trefoil-shaped growth factors, which includes human intestinal trefoil factor (hITF) and human spasmolytic polypeptide (hSP). Although its exact function is unknown, it is believed to be part of a steroid-dependent stimulatory pathway. An estrogen-regulated protein, it has been studied as a marker of an intact estrogen pathway and hence marker hormone sensitivity and favorable prognosis in breast carcinoma. There is growing evidence that members of the trefoil peptide family are involved in active maintenance of the integrity of gastrointestinal mucosa and facilitating its repair.

Applications

1. pS2 positivity is preferentially expressed in hormone-dependent cells in breast cancer. Low concentrations of the protein have been associated with a poor prognosis, while strong expression predicted responsiveness to endocrine treatment. The 5-year recurrence-free survival and overall survival were 85% and 95%, respectively, for estrogen receptor (ER)+/progesterone receptor (PR)+/pS2+ tumors, but only 50% and 54% for patients with ER+/PR+/pS– tumors.

2. pS2 is widely distributed throughout the gastrointestinal tract, particularly adjacent to damaged mucosa. It is consistently expressed in superficial and foveolar epithelium of nonneoplastic gastric mucosa and in 66% of gastric carcinomas but has little value as a prognostic indicator. Colorectal carcinoma stains with pS2 to a lesser extent, but this too lacks statistical significance.

Expression in normal pancreas is usually absent; however, it can be seen focally within occasional ducts in chronic pancreatitis and it is prominent in pancreatic adenocarcinoma and ampullary tumors.

Selected references

May FE, Westley BR. Trefoil proteins: Their role in normal and malignant cells. *J Pathol* 1997;183:4–7.

Poulsom R. Trefoil peptides. *Baillière's Clin Gastroenterol* 1996;10:113–34.

Wysocki SJ, Iacopetta BJ, Ingram DM. Prognostic significance of pS2 mRNA in breast cancer. *Eur J Cancer* 1994;30A:1882–4.

PTEN (phosphatase and tensin homolog deleted on chromosome 10)

Background

Phosphatase and tensin homolog deleted on chromosome 10 (PTEN) is a human protein encoded by the *PTEN* gene.

PTEN is a dual protein/lipid phosphatase and its main substrate, phosphatidylinositol-3,4,5-trisphosphate (PIP3), is the product of PI3 K. Increase in PIP3 recruits Akt to the membrane, where it is activated by other kinases. PTEN contains a tensin-like domain as well as a catalytic domain similar to that of the dual-specificity protein tyrosine phosphatases. *PTEN* is a tumor suppressor gene that is mutated in a large number of cancers and some syndromes (notably Cowden syndrome and Bannayan–Riley–Ruvalcaba syndrome). Unlike most of the protein tyrosine phosphatases, this protein preferentially dephosphorylates phosphoinositide substrates. It negatively regulates intracellular levels of PIP3 in cells and functions as a tumor suppressor by negatively regulating the Akt/PKB signaling pathway. *PTEN* gene mutations have been reported in many types of cancer, and PTEN functional loss has been implicated in pathogenesis of such tumors, particularly endometrial carcinoma. Somatic mutations of PTEN have been described in 34–55% of endometrial cancers, particularly endometrioid type, and many of these are seen in precursor lesions (EIN/ atypical hyperplasia). PTEN immunochemical (IHC) loss in endometrial carcinoma detects not only cases with genetic PTEN loss but also cases with functional PTEN loss, so that there is overall no good correlation between PTEN IHC loss and PTEN mutation. It has also been demonstrated recently that PTEN immunohistochemistry result interpretation is reproducible and can be reported as "positive," "negative," or "heterogeneous" staining.

Reduced expression of PTEN has been reported in a variety of malignancies, including breast, prostate, and endometrial carcinomas. In some cancers, loss of PTEN expression has been shown to correlate with poor prognosis. It has been suggested that PTEN may be a marker of response to progesterone treatment in endometrial hyperplasia and carcinoma.

Applications

1. PTEN IHC loss has been shown in 65% of all endometrial carcinomas, more frequently in endometrioid (75%) than nonendometrioid (45%) type. So, potentially, PTEN can be utilized along with a panel of other IHC markers in the distinction of Grade 3 endometrioid adenocarcinoma from serous carcinomas (which typically show retained expression of PTEN).

   PTEN IHC can help highlight endometrial intraepithelial neoplasia (EIN)/atypical hyperplasia, with PTEN loss described in 63% of EIN cases. However, its use is somewhat limited in that PTEN IHC loss can be seen in normal proliferative and anovulatory endometrium.

2. PTEN IHC can potentially help select patients for targeted therapy in trials involving PI3 K, AKT, and MTOR inhibitors in patients with endometrial carcinoma.

Selected references

Djordjevic B, Hennessy BT, Li J, et al. Clinical assessment of PTEN loss in endometrial carcinoma: Immunohistochemistry outperforms gene sequencing. *Mod Pathol* 2012;25:699–708.

Foo WC, Rashid A, Wang H, et al. Loss of phosphatase and tensin homolog expression is associated with recurrence and poor prognosis in patients with pancreatic ductal adenocarcinoma. *Hum Pathol* 2013; 44: 1024–30.

Govender D, Chetty R. Gene of the month: PTEN. *J Clin Pathol* 2012;65:601–3.

McMenamin ME, Soung P, Perera S, et al. Loss of PTEN expression in paraffin-embedded primary prostate cancer correlates with high Gleason score and advanced stage. *Cancer Res* 1999;59:4291–6.

Perren A, Weng LP, Boag AH, et al. Immunohistochemical evidence of loss of PTEN expression in primary ductal adenocarcinomas of the breast. *Am J Pathol* 1999; 155: 1253–60.

Rabies

Background

Rabies is a rod- or bullet-shaped virus with a single-stranded RNA genome and belongs to the family Rhabdoviridae. It is a highly fatal disease of humans and warm-blooded vertebrates and is usually transmitted via infected saliva following the bite of a diseased animal, most commonly a dog. Virus introduced into the bite wound enters the peripheral nerves and, following an incubation of weeks to months, spreads to the spinal cord and brain. It produces a neurological derangement lasting a few days to weeks and resulting in death.

Antibody C4–62–15–2 to rabies virus is specific to the N-nucleoprotein. It enjoys a wide range of species reactivity and includes mouse, raccoon, skunk, dog/coyote, and bats.

Applications

Antibody to rabies is useful in locating the Negri bodies in sections of brain. During prolonged incubation periods, the sensory neurons of the dorsal root ganglia may be the site of viral sequestration. Efferent spread of virus in the nervous system may extend terminally to the eye and nerve fibers surrounding hair follicles. Hence, demonstration of antigen in corneal impression smears or skin biopsies may be used for confirmation of diagnosis in a live patient. Unless the diagnosis is confirmed during life, an autopsy must be performed with $10-20^3$ mm blocks of cerebrum, cerebellum, hippocampus, medulla, thalamus, and brain stem being taken in duplicate: 50% glycerol-saline for virological examination and 10% buffered formalin for immunohistological examination.

Selected references

Feiden W, Feiden U, Gerhard L, et al. Rabies encephalitis: Immunohistochemical investigations. *Clin Neuropathol* 1985;4:156–64.

Jogai S, Radotra BD, Banerjee AK. Immunohistochemical study of human rabies. *Neuropathology* 2000;20:197–203.

Retinoblastoma gene protein (P110^{Rb}, Rb protein)

Background

The *Rb* gene is located on chromosome 13q14 and spans a region of more than 200 kb, including 27 exons. The Rb gene is the only tumor suppressor that has been shown to directly suppress tumor formation. It is a cell cycle regulator preventing cells from entering the S-phase. The Rb protein has a molecular mass of 105 kD, and a number of antibodies that recognize specific parts of this protein have been developed. Besides loss of function due to chromosomal abnormalities, including chromosomal deletion, translocation, and point mutation, as with p53, phosphorylation may inactivate the Rb protein. In addition, a variety of viral oncoproteins, including simian virus 40 T antigen, El A from adenovirus, and E6 from human papilloma virus, may bind and inactivate the Rb protein.

Immunostaining may be a valid way to assess the presence of normal Rb protein, but several factors affecting staining should be considered before accepting the relevance of the technique. Firstly, it has been observed that the level of expression of Rb protein is not the same in all cells in any individual tissue, e.g., in the epithelium of the cervix, there are low or undetectable levels of staining in the basal layers, and staining increases with cell maturation. In contrast, low or absent anti-Rb protein staining was observed in the well-differentiated epithelial cells of the gastric mucosa, such as the foveolar and mucus cells, compared with the cells in the crypts and neck of the glands. Astrocytes and microglia do not show detectable Rb protein by immunostaining, and other subsets of normal cells, such as some stromal cells, do not display demonstrable Rb protein. The reasons for failure to demonstrate the protein at an equivalent level in all cells may relate to variations in expression as a function of cell cycling activity, cell differentiation, and protein phosphorylation. More importantly, there is a large subset of cells, including endothelial cells, lymphocytes, and stromal cells, in which the ability to demonstrate p11O^{RB} expression is critically dependent on the method of staining used.

Applications

1. Alterations in the *RB* gene have been described in a number of human tumors, including retinoblastoma, osteosarcoma, other sarcomas, leukemias, lymphomas, and certain carcinomas, including those from the breast, prostate, lung, bladder, kidney, and testis. There was loss of immunostaining for Rb protein in ovarian carcinomas compared with benign and borderline tumors and this loss correlated with a higher proliferative index and loss of heterozygosity at the Rb-1 locus. In clear cell renal carcinoma, increased Rb protein and decreased p27 immunoexpression are claimed to be powerful and independent poor prognostic factors.
2. Rb protein loss is seen in spindle cell lipoma, mammary-type myofibroblastoma, and cellular angiofibroma.

Selected references

Cordon-Cardo C, Richon VM. Expression of the retinoblastoma protein is regulated in normal human tissues. Am J Pathol 1994;144:500–10.

S100

Background

S100 protein, so named because of its solubility in a saturated ammonium sulfate solution, occurs as three biochemically distinct forms. Each is a protein dimer of two subunits, designated A and B. The three dimers are $S100A_0$ (A–A), S100A (A–B), and S100B (B–B). The A- and B-subunits each have a molecular weight of approximately 10.5 kDa with extensive amino acid sequence homology between the two subunits. They both have amino acid sequences known to code for the calcium binding sites of the calmodulin family of proteins. S100 is highly acidic and water soluble with varying affinities for calcium, zinc, and manganese. These properties are related to many basic cell functions such as calcium regulation and microtubule assembly. S100 protein is conserved in nature and is present within the cells of all three germ layers in humans, a reflection of its important role in basic cell function. Laboratories use antibodies that recognize all three isotypes and hence, historically, S100 antigen was used as a useful marker of melanocytic lesions, peripheral nerve sheath tumors, and Langerhans cell histiocytosis.

Applications

1. Melanocytic lesions: One of the most useful applications of the S100 protein is its use as a marker of nevus cells and melanomas. Virtually all benign melanocytic lesions contain S100 protein, which is also observed in over 95% of malignant melanomas. But given its relative lack of specificity, other more specific melanoma markers are commonly used in lieu of S100 in establishing the diagnosis of melanoma in a metastatic setting or as part of an immunohistochemistry panel in separating Paget's disease from melanoma. Desmoplastic melanomas are typically positive for S100 and less so for other newer and more specific melanocytic markers, and S100 remains useful in this setting.
2. Normal cartilage and neoplastic cartilaginous (benign and malignant) tumors express S100 protein, which is useful in confirming chondroid differentiation. Chordomas also express S100 but differ from cartilaginous tumors by the presence of cytokeratin, epithelial membrane antigen (EMA), and brachyury in the former and their absence in the latter.
3. S100 is also useful for the labeling of myoepithelial cells in mammary ducts, particularly when distinguishing sclerosing adenosis from tubular carcinomas or for evaluating microinvasion associated with ductal carcinoma in situ. However, more specific myoepithelial markers are preferentially utilized in routine practice, such as p63, smooth muscle myosin, and CK5/6.
4. S100 labels sustentacular cells in paraganglioma, pheochromocytoma, and olfactory neuroblastoma. But the S100 staining can be occasionally absent and incompletely present when the sustentacular cell layer is attenuated.
5. Nerve sheath tumors: S100 is expressed diffusely in schwannomas, and neurofibromas show variable degrees of positivity. Perineuriomas are typically negative for S100. Malignant peripheral nerve sheath tumors (MPNST) usually show patchy and variable positivity for S100 and usually in 50% or fewer tumor cells. The one exception is epithelioid MPNST, which typically is S100 positive.
6. Other soft tissue tumors: Granular cell tumors and myoepitheliomas show S100 positivity consistently. Lipomatous tumors also commonly show S100 positivity, including lipoblasts that can mark with S100.
7. Histiocytes also label with S100 antibody. The interdigitating reticulum cells of the paracortical areas in the lymph node stain with S100 protein antibodies, as do dendritic reticulum cells of the lymphoid follicles. Langerhans cells in skin, mucous membranes, and other sites are also positive for S100. S100 protein is therefore a useful marker for the identification of Langerhans cell histiocytosis, Rosai Dorfman disease, and interdigitating reticulum cell sarcoma. Histiocytic sarcomas do not show strong diffuse positivity and often only in a small number of tumor cells.

8. Tumors of salivary glands also express S100 protein, and the ones that show S100 expression consistently are pleomorphic adenoma, adenoid cystic carcinoma, myoepithelial carcinoma, and mammary analogue secretory carcinoma.

9. Newer entities: S100 expression is reported in newly described entities including biphenotypic sinonasal sarcoma, gastrointestinal neuroectodermal tumor (clear cell sarcoma-like tumor of gastrointestinal tract), and spindle cell tumors coexpressing S100 and CD34 with NTRK1 gene rearrangements.

Selected references

Anstey A, Cerio R, Ramnarain N, et al. Desmoplastic malignant melanoma: An immunocytochemical study of 25 cases. *Am J Dermatopathol* 1994;16(1):14–22.

Daimaru Y, Hashimoto H, Enjoji M. Malignant peripheral nerve sheath tumours (malignant schwannomas):. An immunohistochemical study of 29 cases. *Am J Surg Pathol* 1985;9:434–44.

Loeffel SC, Gillespie GY, Mirmiran SA, et al. Cellular immunolocalisation of S100 protein within fixed tissue sections by monoclonal antibodies. *Arch Pathol Lab Med* 1985;109:117–22.

Suurmeijer AJH, Dickson BC, Swanson D, et al. A novel group of spindle cell tumors defined by S100 and CD34 co-expression shows recurrent fusions involving RAF1, BRAF, and NTRK1/2 genes. *Genes Chromosomes Cancer* 2018;57(12):611–21.

SALL4

Background

SALL4 is a zinc finger transcription factor that shares homology to the Drosophila *spalt*-gene: **spa**l**t**-**l**ike-**4** (*SALL*) gene. The *SALL4* gene is located on chromosome 20q13.13-13.2 and is essential for embryological development. It forms a regulatory circuit with OCT4.

Applications

1. Immunohistochemical staining for SALL4 can be detected in all types of testicular germ cell tumors (GCT), in contrast to OCT4, which only labels intratubular germ cell neoplasia (ITGCN), classic seminoma, and embryonal cell carcinoma (EC). SALL4 is a very sensitive marker for most primary GCT and metastatic tumors including seminomas, EC, and yolk sac tumors (YST) with 100% sensitivity.

   The demonstration of SALL4 in teratomas (intestinal epithelium in mature teratomas also reveals uniform positivity for SALL4) and YST in neonates and infants, classic seminoma and nonseminomatous GCT in post-pubertal patients, and spermatocytic seminoma suggests that SALL4 is a common pathogenetic factor.

2. SALL4 is a helpful stain in the workup of metastatic GCT, especially when limited biopsy material is available and the differential diagnosis includes non-GCT.

   SALL4 is positive in more than 90% of the GCTs and forms an important part of a limited panel along with OCT4 and EMA (epithelial membrane antigen) and/or CK7 (cytokeratin 7). A positive SALL4 rules out non-GCTs (with some exceptions; see later). A positive SALL4 with a negative OCT4 and positive glypican-3 is consistent with YST.

3. While SALL4 is highly expressed in all GCTs, it can be expressed in a variety of poorly differentiated carcinomas as well: 30% of ovarian serous carcinomas; 25% of gastric adenocarcinomas (hepatoid, intestinal-like, or fetal differentiation); 20% of high-grade urothelial carcinomas; cholangiocarcinoma; and pulmonary small cell carcinomas.

SALL4 immunoexpression can also be seen in renal rhabdoid tumors, Wilms tumors, rare cases of desmoplastic small round cell tumors, embryonal rhabdomyosarcomas of uterine cervix, epithelioid sarcomas, lymphoblastic lymphomas, anaplastic large cell lymphomas, and myeloid leukemias.

Selected references

Cao D, Li J, Guo CC, et al. SALL4 is a novel diagnostic marker for testicular germ cell tumors. *Am J Surg Pathol* 2009;33:1065–77.

Cao D, Guo S, Allan RW, et al. SALL4 is a novel sensitive and specific marker of ovarian primitive germ cell tumors and is particularly useful in distinguishing yolk sac tumor from clear cell carcinoma. *Am J Surg Pathol* 2009;33:894–904.

Cao D, Humphrey PA, Allan RW. SALL4 is a novel sensitive and specific marker for metastatic germ cell tumors, with particular utility in detection of metastatic yolk sac tumors. *Cancer* 2009;115:2640–51.

Liu A, Cheng L, Du J, et al. Diagnostic utility of novel stem cell markers SALL4, OCT4, NANOG, SOX2, UTF1, and TCL1 in primary mediastinal germ cell tumors. *Am J Surg Pathol* 2010;34:697–706.

Miettinen M, Wang Z, McCue PA, et al. SALL4 expression in germ cell and non-germ cell tumors: A systematic immunohistochemical study of 3215 cases. *Am J Surg Pathol* 2014;38:410–20.

Ushiku T, Shinozaki A, Shibahara J, et al. SALL4 represents fetal gut differentiation of gastric cancer, and is diagnostically useful in distinguishing hepatoid gastric carcinoma from hepatocellular carcinoma. *Am J Surg Pathol* 2010;34:533–40.

Wang F, Liu A, Peng Y, et al. Diagnostic utility of SALL4 in extragonadal yolk sac tumors: An immunohistochemical study of 59 cases with comparison to placental-like alkaline phosphatase, alpha-fetoprotein, and glypican-3. *Am J Surg Pathol* 2009;33:1529–39.

SATB2

Background

Special AT-rich sequence Binding protein 2 (SATB2) was initially thought to be a novel marker of osteoblastic differentiation. The *SATB2* gene is located on 2q33.1 and its protein attaches to regions of DNA called matrix attachment regions (MARs). In this way chromatin structure is modeled and enables the regulation of gene expression during development. The special AT-rich sequence binding protein (SATB2) is a 733–amino acid–long DNA-binding protein, which preferentially binds to nuclear MARs of DNA. SATB2 is involved in regulation of transcription and chromatin remodeling. It plays a critical role in the transcriptional network regulating craniofacial development and differentiation of cortical neurons. Hence, defects in this gene are associated with isolated cleft palate and mental retardation. The SATB2 protein also plays a role in carcinogenesis; it is selectively expressed in colorectal and esophageal cancers and benign and malignant mesenchymal tumors.

SATB2 protein coordinates the activity of multiple genes, including promoting the maturation of osteoblasts and neurons.

Mutations in the *SATB2* gene cause the *SATB2*-associated syndrome, which is characterized by intellectual disability, cleft palate, dental abnormalities and craniofacial anomalies, and speech problems.

Applications

1. The protein has been used as both a diagnostic and a prognostic marker for colorectal cancer. The main application is in the identification of colorectal cancer (even if poorly differentiated) in a metastatic setting, for example, in the liver. When it is used alone as a marker of colorectal cancer, various studies have reported a positivity rate of 85–90%. In combination with CK20 and CK7, SATB2 is a powerful and specific marker for colorectal

origin of an adenocarcinoma. Gastric, pancreatic, lung, and gynecological adenocarcinomas have low rates of positivity for SATB2. The protein appears to be highly selective and specific for lower gastrointestinal epithelium, including the appendix. It should be noted that some small intestinal adenocarcinomas also stain. Prognosis is better if SATB2 is expressed.

2. In addition to staining colorectal cancers, SATB2 expression has been noted in renal cell cancer (poor prognosis if not expressed).

3. Merkel cell carcinoma, 90% of well-differentiated neuroendocrine tumors of the rectosigmoid, and 80% of appendiceal neuroendocrine tumors.

4. Well-differentiated osteosarcoma, osteoblastic benign bone tumors, and liposarcoma. SATB2 has been noted to stain phosphaturic mesenchymal tumors consistently.

5. SATB2 has also been shown to stain the nuclei of squamous morules associated with endometrioid lesions. It also labels the stromal cells within atypical polypoid adenomyoma while the stroma of other endometrial polypoid lesions (endometrial polyp, adenomyoma, and adenosarcoma) lacks staining.

6. Head and neck squamous cell carcinomas (SCC): SATB2 expression in SCC may confer resistance to chemotherapy while loss of expression in laryngeal SCC is associated with a poorer prognosis (recurrence and high-grade tumors).

Interpretation of staining

SATB2 is a nuclear stain. Staining is intense irrespective of differentiation and site of origin of the colorectal cancer.

Selected references

Agaimy A, Michal M, Chiosea S, et al. Phosphaturic mesenchymal tumors: Clinicopathologic, immunohistochemical and molecular analysis of 22 cases expanding their morphologic and immunophenotypic spectrum. *Am J Surg Pathol* 2017;41:1371–80.

Bellizzi AM. SATB2 in neuroendocrine tumours: Strong expression is restricted to well differentiated tumours of the lower gastrointestinal tract and is most frequent in Merkel cell carcinoma among poorly differentiated carcinomas. *Histopathology* 2020;76:251–64.

Conner JR, Hornick JL. SATB2 is a novel marker of osteoblastic differentiation in bone and soft tissue tumours. *Histopathology* 2013;63:36–49.

Dragomir A, de Wit M, Johansson C, et al. The role of SATB2 as a diagnostic marker for tumors of colorectal origin: Results of a pathology-based clinical prospective study. *Am J Clin Pathol* 2014:141:630–8.

Geng G-J, Li N, Mi Y-J, et al. Prognostic value of SATB2 expression in patients with esophageal squamous cell carcinoma. *Int J Clin Exp Pathol* 2015;8:423–31.

Magnusson K, de Wit M, Brennan DJ, et al. SATB2 in combination with cytokeratin 20 identifies over 95% of all colorectal cancers. *Am J Surg Pathol* 2011;35:937–48.

McCluggage WG, Van der Vijer K. SATB2 is consistently expressed in squamous morules associated with endometrioid proliferative lesions and in the stroma of atypical polypoid adenomyoma. *Int J Gynecol Pathol* 2019;38:397–403.

Serotonin

Background

Serotonin (5-hydroxytryptamine) is a neurotransmitter substance, which is found in a broad range of normal, hyperplastic, and neoplastic tissues, including the gastrointestinal tract, central nervous system, adrenergic nerve fibers, platelets, and basophils. The major use of this marker has been to identify serotonin-secreting carcinoid tumors, which mostly arise from the midgut.

Applications

1. Immunostaining for serotonin has been employed as a marker of neuroendocrine differentiation. However, like other specific neuropeptides such as bombesin, adrenocorticotropic hormone (ACTH), calcitonin, and vasoactive intestinal peptide (VIP), it is of low sensitivity and specificity and should only be employed in a panel of several antibodies with more specific markers such as chromogranin and synaptophysin. The major application of serotonin lies in the detection of carcinoid tumors, particularly as such tumors may respond to specific therapy with the somatostatin analogue octreotide and alpha interferons. Serotonin may also be detected in scattered cells within other neuroendocrine tumors from a variety of sites.

2. Interestingly, using serotonin staining as a marker of neuroendocrine differentiation, it was shown that androgen ablation promotes neuroendocrine cell differentiation in human and dog prostates. Replacement androgens and estrogens after castration restored this cell population to normal values and induced luminal differentiation and basal metaplasia, respectively.

Selected references

Burke AP, Thomas RM, Elsayed AM, et al. Carcinoids of the jejunum and ileum: An immunohistochemical and clinicopathologic study of 167 cases. *Cancer* 1997;79:1086–93.

SF-1

Background

Steroidogenic factor 1 (adrenal 4-binding protein) regulates genes involved in development of gonads/adrenal gland and steroidogenesis, among others. SF-1 is a nuclear transcription factor and a specific marker of ovarian sex cord–stromal tumors (SCSTs) that is seen in all categories, including granulosa cell tumor (adult and juvenile), Sertoli–Leydig cell tumor, steroid cell tumor, fibroma, and fibrothecoma. SF-1 positivity has also allowed confirmation of tumors to be added to the sex cord–stromal tumor family, including uterine tumor resembling ovarian sex cord tumor (UTROSCT), microcystic stromal tumor, and luteinized thecoma (thecomatosis), and this has been used to favor classification of certain tumors, such as female adnexal tumor of probable Wolffian origin (FATWO) (being SF-1 negative), as not being SCST.

Applications

1. SF-1 can be utilized in confirming the diagnosis of SCST of the ovary. Mimics of SCST can pose diagnostic challenges. Examples include:
   a. There can be morphologic overlap between granulosa cell tumor and germ cell tumors like yolk sac tumors. Yolk sac tumors are negative for SF-1.
   b. Endometrioid tumors and carcinoid tumors of the ovary that can morphologically mimic Sertoli cell tumor are SF-1 negative.
   c. Fibromas and fibrothecomas can often be negative for calretinin and inhibin; SF-1 can be useful in this role.
2. Stains luteinizing hormone (LH) and follicle stimulating hormone (FSH)-producing cells in the pituitary.
3. Stains cells of the adrenal cortex.

NOTES

Simian virus 40 (SV40 T antigen)

Background

SV40 T antigen (Ab-3) is a mouse monoclonal antibody with specificity for antigenic determinants unique to the SV40 small T antigen and nonreactive with SV40 large T antigen. Both antigens are encoded by the early region of the SV40 genome.

Simian virus 40 (SV40) large T antigen is an 81 kD multifunctional viral phosphoprotein. Some of its functions are essential to the viral replication in monkey cells. Others contribute to its neoplastic transforming activity.

The large T antigen binds DNA and complexes with p53 protein. It also forms a specific complex with the PI05 product of the retinoblastoma susceptibility gene.

Applications

The use of this antibody has been confined to the research laboratory to define the cellular location of small t antigen in subcellular extracts of SV40-infected cells. Pab280 reacted strongly with a cytoplasmic form of small t antigen that appears to be associated with the cytoskeleton. Small t was found to accumulate late in the SV40 lytic cycle and was localized in both the cytoplasm and the nucleus of cells infected with wild-type SV40.

The demonstration that 60% of human mesotheliomas contain and express SV40 sequences stimulated a great deal of interest. It has also been shown that SV40 large T antigen interferes with the normal expression of the tumor suppressor gene p53 in human mesotheliomas, raising the possibility that SV40 may contribute to the development of human mesotheliomas. The cell cycle inhibitor p21[WAFI], a downstream target of p53, was recently evaluated immunohistochemically and found to show a significant positive correlation with survival, further supporting the role of SV40 in the pathogenesis of mesothelioma. One study has failed to demonstrate SV40 immunocytochemically in mesothelioma effusions and cell block preparations. SV40 has been demonstrated in fixed tissue with the novel application of a DNA thermal cycler for antigen retrieval.

The antigen is nuclear in location.

Selected references

Baldi A, Groeger AM, Esposito V, et al. Expression of p21 in SV40 large T antigen positive human pleural mesothelioma: Relationship with survival. *Thorax* 2002;57:353–6.

Carbone M, Rizzo P, Grimley PM, et al. Simian virus-40 large-T antigen binds p53 in human mesotheliomas. *Nat Med* 1997;3:908–12.

SMARCA4/BRG-1

Background

SMARCA4 is a member of the SWI/SNF (switch/sucrose non-fermentable) chromatin-remodeling gene complex. It is a gene on chromosome 19p, encoding for BRG-1 protein. Mutations in SMARCA4 have been associated with a variety of carcinomas and rhabdoid tumors, and with a high frequency in small cell carcinoma of ovary, hypercalcemic type (SCCOHT). Both somatic and germline mutations are described in tumors with SMARCA4 loss, such as SCCOHT, and in tumors of various sites with an undifferentiated or rhabdoid morphology. This includes soft tissue tumors such as epithelioid sarcoma (with intact SMARCB1) and carcinomas from sinonasal tract, endometrium, and gastrointestinal tract.

Mutations (usually inactivating) in SMARCA4 lead to loss of BRG-1 immunohistochemical (IHC) protein expression.

Applications

1. SMARCA4 IHC loss is sensitive and specific to support the diagnosis of SCCOHT (94% of cases are "positive," showing loss by immunohistochemistry). Other ovarian tumors, including epithelial tumors, and sex cord–stromal tumors (usually differential diagnostic considerations of SCCOHT) express SMARCA4. Pitfalls include that in the presence of an in-frame deletion (which can be seen in rare cases of SCCOHT), there can be retained expression of SMARCA4. Additionally, rare cases of clear cell carcinoma and melanoma of ovary can show loss of SMARCA4 (3% of cases of each).
2. SMARCA4 is useful in the workup of tumors with a rhabdoid morphology in various sites, including:
   a. Lung/ thorax:
      i. Thoracic sarcoma: Such tumors usually have a poorly differentiated epithelioid/rhabdoid morphology and consistently show loss of SMARCA4, and this is useful in excluding other differential diagnoses such as melanoma, germ cell tumor, and poorly differentiated carcinomas.
      ii. Rarely (2%), non-small-cell carcinomas of lung also show loss of SMARCA4, and the histology is such cases usually is that of a recognizable adenocarcinoma.
   b. Gynecologic tract:
      i. Undifferentiated endometrial carcinoma: 50% of these tumors show loss of SWI/SNF proteins, including about 30% showing loss of SMARCA4.
      ii. In dedifferentiated carcinomas, when there is loss of SMARCA4, those cases usually show loss of PAX-8 and estrogen receptor (ER).
      iii. SMARCA4-deficient uterine sarcoma has been described, in which SMARCA4 loss distinguishes it from other uterine sarcomas. However, since undifferentiated carcinomas can share SMARCA4 loss, other epithelial markers such as Claudin-4 and mismatch repair (MMR) IHC markers can be useful in this differential diagnosis, with MMR loss and claudin-4 expression favoring the diagnosis of undifferentiated carcinoma.
   c. Other sites:
      i. SMARCA4-deficient carcinomas with an undifferentiated/rhabdoid phenotype have been described in gastrointestinal tract, sinonasal, and renal cell carcinomas.
3. Other sarcomas: Sarcomas with round cell morphology can be in the differential diagnostic considerations of SCCOHT, such as Ewing sarcoma, undifferentiated "Ewing-like" sarcoma, desmoplastic small round cell tumors, and endometrial stromal sarcomas. Unlike SCCOHT, all such sarcomas express SMARCA4.

Comments

Rare SCCOHT can show retained SMARCA4 expression and in such cases are usually deferred to molecular testing. While the majority of SCCOHT show the classic morphology with small cells, a large cell component or, rarely, tumors comprised entirely of large cells (so-called "large cell variant of SCCOHT") can pose a diagnostic challenge. Other IHC markers in SCCOHT are relatively nonspecific with positivity described for cytokeratin, epithelial membrane antigen (EMA), WT1, and CD10. Neuroendocrine markers can be expressed in some cases.

There can be variable staining for SMARCA4 and hence, caution must be exercised in small samples when evaluating areas devoid of SMARCA4 staining. [3]

Selected references

Agaimy A, Bertz S, Cheng L, et al. Loss of expression of the SWI/SNF complex is a frequent event in undifferentiated/dedifferentiated urothelial carcinoma of the urinary tract. *Virchows Arch* 2016;469(3):321–30.

Conlon N, Silva A, Guerra E, et al. Loss of SMARCA4 expression is both sensitive and specific for the diagnosis of small cell carcinoma of ovary, hypercalcemic type. *Am J Surg Pathol* 2016;40(3):395–403.

Karanian-Philippe M, Velasco V, Longy M, et al. SMARCA4 (BRG1) loss of expression is a useful marker for the diagnosis of ovarian small cell carcinoma of the hypercalcemic type (ovarian rhabdoid tumor): A comprehensive analysis of 116 rare gynecologic tumors, 9 soft tissue tumors, and 9 melanomas. *Am J Surg Pathol* 2015;39(9):1197–205.

Kolin DL, Quick CM, Dong F, et al. SMARCA4-deficient uterine sarcoma and undifferentiated endometrial carcinoma are distinct clinicopathologic entities. *Am J Surg Pathol* 2020;44(2):263–70.

Perret R, Chalabreysse L, Watson S, et al. SMARCA4-deficient thoracic sarcomas: Clinicopathologic study of 30 cases with an emphasis on their nosology and differential diagnoses. *Am J Surg Pathol* 2018;43(4):1.

SMARCB1

Background

SWI/SNF-related, matrix associated, actin-dependent regular of chromatin, subfamily B, member 1 (SMARCB1) is the protein product of the gene *SMARCB1* (also known as *BAF47*, *INI1*, and *SNF5*) located on chromosome 22q11.2. SMARCB1 has functional roles in ATP-dependent chromatin remodeling, cell cycle control, and regulation of the cytoskeleton. SMARCB1 is widely expressed in cell lines and tissues. The *SMARCB1* gene is mutated in varying types of tumors, consistently with a tumor suppressor role for SMARCB1. Loss of SMARCB1 expression correlates with point mutations in the *SMARCB1* gene in malignant rhabdoid tumors and with larger chromosomal deletions in epithelioid sarcoma. Of note, germline mutations in the *SMARCB1* gene have been identified in a subset of the patients with these tumors. In addition, homozygous deficiency for SMARCB1 is lethal in mice with early embryonic death, while SMARCB1 heterozygous mice display a variety of tumors in the soft tissues of the head and neck. SMARCB1 also binds the HIV-1 integrase and stimulates integrase-mediated DNA joining activity. Thus, SMARCB1 is a component of SWI/SNF complexes that may be critical for normal development and tumor suppression, and may also have a role in viral DNA integration into host DNA. The loss of SMARCB1 protein expression in tumor cell nuclei correlates with biallelic deletion or mutations in the *SMARCB1* gene. The absence of nuclear SMARCB1 reactivity is useful diagnostically in a few contexts.

Applications

1. Loss of SMARCB1 expression is present in 98% of malignant rhabdoid tumors and 90% of epithelioid sarcomas, whether conventional or proximal type, and in 50% of epithelioid malignant peripheral nerve sheath tumors. Smaller proportions of other tumors demonstrate SMARCB1 loss of expression including in 40% of pediatric and 10% of adult myoepithelial carcinomas, 15% of extraskeletal myxoid chondrosarcomas, poorly differentiated chordoma, undifferentiated hepatoblastoma, and renal medullary carcinoma.
2. Germline mutations in *SMARCB1* occur in approximately 60% of patients with the rare hereditary syndrome of familial schwannomatosis, associated with a "mosaic" pattern of protein loss by immunochemistry.

Selected references

Biegel JA. Molecular genetics of atypical teratoid/rhabdoid tumor. *Neurosurg Focus* 2006;20:E11.

Bourdeaut F, Lequin D, Brugières L, et al. Frequent hSNF5/INI1 germline mutations in patients with rhabdoid tumor. *Clin Cancer Res* 2011;17:31–8.

Calderaro J, Moroch J, Pierron G, et al. SMARCB1/INI1 inactivation in renal medullary carcinoma. *Histopathology* 2012;61:428–35.

Hollmann TJ, Hornick JL. INI1-deficient tumors: Diagnostic features and molecular genetics. *Am J Surg Pathol* 2011;35:e47–63.

Hornick JL, Dal Cin P, Fletcher CD. Loss of INI1 expression is characteristic of both conventional and proximal-type epithelioid sarcoma. *Am J Surg Pathol* 2009;33:542–50.

Sullivan LM, Folpe AL, Pawel BR, et al. *Mod Pathol* 2013;26:385–92. Epithelioid sarcoma is associated with a high percentage of SMARCB1 deletions.

Smooth muscle actin (SMA)

Background

Cytoplasmic actins vary in amino acid sequences and can be separated by electrophoresis into six different isotopes, all having the same molecular weight of 42 kDa. Alpha-actins are found in muscle cells, while beta- and gamma-actins may be present in muscle cells as well as most other cell types in the body, including nonmuscle cells. Striated and smooth muscle fibers differ in their expression of actin isotypes, and this has formed the basis for the generation of antibodies directed at muscle-specific actin subtypes. HHF35 (muscle-specific actin) identifies all four actin isoforms present in smooth muscle as well as skeletal muscle cells, pericytes, myoepithelial cells, and myofibroblasts. In contrast, antibodies to α-SMA specifically identify the single α-isoform characteristic of smooth muscle cells and those cells with myofibroblastic differentiation.

Applications

Antibodies to α-SMA are used in several diagnostic situations:

1. Identification of myoepithelial cells admixed with epithelial cells in benign proliferative lesions of the breast, salivary, and sweat glands. Myoepithelial cells line benign ductules of the breast, while they are absent in malignant ductal proliferation. So, SMA can be useful in distinguishing benign breast proliferations (such as adenosis) from invasive carcinoma and in evaluating foci of early invasion associated with ductal carcinoma in situ.
2. α-SMA can be used as part of a panel of other markers in confirming the diagnosis of myoepithelioma of various sites such as soft tissue, salivary glands, and skin.
3. α-SMA is also a useful marker to confirm or support myofibroblastic differentiation and is positive in a variety of lesions including nodular fasciitis, inflammatory myofibroblastic tumor, nodal myofibroblastoma, and myofibroblastic sarcoma. However, this rather wide

spectrum of SMA expression limits its utility also. For example, fibromatosis also shows SMA expression, but it is considered nonspecific and is not utilized in supporting the diagnosis.
4. α-SMA is expressed in benign and malignant smooth muscle tumors. However, other markers like desmin and caldesmon are more specific in supporting the diagnosis of a tumor with smooth muscle differentiation.
5. In organ specific spindle cell proliferations, SMA also shows wide expression, and this limits its role in diagnostic pathology. Examples include spindle cell tumors of the female genital tract (the vast majority express SMA) and spindle cell tumors of the breast and the head and neck (where diverse lesions such as sinonasal hemangiopericytoma and nodular fasciitis express SMA).

Comments

Since α-SMA also stains myofibroblasts, in the scenario of problematic breast lesions (separating adenosis from invasive carcinoma), its use has been superseded by other myoepithelial markers such as p63, calponin, CK5, and smooth muscle myosin. Myofibroblastic proliferations may display a characteristic "tram-track" pattern of distribution of muscle actins distributed in a subplasmalemmal location.

While SMA is widely expressed in mesenchymal tumors, some soft tissue tumors that are SMA negative include nuchal fibroma, cellular angiofibroma, and rhabdomyosarcoma.

SMA expression can be seen commonly in other diverse entities such as glomangiopericytoma, biphenotypic sinonasal sarcoma, and fibromatosis. It can also, less commonly, be seen expressed in tumors without smooth muscle differentiation, such as solitary fibrous tumors, gastrointestinal stromal tumor, and even other nonmesenchymal tumors, rarely including melanoma, mesothelioma, and some metastatic carcinomas.

Selected references

Banerjee SS, Harris M. Morphological and immunophenotypic variations in malignant melanoma. *Histopathology* 2000;36:387–402.

Kinner B, Spector M. Smooth muscle actin expression by human articular chondrocytes and their contraction of a collagen–glycosaminoglycan matrix in vitro. *J Orthop Res* 2001;19:233–41.

Kung IT, Thallas V, Spencer EJ, et al. Expression of muscle actins in diffuse mesothelioma. *Hum Pathol* 1995;26:565–70.

Kutzner H, Mentzel T, Kaddu S, et al. Cutaneous myoepithelioma: An under-recognised cutaneous neoplasm composed of myoepithelial cells. *Am J Surg Pathol* 2001;25:348–55.

Leong AS-Y, Milios J, Leong FJ. Patterns of basal lamina immunostaining in soft-tissue and bony tumors. *Appl Immunohistochem* 1997;5:1–7.

Ohta K, Mortenson RL, Clark RA, et al. Immunohistochemical identification and characterization of smooth muscle-like cells in idiopathic pulmonary fibrosis. *Am J Resp Crit Care Med* 1995;152:1659–65.

Raymond WA, Leong AS-Y. Assessment of invasion in breast lesions using antibodies to basement membrane component and myoepithelial cells. *Pathology* 1991;23:291–7.

Santini D, Ceccarelli C, Leone O, et al. Smooth muscle differentiation in normal human ovaries, ovarian stromal hyperplasia and ovarian granulosa-stromal cell tumors. *Mod Pathol* 1995;8:25–30.

Smooth muscle myosin heavy chain

Background

Smooth muscle myosin heavy chain (SMM-HC) is a cytoplasmic structural protein/component of smooth muscle cells. SMM-HC expression is developmentally regulated and appears early in smooth muscle development. Although specific for smooth muscle development, it is not a contractile regulatory protein. SMM-HC exists in two isoforms, MHC-1 (205 kDa) and MHC-2 (200 kDa), and is composed of dimerized heavy chains, which then bind with two pairs of myosin light chains to form myosin polypeptide. SMM-HC is encoded by a single gene through alternative splicing of mRNA. Both isoforms are specific for smooth muscle cells and are considered markers of "terminal" smooth muscle differentiation. In normal breast tissue, SMM-HC highlights vascular smooth muscle and myoepithelial cells in lobules, ducts, and lactiferous ducts. Similarly, periacinar and periductal myoepithelial cells of salivary gland are also immunopositive with SMM-HC, whereas all the acinar/ductal epithelial cells are negative.

Applications

Anti-SMM-HC immunochemistry (IHC) can be used in a panel including other myoepithelial markers in order to demonstrate myoepithelial cells in breast lesions. Some scenarios include radial scar versus tubular carcinoma cancerization of adenosis by ductal carcinoma in situ (DCIS) mimicking microinvasive carcinoma, invasive cribriform carcinoma mimicking noninvasive lesions, papillary carcinoma, nipple adenoma, and syringomatous nipple adenoma versus infiltrating duct carcinoma.

Comments

Anti-SMM-HC has proved to be superior to muscle actin for the demonstration of myoepithelial cells in breast tissue, as the latter also stains the vast number of myofibroblasts in the stroma.

SMM-HC expression has been described in follicular dendritic cells although in routine practice, the gold standard continues to be CD21.

Selected references

Borrione AC, Zanellato AM, Scannapieco G, et al. Myosin heavy-chain isoforms in adult and developing rabbit vascular smooth muscle. *Eur J Biochem* 1989;183:413–17.

Eddinger TJ, Murphy RA. Developmental changes in actin and myosin heavy chain isoform expression in smooth muscle. *Arch Biochem Biophys* 1991;284:232–7.

Ioannidis I, Laurini JA. Use of smooth muscle myosin heavy chain as an effective marker of follicular dendritic cells. *Appl Immunohistochem Mol Morphol* 2019;27(1):48–53.

Savera AT, Gown AM, Zarbo RJ. Immunolocalization of three novel smooth muscle-specific proteins in salivary gland pleomorphic adenoma: Assessment of the morphogenetic role of myoepithelium. *Mod Pathol* 1997;10:1093–100.

Wang NP, Wan BC, Skelly M, et al. Antibodies to novel myoepithelium-associated proteins distinguish benign lesions and carcinoma in situ from invasive carcinoma of the breast. *Appl Immunohistochem* 1997; 5:141–51.

White S, Martin AG, Periasamy M. Identification of a novel smooth muscle myosin heavy chain cDNA: Isoform diversity in the SI head region. *Am J Physiol* 1993;264:1252–8.

Yaziji H, Gown AM, Sneige N. Detection of stromal invasion in breast cancer: The myoepithelial markers. *Adv Anat Pathol* 2000;7:100–9.

SOX9

Background

SOX9 (sex determining region Y-box 9) is a transcription factor associated with the testis-determining factor sex determining region Y (SRY). It is expressed predominantly in adult tissues as well as fetal testis and skeletal tissue. There are two functional domains: a high-mobility group (HMG) DNA-binding domain and a C-terminal transactivation domain. SOX9 plays a major role in cartilage differentiation (chondrogenesis) and early testis development. Mutation of the *SOX9* gene in humans causes campomelic dysplasia, a severe dwarfism syndrome, and autosomal XY sex reversal. Sox9 is thought to be a master regulator of the differentiation of mesenchymal cells into chondrocytes.

Applications

It is a nuclear marker for cartilaginous tumors and has been used to separate mesenchymal chrondrosarcoma from other small round blue cell tumors.

Selected references

Wehrli BM, Huang W, De Crombrugghe B, et al. Sox9, a master regulator of chondrogenesis, distinguishes mesenchymal chondrosarcoma from other small blue round cell tumors. *Hum Pathol* 2003;34:3263–9.

SOX10

Background

The *SOX10* gene encodes a member of the SOX (SRY-related HMG-box) family of transcription factors involved in the regulation of embryonic development and in the determination of cell fate. Mutations are associated with Waardenburg–Shah syndrome, Kallman syndrome, and Hirschsprung disease. The encoded protein acts as a transcriptional activator after forming a protein complex with other proteins. The SOX10 protein serves as a nucleocytoplasmic shuttle protein and is important for neural crest and peripheral nervous system development. SOX10 is therefore a neural crest transcription factor crucial for maturation and maintenance of Schwann cells and melanocytes. Antibodies against SOX10 have been applied to a variety of neural crest–derived tumors and mesenchymal and epithelial neoplasms.

Applications

1. Melanocytic tumors: SOX10 is a very sensitive and specific marker for the diagnosis of malignant melanoma, with more than 90% of melanomas (conventional, spindle cell, desmoplastic, and metastatic) showing SOX10 expression. Variants that can be difficult to diagnose, such as desmoplastic and spindle cell melanomas, are also positive for SOX10 in 97–100% of cases. So, along with S100, SOX10 forms a very useful panel in confirming melanocytic differentiation, and this is one of its most widely employed utilities. However, there are cases (5%) of metastatic melanoma that can be negative for SOX10 and other melanocytic markers. Since SOX10 is expressed in benign nevi, it cannot be used in separating them from melanoma. SOX10 expression is similar to S100, but SOX10 is a more sensitive and specific marker of melanocytic and schwannian tumors than S100 protein.
2. Nerve sheath tumors: SOX10 is useful in supporting the diagnosis of schwannoma and neurofibroma. SOX10 is expressed in the majority (close to 100%) of benign nerve sheath tumors, including neurofibroma and schwannoma. Perineurioma and neurothekeomas are SOX10 negative, and this can be useful in differential diagnosis with nerve sheath myxoma (which expresses SOX10). Malignant peripheral nerve sheath tumors show variable degrees of positivity in up to 30% of cases.
3. Other soft tissue tumors: SOX10 expression is seen in myoepithelioma and granular cell tumor. Additionally, SOX10 is positive in most cases of clear cell sarcoma of soft parts. SOX10 is not usually seen in other mesenchymal tumors and is rarely described in alveolar rhabdomyosarcoma and ossifying fibromyxoid tumor.
4. Salivary gland tumors: SOX10 is seen commonly in both benign (pleomorphic adenoma) and several malignant tumors (adenoid cystic, acinic cell, and myoepithelial carcinoma), which somewhat limits its utility in working up salivary gland tumors (negative for salivary duct carcinoma, lymphoepithelial carcinoma, hyalinizing clear cell carcinoma, and oncocytoma).
5. SOX10 expression can be seen in dermal tumors such as cylindroma and eccrine syringoma, and in 12% of mammary ductal carcinomas.
6. Gastrointestinal tract: SOX10 is a helpful marker to help separate gastrointestinal stromal tumor (GIST) from nerve sheath tumors. Other spindle cell mesenchymal tumors are SOX10 negative.
7. SOX10 positivity is seen in sustentacular cells of paraganglioma and olfactory neuroblastoma.
8. While SOX-10 expression is unusual and rare in carcinomas, 66% of triple-negative mammary carcinomas have been reported positive, which can be a pitfall in separation from malignant melanoma.
9. In cerebello-pontine angle tumors, schwannoma and meningiomas are often differential diagnostic considerations. SOX10 is typically seen in schwannomas and not in meningiomas, although occasional meningiomas (fibrous meningiomas) can express

SOX10 but usually in a weak and focal way, unlike the strong diffuse expression in schwannoma. While SOX10 expression can be seen in gliomas (astrocytoma and oligodendroglioma), given other specific glial markers, it is not typically used in workup of gliomas.

Selected references

Behrens EL, Boothe W, D'Silva N, et al. SOX-10 staining in dermal scars. *J Cutan Pathol* 2019;46(8):579–85.

Cimino-Mathews A, Subhawong AP, Elwood H, et al. Neural crest transcription factor Sox10 is preferentially expressed in triple-negative and metaplastic breast carcinomas. *Hum Pathol* 2013;44(6):959–65.

Miettinen M, McCue PA, Sarlomo-Rikala M, et al. Sox10–a marker for not only schwannian and melanocytic neoplasms but also myoepithelial cell tumors of soft tissue: A systematic analysis of 5134 tumors. *Am J Surg Pathol* 2015;39(6):826–35.

Mohamed A, Gonzalez RS, Lawson D, et al. SOX10 expression in malignant melanoma, carcinoma, and normal tissues. *Appl Immunohistochem Mol Morphol* 2013;21(6):506–10.

Ohtomo R, Mori T, Shibata S, et al. SOX10 is a novel marker of acinus and intercalated duct differentiation in salivary gland tumors: A clue to the histogenesis for tumor diagnosis. *Mod Pathol* 2013;26(8):1041–50.

Rooper LM, Huang SC, Antonescu CR, et al. Biphenotypic sinonasal sarcoma: An expanded immunoprofile including consistent nuclear beta-catenin positivity and absence of SOX10 expression. *Hum Pathol* 2016;55:44–50.

Spectrin/Fodrin

Background

Spectrin is a flexible rod-shaped molecule of 200 nm length found in mammalian and avian erythrocytes. It is composed of two nonidentical subunits, a and p, and linked to the plasma membrane by the protein ankyrin. Along with actin, ankyrin, and band 4.1, spectrin forms a network or membrane skeleton that lies immediately beneath the plasma membrane. The main function of the spectrin cytoskeleton is that of structural support for the bi-lipid layer of the cell membrane, and the spectrin-based membrane skeleton also controls lateral mobility of the erythrocyte membrane proteins. Thermal denaturation of spectrin leads to disintegration of the erythrocytes into vesicles, and deficiencies or structural abnormalities of the membrane skeleton proteins lead to loss of shape or tensile strength of the erythrocytes, resulting in fragmentation and destruction as they pass through the spleen. Defects of spectrin are associated with fragile erythrocytes in hemolytic anemias such as hereditary elliptocytosis, pyropoikilocytosis, and spherocytosis.

Nonerythroid cells also show a membrane skeleton that contains spectrin, although the molecular organization in such cells is less known. Nonerythroid spectrin is known as fodrin, has a molecular weight of 240 kD, exhibits many similarities to spectrin, including immunochemical cross-reactivity, and is found in virtually all nonerythroid cells.

Applications

1. The interest in fodrin lies in its role in cell adhesion during embryogenesis and in neoplasms. In comparison to their nonneoplastic counterparts, neoplastic epithelial cells show elevated levels of fodrin immunostaining regardless of tumor type. There was strong, fragmented, and circumferential staining for fodrin, which often became accentuated with increasing grades of anaplasia, and loss of membrane staining corresponded with loss of tumor cell cohesiveness.
2. There was also accumulation of cytoplasmic fodrin in the invasive cells of squamous cell carcinoma and melanoma.

Selected references

Bennett V. The spectrin-actin junction of erythrocyte membrane skeletons. *Biochem Biophys Acta* 1989;988:107–22.

STAT6

Background

STAT6, which belongs to the STAT (signal transducers and activators of transcription) family of transcriptional factors, modulates signaling that is important for normal cellular processes, including immune function and cell differentiation/ proliferation. The *NAB2-STAT6* fusion gene on chromosome 12q13 has been described as a transcriptional activator, and this rearrangement has been identified in solitary fibrous tumors (SFT). The resultant protein STAT6 is seen by immunochemical (IHC) nuclear expression as a reliable surrogate of this fusion and is a consistent finding in SFT. This finding has also been described in other similar tumors, including meningeal hemangiopericytoma, which is now considered to be a variant of SFT.

Applications

1. STAT6 IHC expression is seen in the majority (86–98%) of SFT from all locations, including in atypical and malignant variants. STAT6 expression usually is diffuse and moderate to strong in SFT and is currently perhaps the single most useful marker in establishing the diagnosis in the appropriate morphology. There seems to be an association between fusion types and morphology, with *NAB2ex4-STAT6ex2/3* associated with classic SFT (usually in pleura of older patients) and the less common *NAB2ex6-STAT6ex16/17* in younger patients (deep soft tissue location and aggressive clinical behavior).
2. STAT6 expression can be seen in some cases of well-differentiated and dedifferentiated liposarcoma (7–15%, usually nuclear and cytoplasmic), and this pitfall has to be a consideration in evaluating tumors in the deep soft tissues or retroperitoneum with an SFT-like growth pattern. However, unlike in SFT, the staining pattern in dedifferentiated liposarcoma usually is variable, and cases that showed distinct/strong nuclear positivity also showed cytoplasmic positivity.
3. STAT6 expression has rarely been described in desmoid tumors, ovarian fibroma, low-grade fibromyxoid sarcoma, myxoid liposarcoma, deep benign fibrous histiocytoma, and unclassified sarcomas and is usually weak and/or focal rather than the strong, diffuse pattern seen in SFT.
4. STAT6 expression is not seen in meningiomas and helps to identify and separate meningeal hemangiopericytoma (which is considered to be an SFT variant).
5. Other tumors with a hemangiopericytoma-like morphology that can be differential diagnostic considerations of SFT, such as glomangiopericytoma (sinonasal hemangiopericytoma), synovial sarcoma, spindle cell lipoma, and malignant peripheral nerve sheath tumor, are negative for STAT6.
6. In addition, STAT6 may be useful in hematopathology. Within Hodgkin disease (HD) nuclear expression of STAT6 is restricted to R-S cells classical HD.

Interpretation

STAT6 is a nuclear stain.

Selected references

Demicco EG, Harms PW, Patel RM, et al. Extensive survey of STAT6 expression in a large series of mesenchymal tumors. *Am J Clin Pathol* 2015;143(5):672–82.

Doyle LA, Tao D, Marino-Enriquez A. STAT6 is amplified in a subset of dedifferentiated liposarcoma. *Mod Pathol* 2014;27(9):1231–7.

Doyle LA, Vivero M, Fletcher CD, et al. Nuclear expression of STAT6 distinguishes solitary fibrous tumor from histologic mimics. *Mod Pathol* 2014;27(3):390–5.

Yoshida A, Tsuta K, Ohno M, et al. STAT6 immunohistochemistry is helpful in the diagnosis of solitary fibrous tumors. *Am J Surg Pathol* 2014;38(4):552–9.

Surfactant apoprotein-A

Background

Pulmonary surfactant apoproteins together with phospholipids play an essential role in maintaining the surface tension of intra-alveolar fluid and preventing the alveoli from collapsing at the end of expiration. Surfactant has been localized in two functionally distinct structures within alveolar type II pneumocytes, i.e., the lamellar bodies and lysosomes, the former probably involved in surfactant secretion and the latter in degradation. Surfactant has also been demonstrated within tracheobronchial epithelial cells by immunostaining.

Applications

1. Except for type II pneumocytes and pulmonary macrophages, and the walls and perivascular connective tissues of small to medium-sized blood vessels of the lung, normal cells or tissues are generally not labeled. In particular, it does not react with type I pneumocytes and mesothelial cells and has been shown to be negative in mesotheliomas, so that it is a useful marker to distinguish pulmonary adenocarcinomas from mesotheliomas.

   Surfactant immunoexpression does not appear to distinguish between type II pneumocyte and Clara cell type adenocarcinomas, perhaps because of a common precursor.
2. The protein has been demonstrated in sclerosing hemangioma of the lung.

Selected references

Braidotti P, Cigala C, Graziani D, et al. Surfactant protein A expression in human normal and neoplastic breast epithelium. *Am J Clin Pathol* 2001;116:721–8.

Yousem SA, Wick MR, Singh G, et al. So-called sclerosing hemangioma of lung: An immunohistochemical study supporting a respiratory epithelial origin. *Am J Surg Pathol* 1988;12:582–90.

Synaptophysin

Background

Synaptophysin is an integral-membrane glycoprotein (38 kD) of presynaptic vesicles. The protein is a component of the classical, locally recycled small synaptic vesicle present in almost all neurons.

Synaptophysin is localized to "empty" vesicles and is both chemically and topographically different from chromogranin (68 kD), a membrane protein of the dense-core neuroendocrine granules.

Antibody (SY38) to synaptophysin has been raised against presynaptic vesicles from bovine brain. Hence, the antibody shows reactivity with neuronal presynaptic vesicles of brain, spinal cord, retina, neuromuscular junctions, and small vesicles of adrenal medulla and pancreatic islets of human, bovine, rat, and mouse origin. In normal tissues, neuroendocrine cells of the human adrenal medulla, carotid body, skin, pituitary, thyroid, lung, pancreas, and gastrointestinal mucosa are labeled with this antibody.

Applications

1. Antibody to synaptophysin allows specific staining of neuronal, adrenal, and neuroepithelial tumors: these include pheochromocytoma, paraganglioma, pancreatic islet cell tumors, medullary thyroid carcinoma, pulmonary/gastrointestinal/mediastinal carcinoid tumors, and pituitary/parathyroid adenomas.
2. Other neural tumors like neuroblastomas, ganglioneuroblastomas, ganglioneuromas, central neurocytoma, and ganglioglioma also demonstrate immunoreactivity with this antibody.

Comments

Synaptophysin is a specific and fairly sensitive marker for neural/neuroendocrine tumors of low and high grades of malignancy.

Selected references

Chejfec G, Falkmer S, Grimelius L, et al. Synaptophysin: A new marker for pancreatic neuroendocrine tumors. *Am J Surg Pathol* 1987;11:241–7.

Gould VE, Lee I, Wiedenmann B, et al. Synaptophysin: A novel marker for neurons, certain neuroendocrine cells, and their neoplasms. *Hum Pathol* 1986;17:979–83.

TAG 72 (B72.3)

Background

Clone B72.3 represents the monoclonal antibody to tumor-associated glycoprotein (TAG-72) (Isotype: IgT1). The immunogen is a membrane-enriched fraction of a breast carcinoma derived from liver metastases. This antibody recognizes a tumor-associated oncofetal antigen (TAG-72) expressed by a wide variety of human adenocarcinomas. It reacts with a sialyl-Tn epitope (72 kD) expressed on mucins. TAG-72 expression in fetal tissue is only observed in tissues of the gastrointestinal tract, including the colon, esophagus, and stomach. Although weak reaction with some tissues of adults has been observed, no reactivity is seen with tissue from organ systems including lymphoreticular, cardiovascular, hepatic, pulmonary, neural, muscular, skin, endocrine, and genitourinary tract.

Applications

1. Immunoreactivity of TAG-72 has been observed in 85% of pulmonary adenocarcinomas while only 15% of mesotheliomas react with this antibody.

2. Adenocarcinomas from a variety sites show strong, usually focal, and predominantly cytoplasmic reactivity with TAG-72: 85% of invasive ductal breast carcinomas and 85–95% of colon, pancreatic, gastric, esophageal, lung, ovarian, and endometrial adenocarcinomas.

Selected references

Galietta A, Pizzi C, Pettinato G, et al. Differential TAG-72 epitope expression in breast cancer and lymph node metastases: A marker of a more aggressive phenotype. *Oncol Rep* 2002;9:135–40.

Sheibani K, Esteban JM, Bailey A, Battifora H, Weiss LM. Immunopathologic and molecular studies as an aid to the diagnosis of malignant mesothelioma. *Hum Pathol* 1992;23:107–16.

Szpak CA, Johnston WW, Roggli V, et al. The diagnostic distinction between malignant mesothelioma of the pleura and adenocarcinoma of the lung as defined by a monoclonal antibody B72.3. *Am J Pathol* 1986;122:252–60.

Tau

Background

The major components of the neuronal cytoskeleton are alpha and beta tubulin, the microfilament associated proteins (MAPs), neurofilaments, and actin. Tau is a neuronal microtubule-associated protein, which is the major antigenic component of neurofibrillary tangles and senile plaques in Alzheimer's disease. Comparison of tau-immunoreactive lesions in three relatively uncommon neurodegenerative diseases, namely, supranuclear palsy, Pick's disease, and corticobasal degeneration, demonstrated unexpected pathological similarities but also fundamental differences between these disorders.

Tau2 was produced using bovine MAP as immunogen. It reacts exclusively with the chemically heterogeneous tau in both the phosphorylated and the nonphosphorylated form. Tau2 does not react with other MAPs or with tubulin and localizes along microtubules in axons, dendrites, somata, and astrocytes, and on ribosomes. Tau2 cross-reacts with bovine, monkey, and chicken tissue. A variety of antibodies to phosphorylated neurofilament proteins have been shown to cross-react with phosphorylated epitopes of tau.

Applications

Applications of tau are mainly in the field of neuropathological research in neurodegenerative disorders. In the diagnostic setting, conventional silver impregnation stains such as Bielchowsky or Bodian are used for the demonstration of neurofibrillary tangles. These can now also be detected with antibodies to phosphorylated tau epitopes and ubiquitin. Tau is not only a basic component of neurofibrillary degeneration but is also an etiologic factor, as demonstrated by mutations on the tau gene responsible for frontotemporal dementias with parkinsonism linked to chromosome 17. The abnormal accumulation of tau protein in glia in many neurodegenerative diseases suggests that in some instances the disease process may also target the glial tau, with neuronal degeneration as a secondary consequence of this process. Prominent filamentous tau pathology and brain degeneration in the absence of extracellular amyloid deposition thus characterize a number of neurodegenerative disorders other than Alzheimer's disease, including progressive supranuclear palsy, corticobasal degeneration, and Pick's disease, collectively referred to as the tauopathies. Tau protein has also been demonstrated in gastrointestinal stromal tumors in an intense diffuse staining pattern in both epithelioid and spindle cell tumors in as many as 76% of both gastric and small bowel tumors. Tau also immunostained other intra-abdominal tumors including neuroendocrine carcinomas, paragangliomas, and desmoplastic round cell tumors.

Selected references

Cork LC, Sternberger NH, Sternberger LA, et al. Phosphorylated neurofilament antigens in neurofibrillary tangles in Alzheimer's disease. *J Neuropathol Exp Neurol* 1986;45:56–64.

Feany MB, Dickson DW. Neurodegenerative disorders with extensive tau pathology: A comparative study and review. *Ann Neurol* 1996;40:139–48.

Joachim CL, Morris JH, Kosik KS, Selkoe DJ. Tau antisera recognize neurofibrillary tangles in a range of neurodegenerative disorders. *Ann Neurol* 1987;22:514–20.

TCL1

Background

T-cell leukemia/lymphoma 1 (TCL1) is an oncoprotein encoded by the *TCL1* gene on chromosome 14q32.1. It acts as an AKT kinase coactivator and promotes cell survival and proliferation. Expressed during early embryogenesis and in fetal lymphoid tissues, TCL1 expression is restricted to germ cells in the testis, B- and T-lymphoid precursors, and plasmacytoid dendritic cells in adults. In B cells, TCL1 is expressed from pro-B cells to naïve B cells, downregulated in the germinal center (GC) B cells, and silenced in post-GC memory B cells and plasma cells. In T cells, TCL1 expression is limited to surface CD3−, CD4−, CD8− thymocytes.

Applications

TCL1 is overexpressed in T-cell prolymphocytic leukemia (T-PLL) mainly due to the chromosome rearrangements juxtaposing the regulatory elements of the T-cell receptor locus to the *TCL1* gene. By immunohistochemistry analysis, TCL1 is positive in about 70–80% of T-PLL and can be used to differentiate it from other T-cell leukemia/lymphomas in which it is not expressed.

TCL1 is positive in almost all blastic plasmacytoid dendritic cell neoplasm cases and is negative in myelomonocytic blasts. TCL1 is therefore a good marker for plasmacytoid dendritic cell neoplasm.

TCL1, expressed in most B cells, is also positive in B-cell lymphoma but is not routinely used for diagnosis of B-cell lymphoma. Burkitt lymphoma has been shown to be homogeneously strongly positive for TCL1, and multiple other B-cell lymphomas, including follicular lymphoma (FL), chronic lymphocytic leukemia/small lymphocytic lymphoma (CLL/SLL), mantle cell lymphoma (MCL), marginal zone lymphoma (MZL), hairy cell leukemia (HCL), and diffuse large B-cell lymphoma (DLBCL), display variable intensity of TCL1 staining. TCL1 expression has been associated with adverse clinical outcome in CLL, MCL, and DLBCL.

While *TCL1* expression is detectable in the testis by reverse transcription-polymerase chain reaction (RT-PCR), normal germ cells are TCL1 negative by immunohistochemical analysis. However, TCL1 is positive in intratubular germ cell neoplasia (IGCNU), testicular seminoma (80–100% cases positive), and ovarian dysgerminoma. A small subset of embryonal carcinoma and spermatocytic seminoma cases may show very focal and weak staining. TCL1 is negative in testicular yolk sac tumor, teratoma, and choriocarcinoma. A subset of yolk sac tumor in the ovary was reported to be positive. The percentage of mediastinal dysgerminoma positive for TCL1 varies in different studies. A small percentage of nonlymphoid non–germ cell tumors show weak TCL1 staining. Overall, TCL1 is a useful marker for IGCNU and seminoma diagnosis.

Interpretation

Positive staining is mainly nuclear with some cytoplasmic staining.

Selected references

Aggarwal M, Villuendas R, Gomez G, et al. TCL1A expression delineates biological and clinical variability in B-cell lymphoma. *Mod Pathol* 2009;22(2):206–15.

Cao D, Lane Z, Allan RW, et al. TCL1 is a diagnostic marker for intratubular germ cell neoplasia and classic seminoma. *Histopathology* 2010;57(1):152–7.

Laine J, Kunstle G, Obata T, et al. The protooncogene TCL1 is an Akt kinase coactivator. *Mol Cell* 2000;6:395–407.

Sangle NA, Schmidt RL, Patel JL, et al. Optimized immunohistochemical panel to differentiate myeloid sarcoma from blastic plasmacytoid dendritic cell neoplasm. *Mod Pathol* 2014;27(8):1137–43.

Sun Y, Tang G, Hu Z, et al. Comparison of karyotyping, TCL1 fluorescence in situ hybridisation and TCL1 immunohistochemistry in T cell prolymphocytic leukaemia. *J Clin Pathol* 2018;71(4):309–15.

Trinh DT, Shibata K, Hirosawa T, et al. Diagnostic utility of CD117, CD133, SALL4, OCT4, TCL1 and glypican-3 in malignant germ cell tumors of the ovary. *J Obstet Gynaecol Res* 2012;38(5):841–8.

Weissferdt A, Rodriguez-Canales J, Liu H, et al. Primary mediastinal seminomas: A comprehensive immunohistochemical study with a focus on novel markers. *Hum Pathol* 2015;46(3):376–83.

Tenascin

Background

Tenascin is a large glycoprotein of the extracellular matrix with a unique six-armed multidomain macromolecular structure. It is expressed in fibroblasts and the extracellular matrix during embryogenesis and growth. Tenascin is synthesized by fibroblasts and is believed to have active functions in epithelial–mesenchymal interactions.

Tenascin expression is also induced during wound healing and inflammatory processes. The amino acid sequence of tenascin comprises epidermal growth factor (EGF)-like repetitions, which bind to EGF receptors of tumor cells, implying that tenascin may play a role in tumor invasion and metastasis. Tenascin has also been demonstrated in the extracellular matrix of mature tissue and benign and malignant neoplasms.

Hence, tenascin has been demonstrated to be a stromal marker of malignancy in breast carcinoma, with a positive correlation between tenascin expression, 5-year disease-free survival, and distant metastases in breast carcinomas. Increased tenascin immunoexpression has also been demonstrated in the stroma of gastric, endometrial, and colon carcinomas. In comparison to normal tissue and benign tumors, increased tenascin expression has therefore been regarded as a stromal marker of tumor progression.

Tenascin immunoexpression has also been demonstrated in mesenchymal tumors, including schwannomas, leiomyosarcomas, fibromas, liposarcomas, and other fibrohistiocytic tumors. The corona-like expression of tenascin around lymphofollicular infiltrates appears to be a distinctive feature of lymphocytic thyroiditis. A similar pattern of tenascin staining has been described in lymphoid hyperplasia of the thymus associated with myasthenia gravis, another autoimmune disorder. This has been interpreted as the lymphoid follicles stimulating/activating the surrounding mesenchyme to produce tenascin as part of the extracellular matrix during the course of the autoimmune disease process.

Recently, it was demonstrated that tenascin is an extracellular matrix glycoprotein that plays a role in endometrial proliferation and possibly endometrial carcinogenesis.

Application

1. Tenascin immunopositivity at the dermal–epidermal junction overlying dermatofibroma but not dermatofibrosarcoma protuberans has been shown to be useful to distinguish between these skin tumors.
2. Malignant pheochromocytomas (defined by the presence of metastases) demonstrated strong stromal tenascin positivity, whilst pheochromocytomas that had not metastasized were negative; the adrenal medulla was negative. In contrast, paragangliomas showed a heterogeneous pattern with no difference between "benign" and malignant paragangliomas.

Selected references

Erickson HP, Bourdon MA. Tenascin: An extracellular matrix protein prominent in specialized embryonic tissues and tumors. *Ann Rev Cell Biol* 1989;5:71–92.

Koukoulis GK, Gould VE, Bhattacharyya A, et al. Tenascin in normal, reactive, hyperplastic and neoplastic tissues: Biologic and pathologic implications. *Hum Pathol* 1991;22:636–43.

Sedele M, Karaveli S, Pestereli HE, et al. Tenascin expression in normal, hyperplastic and neoplastic endometrium. *Int J Gynecol Pathol* 2002;12:161–6.

Terminal deoxynucleotidyl transferase (TdT)

Background

Terminal deoxynucleotidyl transferase (TdT) is a 58 kD protein encoded by a 35 kb gene on chromosome 10q23–25. It is a nuclear enzyme that catalyzes the random addition of deoxynucleotidyl residues on the 3'OH termini of single-stranded DNA and of oligo-deoxynucleotide primers and differs from other DNA polymerases by not requiring template instruction for polymerization.

TdT is recognized to exert its DNA polymerase function during the early variation of genes coding for T and B cells, perhaps by resulting in the addition of non-germline-encoded nucleotides (N-regions), although its function is still debated.

TdT is normally present only in hematopoietic tissues such as thymus and bone marrow, where it is restricted to a proportion of multipotent cell precursors and immature T and B lymphocytes. TdT positivity is never observed in normal peripheral blood cells.

Approximately 1–2% (more in young individuals) of bone marrow cells show TdT positivity, and these mostly express B-cell precursor phenotype in cell suspension studies. In trephine biopsies, TdT-positive cells do not display preferential localization and are sparsely dispersed in interstitial spaces.

In the thymus, T lymphocytes can be defined into three maturation stages corresponding to their microenvironment. Stage I thymocytes, accounting for 0.5–5% of thymocytes, reside in the subcapsular zone of the thymus and comprise large TdT blast cells, which express CD7, CD2, CD5, and cCD3 (cytoplasmic). Stage II thymocytes, accounting for 60–80% of thymocytes, are TdT and express CD7, CD5, cCD3, CD2, CD1, CD4, and CD8. Stage II thymocytes, accounting for 15–20% of thymocytes, reside in the medulla, do not express TdT or CD1, and show differentiation into either CD4+ or CD8+ cells.

Applications

1. TdT as a marker is mostly used in the diagnosis of lymphomas and leukemias. TdT activity is seen in acute lymphoblastic leukemias (ALL) of both B- and T-cell lineages, so that TdT is a useful diagnostic marker for lymphoblastic leukemias. In addition, as many as 30% of patients with chronic granulocytic leukemia develop a lymphoid blast crisis, which is characterized by a lymphoblastic phenotype with nuclear TdT expression. These TdT lymphoblastic crises have a better prognosis than TdT-nonlymphoid blast crisis and respond to ALL-like therapy.

2. There are about 20% of cases of acute nonlymphoid leukemias that also express TdT and in which the proportion of TdT blasts coexpressing various myeloid markers is variable. It has been suggested that the expression of TdT in such cases is a marker of poor prognosis, but this is controversial. Such cases often show the phenomenon of phenotypic and genotypic "lineage infidelity," in which there is expression of lymphoid antigens such as CD7 and there is rearrangement of Ig and T-cell receptor genes.

The L3 ALL in the French–American–British (FAB) classification, which represents Burkitt-type leukemia, is an exception, as the blast cells of this type of leukemia represent a "mature" B-cell phenotype with surface immunoglobulin expression.

TdT is a reliable marker to distinguish lymphoblastic lymphoma (LL) from other lymphomas that are always TdT negative. LLs are related to T-ALL and their distinction from the latter can be difficult; nevertheless, clinical and phenotypic differences have been observed, with the latter tending to show a more immature immunophenotype. While LL is frequent in children, forming about one-third of all non-Hodgkin's lymphoma, it also makes up about 5% of cases in adults, and cases of non-T, non-B, or pre-B-cell LL have been reported in extranodal sites in both children and adults. TdT is particularly useful for the separation of LL from the other small cell tumors of childhood.

TdT is thus a useful marker for diagnosis as well as for staging, as it helps identify tumor cells from reactive lymphocytes. TdT staining can be used for the detection of early involvement and in staging, especially in extranodal sites such as the testes, central nervous system (CNS) (through cerebrospinal fluid examination), skin, liver, kidney, and other sites of extramedullary involvement, and for monitoring minimal residual disease following chemotherapy. In the assessment of residual LL, it should be noted that a small population of TdT+ lymphoblasts resides in benign lymph nodes and tonsils. In benign lymph nodes from 26 consecutive pediatric patients TdT-positive cells were found adjacent to medullary and cortical sinuses in a frequency of 1 to 180 cells per high power field, as single cells or small clusters. These cells had a B precursor phenotype staining for CD79a, CD34, and CD10. In the tonsil, TdT-positive cells were demonstrated in all 15 adults and children studied by immunostaining, indicating that tonsils, like bone marrow and thymus, are sites of lymphopoiesis.

3. In the identification of thymomas, particularly when sited in unusual sites such as the pleura, the presence of TdT-positive, CD1a+, Cd2+, CD99+ phenotype in the associated lymphoid population is supporting evidence of thymoma, as is the aberrant expression of CD20 in the cytokeratin-positive neoplastic cells.

Selected references

Chilosi M, Pizzolo G. Review of terminal deoxynucleotidyl transferase: Biological aspects, methods of detection, and selected diagnostic applications. *Appl Immunohistochem* 1995;3:209–21.

Onciu M, Lorsbach RB, Henry EC, et al. Terminal deoxynucleotidyl transferase-positive lymphoid cells in reactive lymph nodes from children with malignant tumor: Incidence, distribution pattern, and immunophenotype in 26 patients. *Am J Clin Pathol* 2002;118:248–54.

Orazi A, Cattoretti G, Joh K, et al. Terminal deoxynucleotidyl transferase staining of malignant lymphomas in paraffin sections. *Mod Pathol* 1994;7:582–6.

TFE3

Background

The transcription factor for immunoglobulin heavy chain enhancer region 3 (TFE3) is a member of the microphthalmia transcription factor (MiTF) family that is ubiquitously expressed in humans and is presumed to regulate many genes. Genetic translocations involving the *TFE3* gene on the X chromosome (Xp11.2) include the *ASPL:TFE3* translocation characteristic of alveolar soft part sarcoma, and several different translocation partners present in Xp11 translocation renal cell carcinomas. *TFE3* gene translocation results in the activation of the *MET* oncogene with activation of the rapamycin intracellular signaling pathway. Furthermore, with the potential role of targeted therapies (such as MET inhibitors and vascular endothelial growth factor [VEGF] blockade clinical trials), the recognition and accurate classification of such tumors become important.

Applications

1. Antibodies to TFE3 are used in several diagnostic situations, since it is expressed in almost all tumors featuring TFE3 gene fusions:
   a. Soft tissue tumors: Moderate to strong nuclear TFE3 reactivity is detected in virtually all alveolar soft part sarcomas. This can be confirmed by molecular testing for ASPSCRI:TFE3 fusion.
   b. A subset of PEComas with TFE3 translocation show diffuse TFE3 expression.
   c. Xp11.2 translocation renal cell carcinomas and melanotic Xp11 tumors also consistently express TFE3.
   d. There have been other tumors including epithelioid hemangioendothelioma with YAP1-TFE3 gene fusions that show TFE3 positivity.
   e. Ossifying fibromyxoid tumor.
   f. Rare cases of malignant chondroid syringoma.
2. Nuclear TFE3 immunoreactivity is present in some types of tumors that lack the *TFE3* gene translocation. Owing to their scarcity, these tumors have been studied in small numbers. Almost all granular cell tumors are TFE3 positive, with most showing weak to moderate TFE3 reactivity. TFE3 has been reported consistently in epithelioid hemangioendothelioma (even in the absence of TFE3 rearrangements). TFE3 expression can be detected in tumors with melanocytic or myomelanocytic differentiation, including angiomyolipoma (80%), melanoma (55%), and clear cell sarcoma (70%).

Scattered weak to focally moderate staining intensity of native TFE3 protein has been reported in nontumor cells.

Other tumors staining with TFE3 but lacking mutations: solid pseudopapillary neoplasm of pancreas, ovarian sclerosing stromal tumor.

Comments

Sporadic PEComas frequently harbor TSC2 mutation and loss of heterozygosity (LOH), which forms the basis of mTOR inhibitor therapy. TFE-3 rearranged tumors were shown to lack these alterations and hence, recognizing such PEComa variants potentially has implications in clinical management. Among gynecologic PEComas, the conventional ones (with epithelioid and spindle cell morphology) show patchy reactivity with HMB45 and Melan A and are negative or weakly positive for TFE3. The translocation-associated PEComas show strong diffuse TFE3 positivity along with HMB45 with negative Melan A. Conventional PEComas are only focally/weakly HMB45 positive.

Selected references

Argani P, Aulmann S, Illei PB, et al. A distinctive subset of PEComas harbors TFE3 gene fusions. *Am J Surg Pathol* 2010;34:1395–406.

Argani P, Lal P, Hutchinson B, et al. Aberrant nuclear immunoreactivity for TFE3 in neoplasms with TFE3 gene fusions: A sensitive and specific immunohistochemical assay. *Am J Surg Pathol* 2003;27:750–61.

Thrombomodulin

Background

Thrombomodulin (TM) is a transmembrane glycoprotein composed of 575 amino acids (molecular weight 75 kD) with natural anticoagulant properties. It is normally expressed by a restricted number of cells, such as endothelial and mesothelial cells. In addition, synovial lining and syncytiotrophoblasts of human placenta express TM. Although TM contains six domains that are structurally similar to epidermal growth factor (EGF), there is no cross-reaction of anti-TM with EGF. The anticoagulant activity of TM results from the activation of protein C and the subsequent action on factors Va and VIIIa, and from the binding of thrombin.

Applications

1. TM stains blood and lymphatic channels and their corresponding channels consistently: 95% of benign lymphatic lesions (including lymphangioma and lymphangiectasia), 100% of benign vascular tumors (pyogenic granuloma and hemangioma), and 95% of malignant vascular tumors (Kaposi's sarcoma, angiosarcoma, and epithelioid hemangioendothelioma).
2. It is an immunohistochemical marker for mesothelial cells and malignant mesotheliomas. The results have been rather variable, with some studies claiming high specificity whilst others showed lower specificity in its role of distinguishing mesothelioma from adenocarcinoma.
3. TM is immunoexpressed in a variety of tumors, including squamous cell carcinomas of the lung, synovial sarcoma, angiosarcoma, transitional cell carcinoma, renal cell carcinomas, and thymomas.

Selected references

Appleton MAC, Attanoos RL, Jasani B. Thrombomodulin as a marker of vascular and lymphatic tumors. *Histopathology* 1996;29:153–7.

Attanoos RL, Goddard H, Gibbs AR. Mesothelioma-binding antibodies: Thrombomodulin, OV632 and HBME-1 and their use in the diagnosis of malignant mesothelioma. *Histopathology* 1996;29:209–15.

Collins CL, Ordonez NG, Schaefer R, et al. Thrombomodulin expression in malignant pleural mesothelioma and pulmonary adenocarcinoma. *Am J Pathol* 1992;141:827–33.

Ordonez NG. Value of thrombomodulin immunostaining in the diagnosis of mesothelioma. *Histopathology* 1997;31:25–30.

Thyroglobulin

Background

DAK-Tg6 (IgG1, Kappa) and 1D4 (IgG2a) were raised against purified human thyroglobulin. These antibodies react with thyroglobulin (300 kD) in normal, hyperplastic, and neoplastic thyroid glands. Circulating iodide, derived from dietary sources and deiodination of thyroid hormones, is selectively trapped by the thyroid gland. Oxidation of iodine to the organic form is then effected by a thyroid peroxidase enzyme, which is sited at the apical border of the follicular cell. This is now recognized as the antigen to thyroid antimicrosomal antibody in autoimmune disease. Organic iodide is incorporated into mono- and di-iodotyrosine by binding to tyrosine residues on thyroglobulin stored in colloid. Thyroglobulin contains 140 tyrosine residues but not all of these are iodinated, and T4 and T3 synthesis occurs only at specific sites. Hormone release is brought about by endocytosis of thyroglobulin at the apical pole of the follicular stem cell, fusion of endocytotic vesicles with lysosomes, and release of T3 and T4 by the proteolytic cleavage of thyroglobulin. These hormones are then secreted into the peripheral blood via the basal pole.

Applications

Apart from being immunoexpressed in all papillary and follicular carcinomas, thyroglobulin may also be useful in poorly differentiated and anaplastic carcinomas. Although both latter entities have been shown biochemically to synthesize 19S thyroglobulin, immunohistochemistry often fails to detect thyroglobulin in these tumors. Hürthle cell tumors also demonstrate immunopositivity with thyroglobulin. The other major role of antibodies to thyroglobulin is in the identification of metastatic thyroid carcinomas. A note of caution is necessary, since thyroglobulin may be demonstrated in medullary carcinoma of the thyroid gland. Antibodies to thyroglobulin do not react with epithelial cells from the gastrointestinal tract, pancreas, kidney, lung, and breast or the malignancies that arise in these organs.

Selected references

De Micco C, Ruf J, Carayon P, et al. Immunohistochemical study of thyroglobulin in thyroid carcinomas with monoclonal antibodies. *Cancer* 1987;59:471–6.

Wilson NW, Pambakian H, Richardson TC, et al. Epithelial markers in thyroid carcinoma: An immunoperoxidase study. *Histopathology* 1986;10:815–29.

Thyroid transcription factor-1 (TTF-1)

Background

Thyroid transcription factor- 1 (TTF-1) is a homeodomain-containing regulator of nuclear transcription in the thyroid gland, forebrain, and lung. It belongs to the NKx2 family of transcription factors and is expressed in the nuclei of thyroid follicular and para-follicular C cells and type II pneumocytes in the lung. It has also been found to be expressed in the pituitary and parathyroid glands.

Application

TTF-1 is expressed in the entire range of differentiated thyroid neoplasms: follicular adenoma, carcinoma, papillary carcinoma, and medullary carcinoma. About 30% of Hurthle cell carcinomas are positive. Anaplastic thyroid carcinomas are generally negative.

In the lung, up to 85% of lung adenocarcinomas are positive. Up to 25% of mucinous bronchioloalveolar carcinomas, 30% of sarcomatoid carcinomas, and 40% of large cell carcinomas are TTF-1 positive, while 5% of squamous carcinomas have shown TTF-1 positivity. Up to 10% of gastrointestinal tract adenocarcinomas are positive for TTF-1 when using the SPT24 antibody. In general, nonpulmonary adenocarcinomas are rarely TTF-1 positive.

Over 90% of small-cell lung carcinomas are TTF-1 positive, while lower grades of neuroendocrine tumors in the lung show varying degrees of positivity (35–50%). Up to 40% of extrapulmonary small-cell carcinomas can also express TTF-1. Lower-grade neuroendocrine tumors from outside the lung rarely express TTF-1.

In sclerosing pneumocytomas in the lung, both the lining surface cells and the stromal cells are TTF-1 positive.

Rare cases of endometrioid cancer and ductal and ductal in situ breast cancer have been noted to be TTF-1 positive.

Interpretation of staining

TTF-1 is a nuclear transcription factor; hence, tumor labeling with be nuclear. Normal lung tissue may be used as a positive control. The most commonly used TTF-1 antibody clones are 8G7G3/1 and SPT24; the latter stains a higher percentage of extrapulmonary tumors. Some cytoplasmic positivity has been noted in lung adenocarcinomas with clone 8G7G3/1, but these should be interpreted as negative.

Selected references

Agoff SN, Lamps LW, Philip AT, et al. Thyroid transcription factor-1 is expressed in extrapulmonary small cell carcinomas but not in other extrapulmonary neuroendocrine tumors. *Mod Pathol* 2000,13:238–42.

Bingle CD. Thyroid transcription factor-1. *Int J Biochem Cell Biol* 1997;29:1471–3.

Comperat E, Zhang F, Perrotin C, et al. Variable sensitivity and specificity of TTF1 antibodies in lung metastatic adenocarcinoma of colorectal origin. *Mod Pathol* 2005;18: 1371–6.

TLE1

Background

Transducin-like enhancer of split 1 (TLE1) is one of the four TLE genes that encode human transcriptional repressors, which are homologs for the Drosophila corepressor groucho protein, and an important component of the Wnt signaling pathway. It acts as a transcriptional corepressor implicated in the regulation of hematopoietic, neuronal, and epithelial differentiation. Analysis of the differential expression of TLE1 mRNA demonstrates wide expression in fetal and adult tissues, and synovial sarcoma has been shown to have overexpression of TLE1 in gene profiling studies. In synovial sarcoma, TLE proteins act through the Wnt/B-catenin pathway. Gene expression profiling studies show significant overexpression of TLE1 in synovial sarcoma. The synovial sarcoma fusion protein SS18-SSX appears to perform a bridging function between activating transcription factor 2 (ATF2) and TLE1, resulting in repression of ATF2 target genes. Blocking this pathway results in growth suppression and apoptosis, which supports a pathogenetic role for TLE1 and ATF2 in synovial sarcoma.

TLE1 was first described as a diagnostic immunohistochemical marker for synovial sarcoma from gene expression profiling studies showing expression in 97% of cases including both epithelial and spindle cell components as well as in poorly differentiated synovial sarcomas. Nuclear TLE1 reactivity is present in basal keratinocytes, adipocytes, perineurial cells, endothelial cells, and mesothelial cells.

Applications

1. The majority of synovial sarcomas exhibit moderate to strong nuclear TLE1 reactivity, but the sensitivity (90–100%) and specificity are variably reported. The vast majority of synovial sarcomas (in particular the poorly differentiated type) show moderate to strong TLE1 positivity, although this has been disputed in studies using whole-mount sections. The reported positivity ranges from 82% to 96%, although there are other studies showing fewer than 50% of synovial sarcomas staining with TLE1. A more recent meta-analysis showed TLE1 to have a mean sensitivity and specificity of 94% and 81%, respectively, in detection of synovial sarcoma. Both epithelial and spindle cell components stain for TLE1, and positivity is reported in poorly differentiated synovial sarcoma as well.

2. TLE1 expression has been described in other sarcomas that may mimic synovial sarcoma: malignant peripheral nerve sheath tumor (2–60%), solitary fibrous tumors (8–20%), Ewing sarcoma, BCOR-CCNB3 sarcoma, and cutaneous spindle cell malignant melanoma. Typically these tumors do not show moderate to strong positivity. Perineuriomas are TLE1 negative.

3. Carcinomas that can be in the differential diagnosis of synovial sarcoma can rarely show TLE1 positivity: 7% of carcinomas (prostatic, esophageal, endometrial adenocarcinomas, ovarian serous carcinoma, basal cell and small cell carcinoma).

4. TLE1 expression has also been described in a minority of tumors that might or might not be in the differential diagnosis of synovial sarcoma, including endometrial stromal sarcoma, leiomyosarcoma, liposarcoma, rhabdomyosarcoma, epithelioid sarcoma, undifferentiated sarcoma and atypical fibroxanthoma, benign nerve sheath tumors including schwannoma and neurofibroma, gastrointestinal stromal tumor, and malignant mesothelioma.

5. TLE1 has been more recently described in atypical teratoid/rhabdoid tumor, clear cell sarcoma of kidney, and malignant rhabdoid tumor.

Selected references

Chen G, Courey AJ. Groucho/TLE family proteins and transcriptional repression. *Gene* 2000;249:1–16.

Duncan VE, Wicker JA, Kelly DR, et al. TLE1 expression in malignant rhabdoid tumor and atypical teratoid/rhabdoid tumor. *Pediatr Dev Pathol* 2018;21(6):522–7.

El Beaino M, et al. Diagnostic value of TLE1 in synovial sarcoma: A systematic review and meta-analysis. *Sarcoma* 2020:7192347.

Foo WC, Cruise MW, Wick MR, et al. Immunohistochemical staining for TLE1 distinguishes synovial sarcoma from histologic mimics. *Am J Clin Pathol* 2011;135:839–44.

Jagdis A, Rubin BP, Tubbs RR, et al. Prospective evaluation of TLE1 as a diagnostic immunohistochemical marker in synovial sarcoma. *Am J Surg Pathol* 2009;33:1743–51.

Kosemehmetoglu K, Vrana JA, Folpe AL. TLE1 expression is not specific for synovial sarcoma: A whole section study of 163 soft tissue and bone neoplasms. *Mod Pathol* 2009;22(7):872–8.

Li WS, Liao IC, Wen MC, et al. BCOR-CCNB3-positive soft tissue sarcoma with round-cell and spindle-cell histology: A series of four cases highlighting the pitfall of mimicking poorly differentiated synovial sarcoma. *Histopathology* 2016;69(5):792–801.

Pukhalskaya T, Smoller BR. TLE1 expression fails to distinguish between synovial sarcoma, atypical fibroxanthoma, and dermatofibrosarcoma protuberans. *J Cutan Pathol* 2020;47(2):135–8.

Terry J, Saito T, Subramanian S, et al. TLE1 as a diagnostic immunohistochemical marker for synovial sarcoma emerging from gene expression profiling studies. *Am J Surg Pathol* 2007;31(2):240–6.

Zaccarini DJ, Deng X, Tull J, et al. Expression of TLE-1 and CD99 in carcinoma: Pitfalls in diagnosis of synovial sarcoma. *Appl Immunohistochem Mol Morphol* 2018;26(6):368–73.

Topoisomerase II alpha

Background

The phylogenetic antiquity of DNA topoisomerases indicates their vital function in the cell. The structure and maintenance of genomic DNA depend on the activity of these enzymes, without which replication and cell division are impossible. DNA topoisomerase type II activity is required to change DNA topology and it is important in the relaxation of DNA supercoils generated by cellular processes such as transcription and replication. It is also essential for the condensation of chromosomes and their segregation during mitosis. In mammals this activity is derived from at least two isoforms, namely, topoisomerase II alpha (Topo II alpha) and beta. Because of its essential role in cell replication, Topo II alpha is the target for many drugs used for cancer therapy. Reduced expression of this enzyme is the predominant mechanism of resistance to several chemotherapeutic agents, and a wide variation in the range of expression of this protein is noted in many different tumors. The immunostaining pattern of Topo II alpha is similar to that of the cell cycling marker Ki-67, so that immunostaining of this protein has also been employed as a cell proliferation marker.

Applications

1. As a predictor of chemotherapeutic response to enzyme inhibitors and in the determination of tumor cell proliferation. Increased Topo II alpha immunostaining has been shown to correlate with recurrent colon cancers, with chemosensitivity in ovarian and endometrial carcinomas, and with anthracycline-based adjuvant therapy in node-positive breast cancer. Topo II alpha cell counts have been shown to correlate well with Ki-67 counts in meningiomas, multiple myeloma, adrenocortical tumors, and pituitary adenomas and are a predictor of survival in patients with astrocytoma and ovarian cancer.

Selected references

Di Leo A, Larsimont D, Gancberg D, et al. HER-2 and topoisomerase II alpha as predictive markers in a population of node-positive breast cancer patients randomly treated with adjuvant CMF or epirubicin plus cyclophosphamide. *Ann Oncol* 2001;12:1081–9.

Gotleib WH, Goldberg I, Weisz B, et al. Topoisomerase II immunostaining as a prognostic marker for survival in ovarian cancer. *Gynecol Oncol* 2001;82:99–104.

Toxoplasma gondii

Background

T. gondii is a protozoan parasite, which causes a mild and self-limiting infection in adults. Toxoplasmosis occurs in patients who eat raw or partially cooked meat, reflecting the widespread presence of this protozoan in animals used as food sources. Following gastrointestinal infection, active toxoplasmosis is accompanied by fever with enlargement of lymph nodes and spleen. The immune reactions cause the intracellular Toxoplasma to adopt a cystoid form in which they can persist for a lifetime. However, infections in immunocompromised patients may be fatal, causing acute toxoplasmosis, including toxoplasmosis encephalitis. Activation of a latent infection during pregnancy may lead to intrauterine transmission of the organism to the fetus, resulting in spontaneous abortion, stillbirth, or severe central nervous system damage.

The polyclonal antibody was raised against formalin-fixed tachyzoites of *T. gondii* isolated and purified from infected mice. This latter antibody does not cross-react with the following organisms: Cryptosporidia, Microsporidia, *Histoplasma capsulatum*, Candida, Blastomyces, *Pneumocystis carinii*, *Entamoeba histolytica*, Aspergillus, *Cryptococcus neoformans*, and *Mycobacterium tuberculosis*.

Applications

Both tachyzoites (or trophozoites) and encysted bradyzoite forms of *T. gondii* are demonstrated with these antibodies. Infected Toxoplasma tissue including brain, lung, spleen, and lymph nodes may be positively identified with these antibodies. This is particularly pertinent when examining tissue from immunocompromised patients, e.g., in AIDS, where a high index of suspicion along with application of anti-Toxoplasmosis antibody may help arrive at a definite diagnosis.

Selected references

Conley FK, Jenkins KA, Remington JS. *Toxoplasma gondii* infection of the central nervous system: Use of the peroxidase-antiperoxidase method to demonstrate *Toxoplasma* in formalin-fixed, paraffin-embedded tissue sections. *Hum Pathol* 1981;12:690–8.

Kriek JA, Remington JS. Toxoplasmosis in the adult – an overview. *N Engl J Med* 1978;298:550–3.

NOTES

Tyrosinase

Background

Tyrosinase is an enzyme involved in the initial stages of melanin biosynthesis.

Applications

1. Tyrosinase is useful in the diagnosis of both primary and metastatic melanomas. It is less useful in the identification of spindled melanomas, especially desmoplastic melanomas.
2. Tyrosinase has also been demonstrated to be a sensitive and specific marker to distinguish epithelioid melanocytic nevi from epithelioid histiocytic tumors. Tyrosinase has not been recommended for routine use in the diagnosis of renal and hepatic angiomyolipomas.
3. Pigmented neurofibromas stained positive for tyrosinase were immunopositive.

Selected references

Hofbauer GF, Kamarashev J, Geertsen R, et al. Tyrosinase immunoreactivity in formalin-fixed, paraffin-embedded primary and metastatic melanoma: Frequency and distribution. *J Cutan Pathol* 1998;25:204–9.

Jungbluth AA, Iversen K, Copian K, et al. T311 – an anti-tyrosinase monoclonal antibody for the detection of melanocytic lesions in paraffin embedded tissues. *Pathol Res Pract* 2000;196:235–42.

Kaufmann O, Koch S, Burghardt J, et al. Tyrosinase, Melan-A, and KBA62 as markers for the immunohistochemical identification of metastatic amelanotic melanomas on paraffin sections. *Mod Pathol* 1998;11:740–6.

NOTES

Tyrosine hydroxylase

Background

Tyrosine hydroxylase (TH) plays an important role in the physiology of adrenergic neurons. It belongs to the biopterin-dependent aromatic amino acid hydroxylase family and is the rate-limiting enzyme of catecholamine biosynthesis; it uses tetrahydrobiopterin and molecular oxygen to convert tyrosine to DOPA. Its amino-terminal 150 amino acids comprise a domain whose structure is involved in regulating enzyme activity. The gene is located in the short arm of chromosome 11 at position 15.5 (11p15.5). The protein consists of 528 amino acids and has a molecular weight of 62 kDa. There are four potential splice variants.

Applications

1. TH is strongly localized in adrenal medulla, pheochromocytomas, and paragangliomas and patchily expressed in neuroblastoma. TH activity is high in pheochromocytomas and paragangliomas as compared with the normal adrenal gland, whereas it is low in a neuroblastoma and is undetectable in other tumors. Immunostaining of TH and the measurement of its activity in adreno-medullary and related tumors may provide some information about the process of cell differentiation in these tumors.

   Immunostaining for TH in paragangliomas is present in the majority of tumor cells in their cytoplasm with variable intensity regardless of their cytological features, such as cellular and nuclear pleomorphism; loss of immunostaining for TH may be observed in metastatic tumors.

2. TH is also positive in esthesioneuroblastomas, nasal catecholamine-producing tumors of neural crest origin, which might be derived from certain sympathetic neuronal cell nests in the superior nasal cavity.

3. TH is mostly localized on the cytoplasm of the differentiating neuroblasts of neuroblastic tumors of infancy, while immature elements are rarely positive. Although no correlation is found between the immunoreactive pattern and the site of origin or the staging of the neuroblastic tumors, there is a positive relationship between the urinary catecholamine output and the density of tyrosine hydroxylase–immunoreactive cells. TH is positive in 43% of midgut carcinoid tumors.

Selected references

Ceccamea A, Carlei F, Dominici C, et al. Correlation between tyrosine hydroxylase immunoreactive cells in tumors and urinary catecholamine output in neuroblastoma patients. *Tumori* 1986 31;72(5):451–7.

Iwase K, Nagasaka A, Nagatsu I, et al. Tyrosine hydroxylase indicates cell differentiation of catecholamine biosynthesis in neuroendocrine tumors. *J Endocrinol Invest* 1994;17:235–9.

Meijer WG, Copray SC, Hollema H, et al. Catecholamine-synthesizing enzymes in carcinoid tumors and pheochromocytomas. *Clin Chem* 2003;49:586–93.

Takahashi H, Wakabayashi K, Ikuta F, et al. Esthesioneuroblastoma: A nasal catecholamine-producing tumor of neural crest origin. Demonstration of tyrosine hydroxylase-immunoreactive tumor cells. *Acta Neuropathol* 1988;76:522–7.

Ubiquitin

Background

Ubiquitin is an 8.5 kD polypeptide found almost universally in plants and animals. The best-documented function for ubiquitin involves its conjugation to proteins as a signal to initiate degradation via the ubiquitin-mediated proteolytic pathway. Ubiquitin-mediated proteolysis is involved in the turnover of many short-lived regulatory proteins. This pathway leads to the covalent attachment of one or more multiubiquitin chains to target substrates, which are then degraded by the 26S multicatalytic proteasome complex. Ubiquitin modification of a variety of protein targets within the cells also plays an important role in many cellular processes: regulation of gene expression, regulation of cell cycle and division, involvement in the cellular stress response, modification of cell surface receptors, DNA repair, import of proteins into mitochondria, uptake of precursors into neurons, and biogenesis of mitochondria, ribosomes, and peroxisomes.

Applications

1. Ubiquitin immunostaining has been shown to be a highly sensitive and specific method for the detection of Mallory bodies, thereby making it a valuable tool in the study of alcoholic liver disease.
2. In human spongiform encephalopathies, ubiquitin immunoreactivity has been demonstrated in a punctate distribution at the periphery of prion protein amyloid plaques and in a finely granular pattern in the neuropil around and within areas of spongiform change. Analysis of the relationship of ubiquitin-positive dots and granular structures with pretangle neurons and neurofibrillary tangles suggested that the ubiquitin-positive structures are the result of degeneration and might be related to the initiation of neurofibrillary degeneration.
3. Ubiquitin-positive neuronal and tau 2-positive glial inclusions may prove to be a marker of frontotemporal dementia of motor neuron type.
4. Ubiquitin has also been simultaneously present with glial fibrillary acidic protein (GFAP) in the cytoplasm and cell processes of tumor cells of astrocytomas.
5. The demonstration of ubiquitin immunolabeling in both ductus efferentes and ductus epididymidis epithelia has concluded that ubiquitinated proteins are secreted into the epididymal lumen.

Selected references

Ciechanover A, Schwartz AL. The ubiquitin-mediated proteolytic pathway: Mechanisms of recognition of the proteolytic substrate and involvement in the degradation of native cellular proteins. *FASEB J* 1994;8:182–91.

Ulex europaeus agglutinin 1 lectin (UEA-I)

Background

UEA-1 is a plant lectin isolated from *Ulex europaeus* seeds (gorse seed) by affinity chromatography. The lectin is homogeneous. containing 4.2% neutral sugar and 1.4% glucosamine. Its molecular weight is approximately 110 kD, comprising two covalently bound basic subunits. UEA-1 is specific to certain terminal α-L-fucosyl residues of glycoconjugates and also detects blood group H antigen.

Applications

1. UEA-1 has been used successfully as a marker for endothelial cells. It has been shown to be more sensitive for benign vascular tumors than thrombomodulin or Factor VIII-related antigen. UEA-I does not distinguish between the endothelial cells of blood vessels and lymphatics.

3. UEA-1 demonstrates specific binding to collecting duct carcinoma of the kidney, enabling distinction from other types of renal cell carcinoma.

Selected references

Holthofer H, Virtanen I, Kariniemi AL, et al. *Ulex europaeus* I lectin as a marker for vascular endothelium in human tissues. *Lab Invest* 1982;47:60–6.

Meittinen M, Holthofer H, Lehto VP, et al. *Ulex europaeus* I lectin as a marker for tumors derived from endothelial cells. *Am J Clin Pathol* 1983;79:32–6.

Ordonez NG, Batsakis JG. Comparison of *Ulex europaeus* I lectin and Factor VII-related antigen in vascular lesions. *Arch Pathol Lab Med* 1984;108:129–32.

VEGF (vascular endothelial growth factor)

Background

Vascular endothelial growth factor (VEGF) is a dimeric 46 kD, endothelial cell–specific, glycosylated, heparin-binding cytokine. It has both angiogenic and vascular permeability factor functions. VEGF exerts paracrine effects by binding to specific tyrosine kinase receptors on vascular endothelial cells. It may also exert autocrine effects by stimulating tumor growth. Hence, VEGF is one of the most potent, highly specific angiogenic factors.

VEGF is synthesized by both tumor and normal cells and acts specifically on endothelial cells. VEGF stimulates and induces migration and proliferation of endothelial cells. Hence, VEGF is a useful marker of tumor angiogenesis.

Applications

1. Cytoplasmic immunoreactivity for VEGF has been demonstrated in 42% of melanomas but not in atypical compound melanocytic nevi, cellular blue nevi, or Spitz nevi. Further immunoreactivity for VEGF was related to tumor thickness and to the absence of regression. Hence, although VEGF is not a useful prognostic indicator for malignant melanoma, it may be useful in discriminating between melanoma and benign melanocytic lesions.
2. VEGF immunoexpression was also not found to be a prognostic marker for head and neck squamous cell carcinomas. However, tumor-associated inflammatory cells showed high levels of VEGF expression in all carcinomas studied, suggesting a possible role in tumor angiogenesis.
3. The immunohistochemical localization of VEGF (comparable to the localization of VEGF mRNA) was expressed in all thyroid tumors, including all types of thyroid carcinomas (including papillary, follicular, medullary, and anaplastic) and follicular adenomas. In contrast, in the normal thyroid, VEGF was identified in epithelium of isolated follicles. It was concluded that the histological type of thyroid tumor may determine the vascular pattern through a paracrine mechanism involving VEGF.
4. The characteristic vasculature and edema of sclerosing stromal tumors of the ovary has been demonstrated to be associated with the expression of VEGF.
5. In the prostate gland, VEGF expression was confined to the basal cell layer in benign glands. In high-grade prostatic intraepithelial neoplasia, immunolabeling was seen in all neoplastic secretory cells. All carcinomas were immunopositive for VEGF. Hence, there was a trend for increasing immunolabeling intensity with increasing cellular dedifferentiation.
6. Strong VEGF immunoexpression in malignant chondrocytes was confined exclusively to high-grade chondrosarcomas.
7. It may be useful in distinguishing between melanomas and melanocytic nevi. VEGF immunoexpression may also be predictive of potential metastasizing cartilaginous tumors. VEGF expression correlates with vascularity, metastasis, and proliferation of tumors and may therefore prove to be a useful prognostic marker.

Selected references

Mattern J, Koomagi R, Volm M. Association of vascular endothelial growth factor expression with intratumoral microvessel density and tumour cell proliferation in human epidermoid lung carcinoma. *Br J Cancer* 1996;72:931–4.

Salven P, Keikkila P, Anttonen A, et al. Vascular endothelial growth factor in squamous cell head and neck carcinoma: Expression and prognostic significance. *Mod Pathol* 1997;10:1128–33.

Toi M, Inada K, Suzuki H, et al. Tumor angiogenesis in breast cancer: Its importance as a prognostic indicator and the association with vascular endothelial growth factor expression. *Breast Cancer Res Treat* 1995;36:193–204.

Zymed Laboratories. Polyclonal rabbit anti-VEGF (data sheet).

Villin

Background

Microvilli increase the absorptive surface of epithelial cells by as much as 20 times. They comprise a highly specialized plasma membrane consisting of a thick extracellular coat of polysaccharide and digestive enzymes and a core comprising a central rigid bundle of 20–30 parallel actin filaments that extend from the tip of the microvillus down to the cell cortex. The actin filaments are all oriented with their plus ends pointing away from the cell body and are held together at regular intervals by actin-bundling proteins. Besides fimbrin, which occurs in microspikes and filopodia, the most important bundling protein is villin, which is found only in microvilli. Like fimbrin, villin cross-links actin filaments into tight parallel bundles, but in a different actin-binding sequence, and is capable of stimulating the formation of long microvilli in cultured fibroblasts, which do not normally contain villin and have only a few small microvilli.

Villin, a 95 kD, Ca^{2+}-regulated actin-binding protein, is found in absorptive cells that develop a brush border, such as those of the small and large intestines, ductal cells of the pancreas and biliary system, and cells of the proximal renal tubules. Villin is also found in undifferentiated normal and tumoral cells of intestinal origin in vivo and in cell culture, so that its expression is seen in cells that do not necessarily display microvilli-lined brush borders.

Applications

1. Villin has been employed as a marker of gastrointestinal tumors, particularly those from the colon, stomach, and pancreas. Gallbladder and hepatocellular carcinomas were also demonstrated to express villin.

2. A subset of nongastrointestinal tumors, including some adenocarcinomas of the ovary, endometrium, and kidney, were also positive. About 30% of signet ring cell carcinomas of the lung are positive.

3. The presence of villin in renal carcinomas is variable and is frequently seen in clear cell and chromophilic tumors but not in chromophobe cell tumors. Villin also appears to be expressed in the tubular and glandular areas of better-differentiated tumors and is not observed in sarcomatoid renal carcinoma, leading to the suggestion that villin may be a potential grading marker. Its expression in renal carcinomas suggests that they display proximal rather than distal tubular differentiation. It is also observed in the glandular areas of Wilm's tumor.

4. Villin immunoexpression was shown in 85% of gastrointestinal neuroendocrine tumors and small cell carcinomas of the lung and in 40% of lung carcinoids, where they show a characteristic apical membranous staining pattern. Villin has also been demonstrated in Merkel cells, highlighting their microvilli.

Selected references

Bacchi CE, Gown AM. Distribution and pattern of expression of villin, a gastrointestinal-associated cytoskeletal protein, in human carcinomas: A study employing paraffin-embedded tissue. *Lab Invest* 1991;64:418–24.

Vinculin

Background

Vinculin is a cytoskeletal protein of 117–130 kD. Its gene is encoded on chromosome 10q11.2-qter. It is involved in the indirect binding of intracellular actin filaments to extracellular fibronectin. Vinculin is widely distributed in tissue with expression especially where smooth muscle actin and fibroblasts attach to the extracellular matrix. Therefore, vinculin is a cytoskeletal protein associated with membrane actin filament attachment sites of cell–cell and cell–matrix adherens-type junctions. Hence, as an adhesion-associated protein, reduced or altered expression of vinculin has been associated with the acquisition of an invasive or metastatic phenotype in malignant transformation of cells. These workers demonstrated that the level of vinculin immunoexpression in low-malignancy, nonmetastasizing squamous epithelial lesions was similar to that observed in normal squamous epithelia. In contrast, in squamous cell carcinomas, which are invasive and possess metastatic potential, immunolabeling for vinculin was negative or weak; they concluded that vinculin immunoexpression in tumors arising from stratified squamous epithelia may be predictive of the metastatic potential.

It was previously reported that vinculin was distributed in renal tubular epithelium.

Applications

The use of vinculin immunoexpression in diagnostic surgical pathology is somewhat limited. It may have a predictive role in the biological behavior of tumors of squamous epithelial origin and may also be useful for the identification of renal tumors with a collecting duct phenotype.

The staining pattern of vinculin is membranous. Normal skin is a useful positive control.

Selected references

Burridge K, Feramisco JR. Microinjection and localization of a 130 K protein in living fibroblasts: A relationship to actin and fibronectin. *Cell* 1980;19:587–95.

Kuroda N, Naruse K, Miyazaki E, et al. Vinculin: Its possible use as a marker of normal collecting ducts and renal neoplasms with collecting duct system phenotype. *Mod Pathol* 2000;13:1109–14.

VS38

Background

VS38 was shown to detect a protein similar to the p63 protein. The latter is a nonglycated, reversibly palmitoylated type II transmembrane protein, which is found in rough endoplasmic reticulum. VS38 was originally described as a marker of neoplastic and nonneoplastic plasma cells.

Applications

1. The protein detected by VS38 is not exclusive to plasma cells but serves to distinguish plasma cells from other lymphoid cells because of their high secretory activity. It has been recommended for inclusion in a panel of antibodies for the immunostaining of bone marrow trephines fixed in common fixatives, including Bouin's solution.

2. VS38 immunostaining has been reported in neuroendocrine tumors and in melanocytic lesions, frequently positive in primary and metastatic melanomas. Caution should be exercised when using this marker to identify plasma cell lineage. VS38 is also immunoexpressed in osteoblasts and stromal cells of bone tumors.

Selected references

Banham AH, Turley H, Pulford K, et al. The plasma cell associated antigen detectable by antibody VS38 is the p63 rough endoplasmic reticulum protein. *J Clin Pathol* 1997;50:485–9.

Turley H, Jones M, Erber W, et al. VS38: A new monoclonal antibody for detecting plasma cell differentiation in routine sections. *J Clin Pathol* 1994;47:418–22.

WT1

Background

Wilms tumor gene (WT1) is a tumor suppressor gene located on chromosome 11p13. It encodes for WT1 protein, which is expressed in the developing genitourinary tract, developing spleen, and fetal coelomic lining cells, including mesothelium. WT1 is expressed in benign mesothelial cells, ovarian surface epithelium, inclusion cysts, and tubal epithelium but not in cervical or endometrial epithelium.

Applications

1. Stains Wilms' tumors (nephroblastoma) and malignant rhabdoid tumors of the kidney.
2. Distinction between malignant mesothelioma and adenocarcinoma: WT1 is usually negative in the majority of adenocarcinomas of various sites, the exception being serous carcinomas of the adnexa and peritoneum. In malignant mesothelioma, WT1 is expressed in 94% of all cases: 96% of epithelioid, 84% of biphasic, and 100% of well-differentiated papillary mesothelioma. WT1 is commonly expressed in mesothelial cells, mesothelioma, and tubo-ovarian/peritoneal serous carcinomas, and hence should not be part of a panel of immunohistochemical markers in the workup of peritoneal/abdominal tumors in women for excluding mesothelioma. In patients treated with neoadjuvant chemotherapy for high-grade tubo-ovarian serous carcinoma, WT1 immunohistochemical expression is retained but can show a significant decrease in intensity of staining. Benign mesothelial cells and malignant mesotheliomas are positive. Adenomatoid tumors are WT1 positive.
3. Soft tissue tumors: WT1 is useful in a panel of antibodies to establish the diagnosis of DSRCT (desmoplastic small round cell tumor), using the c-terminus antibody. In more recently described "Ewing-like sarcomas," WT1 is expressed in CIC-DUX4 translocation sarcomas (more than 90%), unlike other differential diagnoses (Ewing sarcoma, synovial sarcoma, BCOR-rearranged sarcoma), which are negative for WT1.

4. Distinction of ovarian from endometrial serous carcinoma: the vast majority (more than 90%) of ovarian serous carcinomas are positive for WT1, and only a small percentage of endometrial serous carcinomas are positive (up to 20%). While WT1 shows diffuse strong positivity in serous carcinomas of ovary and fallopian tube, this is not absolute, and rarely, ovarian serous carcinomas can be negative for WT1. WT1 can be useful in the setting of uterine surface serous carcinoma (endometrial intraepithelial carcinoma) with coexistent extrauterine serous carcinoma. Peritoneal serous carcinomas without coexistent serous carcinoma in an endometrial polyp have a WT1 expression pattern similar to ovarian serous carcinoma, while peritoneal serous carcinomas with coexistent serous carcinoma in an endometrial polyp have a staining pattern similar to uterine serous carcinoma. WT1 may also be helpful in differentiating poorly differentiated ovarian serous carcinoma from poorly differentiated ovarian endometrioid carcinoma. Clear cell carcinoma of ovary is WT1 negative. But WT1 expression is not specific to serous carcinomas and can be seen in other gynecologic tumors, including sex cord–stromal tumors (SCST), being expressed in the majority of all SCST with the exception of steroid cell tumors and Leydig cells in Sertoli–Leydig cell tumor.
5. WT1 is expressed in the majority of benign and malignant vascular neoplasms and also occasionally in glomus tumors. Usually, vascular malformations are negative for WT1.
6. Miscellaneous: breast, lung, colon, and pancreatic cancers, melanomas, cytoplasmic staining in peripheral nerve sheath tumors, rhabdomyosarcoma.

Interpretation

It is a nuclear antigen and hence produces nuclear staining; cytoplasmic positivity for WT1 represents cross-reactivity and not true positivity. However, some have used cytoplasmic staining as the basis for future immune therapy.

The utility of WT1 is somewhat limited as a soft tissue marker since it is expressed in a variety of soft tissue tumors, including rhabdomyosarcoma, and even occasionally in Ewing sarcoma.

Likewise, with newer and more specific endothelial markers, including CD31, ERG, and Claudin-5, WT1 plays a limited role in the workup of vascular tumors.

WT1 expression has also been described in other adenocarcinomas (*see earlier*), but rarely (5–15% of gastric, lung, urothelial, and breast carcinomas).

Selected references

Al-Hussaini M, Stockman A, Foster H, et al. WT-1 assists in distinguishing ovarian from uterine serous carcinoma and in distinguishing between serous and endometrioid ovarian carcinoma. *Histopathology* 2004;44:109–15.

Euscher ED, Malpica A, Deavers MT, et al. Differential expression of WT-1 in serous carcinomas in the peritoneum with or without associated serous carcinoma in endometrial polyps. *Am J Surg Pathol* 2005:29: 1074–8.

McCluggage WG. WT-1 immunohistochemical expression in small round blue cell tumours. *Histopathology* 2008;52:631–2.

Pu RT, Pang Y, Michael CW. Utility of WT-1, p63, MOC31, mesothelin, and cytokeratin (K903 and CK5/6) immunostains in differentiating adenocarcinoma, squamous cell carcinoma, and malignant mesothelioma in effusions. *Diagn Cytopathol* 2008;36:20–5.

Salvatorelli L, Calabrese G, Parenti R, et al. Immunohistochemical expression of Wilms' tumor 1 protein in human tissues: From ontogenesis to neoplastic tissues. *Appl Sci* 2020;10:40–67.

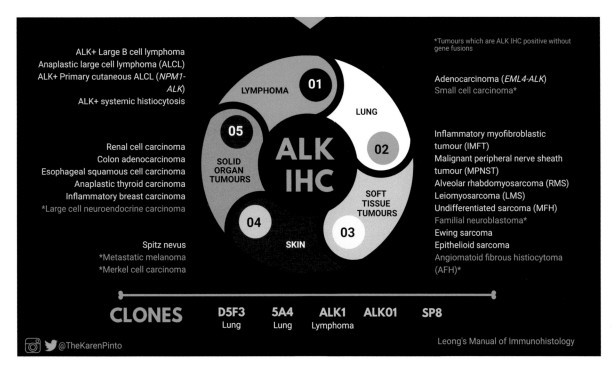

ALK diseases

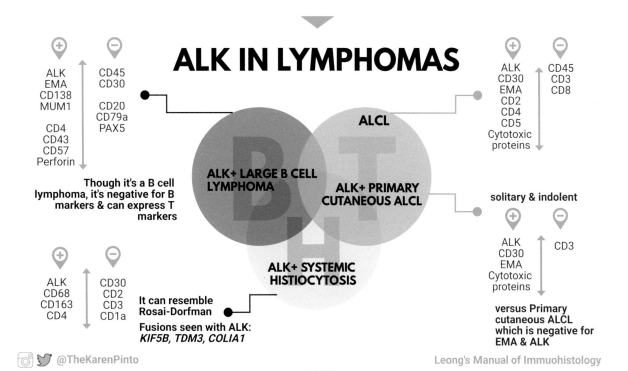

ALK in lymphomas

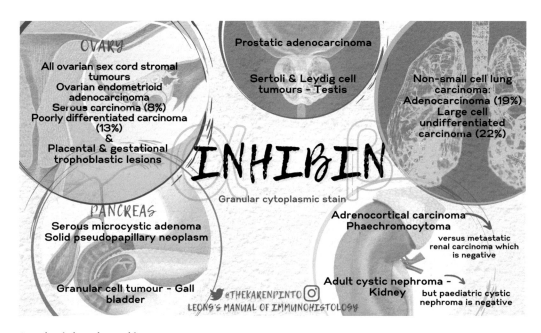

OVARY
All ovarian sex cord stromal tumours
Ovarian endometrioid adenocarcinoma
Serous carcinoma (8%)
Poorly differentiated carcinoma (13%)
&
Placental & gestational trophoblastic lesions

Prostatic adenocarcinoma

Sertoli & Leydig cell tumours - Testis

Non-small cell lung carcinoma:
Adenocarcinoma (19%)
Large cell undifferentiated carcinoma (22%)

INHIBIN

Granular cytoplasmic stain

PANCREAS
Serous microcystic adenoma
Solid pseudopapillary neoplasm

Adrenocortical carcinoma
Phaechromocytoma

versus metastatic renal carcinoma which is negative

Granular cell tumour - Gall bladder

Adult cystic nephroma - Kidney

but paediatric cystic nephroma is negative

@THEKARENPINTO
LEONG'S MANUAL OF IMMUNOHISTOLOGY

Anaplastic lymphoma kinase

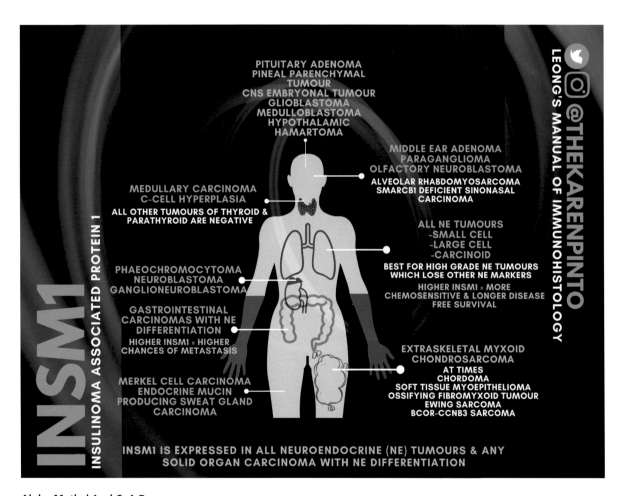

INSM1

INSULINOMA ASSOCIATED PROTEIN 1

PITUITARY ADENOMA
PINEAL PARENCHYMAL
TUMOUR
CNS EMBRYONAL TUMOUR
GLIOBLASTOMA
MEDULLOBLASTOMA
HYPOTHALAMIC
HAMARTOMA

MIDDLE EAR ADENOMA
PARAGANGLIOMA
OLFACTORY NEUROBLASTOMA

ALVEOLAR RHABDOMYOSARCOMA
SMARCB1 DEFICIENT SINONASAL
CARCINOMA

MEDULLARY CARCINOMA
C-CELL HYPERPLASIA

ALL OTHER TUMOURS OF THYROID &
PARATHYROID ARE NEGATIVE

ALL NE TUMOURS
-SMALL CELL
-LARGE CELL
-CARCINOID

BEST FOR HIGH GRADE NE TUMOURS
WHICH LOSE OTHER NE MARKERS

HIGHER INSM1 = MORE
CHEMOSENSITIVE & LONGER DISEASE
FREE SURVIVAL

PHAEOCHROMOCYTOMA
NEUROBLASTOMA
GANGLIONEUROBLASTOMA

GASTROINTESTINAL
CARCINOMAS WITH NE
DIFFERENTIATION

HIGHER INSM1 = HIGHER
CHANCES OF METASTASIS

EXTRASKELETAL MYXOID
CHONDROSARCOMA

AT TIMES
CHORDOMA
SOFT TISSUE MYOEPITHELIOMA
OSSIFYING FIBROMYXOID TUMOUR
EWING SARCOMA
BCOR-CCNB3 SARCOMA

MERKEL CELL CARCINOMA
ENDOCRINE MUCIN
PRODUCING SWEAT GLAND
CARCINOMA

INSM1 IS EXPRESSED IN ALL NEUROENDOCRINE (NE) TUMOURS & ANY
SOLID ORGAN CARCINOMA WITH NE DIFFERENTIATION

Alpha Methyl Acyl CoA Racemase

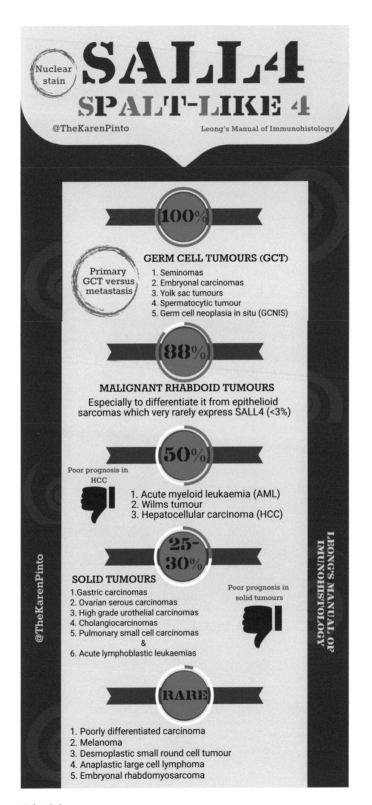

Calretinin

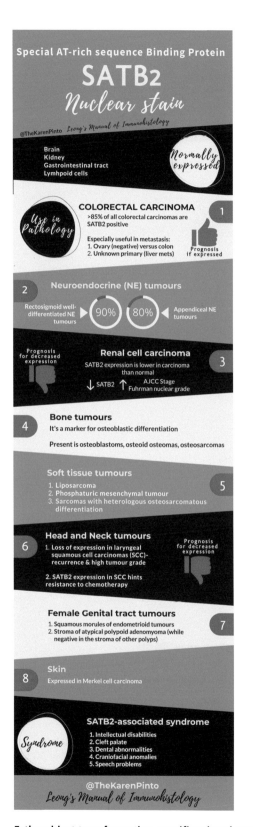

Erthyroblast transformation-specific related gene

Nuclear stain

SOX10

SRY RELATED HMG-BOX 10

ROLE

 Maturation & maintenance of melanocytes and Schwann cells

 Also expressed in myoepithelial cells & neural crest cells

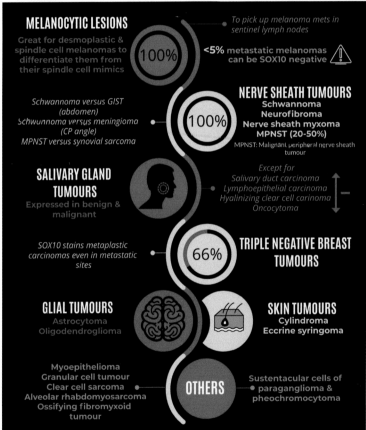

MELANOCYTIC LESIONS

Great for desmoplastic & spindle cell melanomas to differentiate them from their spindle cell mimics

To pick up melanoma mets in sentinel lymph nodes

100%

<5% metastatic melanomas can be SOX10 negative ⚠

Schwannoma versus GIST (abdomen)
Schwannoma versus meningioma (CP angle)
MPNST versus synovial sarcoma

100%

NERVE SHEATH TUMOURS
Schwannoma
Neurofibroma
Nerve sheath myxoma
MPNST (20-50%)
MPNST: Malignant peripheral nerve sheath tumour

SALIVARY GLAND TUMOURS

Expressed in benign & malignant

Except for
Salivary duct carcinoma
Lymphoepithelial carcinoma
Hyalinizing clear cell carinoma
Oncocytoma

SOX10 stains metaplastic carcinomas even in metastatic sites

66%

TRIPLE NEGATIVE BREAST TUMOURS

GLIAL TUMOURS
Astrocytoma
Oligodendroglioma

SKIN TUMOURS
Cylindroma
Eccrine syringoma

Myoepithelioma
Granular cell tumour
Clear cell sarcoma
Alveolar rhabdomyosarcoma
Ossifying fibromyxoid tumour

OTHERS

Sustentacular cells of paraganglioma & pheochromocytoma

MUTATIONS

Waardenburg - Shah syndrome
Hirschsprung disease
Kallman syndrome

📷 🐦 @TheKarenPinto   Leong's Manual of Immunohistology

Friend Leukaemia Integration 1

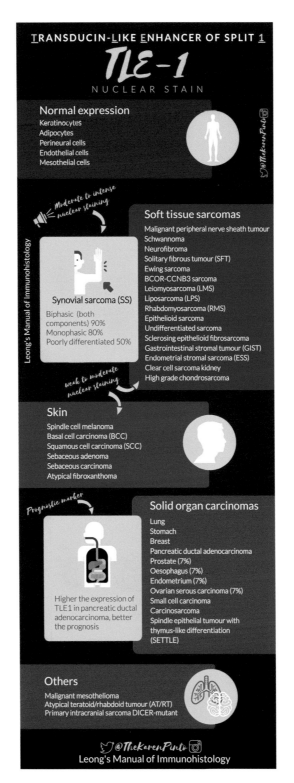

Forkhead box protein 2

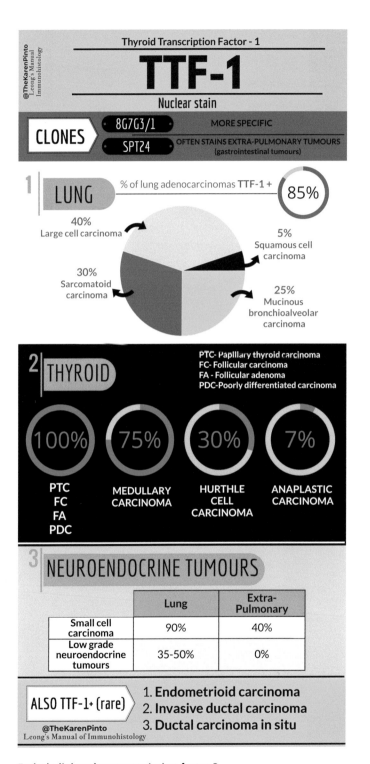

Thyroid Transcription Factor - 1

TTF-1

Nuclear stain

CLONES

8G7G3/1 — MORE SPECIFIC

SPT24 — OFTEN STAINS EXTRA-PULMONARY TUMOURS (gastrointestinal tumours)

1 LUNG

% of lung adenocarcinomas **TTF-1 +** — 85%

- 40% Large cell carcinoma
- 30% Sarcomatoid carcinoma
- 5% Squamous cell carcinoma
- 25% Mucinous bronchioalveolar carcinoma

2 THYROID

PTC- Papillary thyroid carcinoma
FC- Follicular carcinoma
FA - Follicular adenoma
PDC-Poorly differentiated carcinoma

100%	75%	30%	7%
PTC FC FA PDC	MEDULLARY CARCINOMA	HURTHLE CELL CARCINOMA	ANAPLASTIC CARCINOMA

3 NEUROENDOCRINE TUMOURS

	Lung	Extra-Pulmonary
Small cell carcinoma	90%	40%
Low grade neuroendocrine tumours	35-50%	0%

ALSO TTF-1+ (rare)
1. Endometrioid carcinoma
2. Invasive ductal carcinoma
3. Ductal carcinoma in situ

Endothelial nuclear transcription factor 3

WT1

WILMS TUMOUR : NUCLEAR STAIN : IMMUNOTHERAPY ANTIGEN

EXPRESSION

NORMAL		TUMOUR

MESOTHELIUM

Growth & differentiation of normal mesothelium. It's expressed in both benign and malignant

-All mesotheliomas express WT1 Used to differentiate it from lung adenocarcinomas
-Adenomatoid tumours

OVARY

Expressed in nearly all cells of the ovary including granulosa & Sertoli cells, but not Leydig cells

-High grade serous carcinoma (ovary, fallopian tube & peritoneum)
-All sex cord stromal tumours (except Steroid cell)
_Endometrial serous carcinoma (<20%)
-Uterine sarcomas (endometrial stromal, carcinosarcoma, leiomyosarcoma, undifferentiated)

KIDNEY

WT1 plays a vital role in nephrogenesis & is expressed in podocytes

_Wilms tumour
-Cystic partially differentiated nephroblastoma
-Metanephric adenoma
-Nephrogenic rests
-Malignant rhabdoid tumour

SOFT TISSUE TUMOURS

Is expressed in a number of high grade soft tissue sarcomas

↑expression ↓prognosis

-DSRCT
-CIC-DUX4 "Ewing-like" sarcoma (unlike Ewing & BCOR-rearranged sarcoma which are WT1 negative)
-Vascular tumours (benign & maignant)

WT1 PEPTIDE BASED IMMUNOTHERAPY

WT1 protein expression (including cytoplasmic positivity) in cancer cells has been used as a targeted antigen to induce CD8+ T cells to elicit an immunological response against the cancer cell. Used for treating:

-Acute myeloid leukaemia -Myelodysplastic syndrome -Chronic myeloid leukaemia -Multiple myeloma -Acute lymphoblastic leukaemia	Solid organ carcinomas like -colon -lung -breast -thymic cancers	WT1 levels are also measured in peripheral blood to assess minimal residual disease

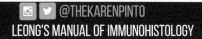

Inhibin: granular cytoplasmic stain

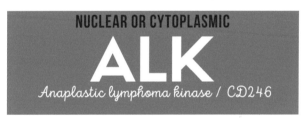

ALK

Anaplastic lymphoma kinase / CD246

NORMALLY ONLY PRESENT IN THE BRAIN

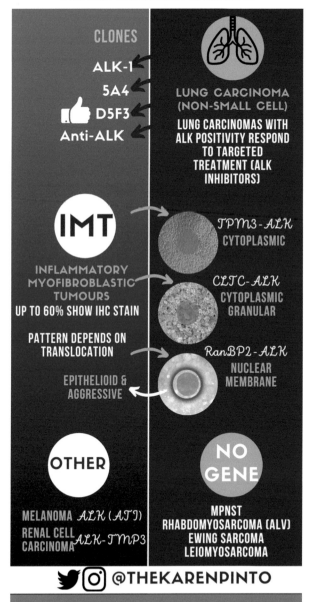

CLONES

ALK-1

5A4

D5F3

Anti-ALK

LUNG CARCINOMA
(NON-SMALL CELL)

LUNG CARCINOMAS WITH
ALK POSITIVITY RESPOND
TO TARGETED
TREATMENT (ALK
INHIBITORS)

IMT

INFLAMMATORY
MYOFIBROBLASTIC
TUMOURS

UP TO 60% SHOW IHC STAIN

PATTERN DEPENDS ON
TRANSLOCATION

EPITHELIOID &
AGGRESSIVE

TPM3-ALK
CYTOPLASMIC

CLTC-ALK
CYTOPLASMIC
GRANULAR

RanBP2-ALK
NUCLEAR
MEMBRANE

OTHER

MELANOMA   ALK (ATI)
RENAL CELL   ALK-TMP3
CARCINOMA

NO
GENE

MPNST
RHABDOMYOSARCOMA (ALV)
EWING SARCOMA
LEIOMYOSARCOMA

@THEKARENPINTO

LEONG'S MANUAL OF IMMUNOHISTOLOGY

Insulinoma associated protein 1

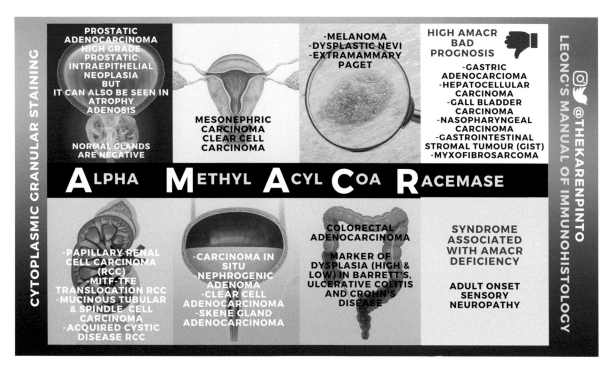

CYTOPLASMIC GRANULAR STAINING

PROSTATIC ADENOCARCINOMA HIGH GRADE PROSTATIC INTRAEPITHELIAL NEOPLASIA BUT IT CAN ALSO BE SEEN IN ATROPHY ADENOSIS

NORMAL GLANDS ARE NEGATIVE

MESONEPHRIC CARCINOMA CLEAR CELL CARCINOMA

-MELANOMA
-DYSPLASTIC NEVI
-EXTRAMAMMARY PAGET

HIGH AMACR BAD PROGNOSIS

-GASTRIC ADENOCARCIOMA
-HEPATOCELLULAR CARCINOMA
-GALL BLADDER CARCINOMA
-NASOPHARYNGEAL CARCINOMA
-GASTROINTESTINAL STROMAL TUMOUR (GIST)
-MYXOFIBROSARCOMA

ALPHA METHYL ACYL COA RACEMASE

-PAPILLARY RENAL CELL CARCINOMA (RCC)
-MITF-TFE TRANSLOCATION RCC
-MUCINOUS TUBULAR & SPINDLE CELL CARCINOMA
-ACQUIRED CYSTIC DISEASE RCC

-CARCINOMA IN SITU
-NEPHROGENIC ADENOMA
-CLEAR CELL ADENOCARCINOMA
-SKENE GLAND ADENOCARCINOMA

COLORECTAL ADENOCARCINOMA

MARKER OF DYSPLASIA (HIGH & LOW) IN BARRETT'S, ULCERATIVE COLITIS AND CROHN'S DISEASE

SYNDROME ASSOCIATED WITH AMACR DEFICIENCY

ADULT ONSET SENSORY NEUROPATHY

Spalt-like 4

CALRETININ

POSITIVE

NEGATIVE

MOST MESOTHELIOMAS ARE POSITIVE, INCLUDING EPITHELIOID & SARCOMATOID

ONLY <5% OF SOLID ORGAN CARCINOMAS (LUNG, OVARIAN SEROUS PAPILLARY) MAY EXPRESS CALRETININ

ESPECIALLY USEFUL IN EFFUSION SPECIMENS

-SERTOLI LEYDIG TUMOURS

-FEMALE ADNEXAL TUMOUR OF PROBABLE WOLFFIAN ORIGIN

-CERVIX MESONEPHRIC ADENOCARCINOMA

-SERTOLIFORM ENDOMETRIOID CARCINOMA

-FIBROTHECOMA
-GRANULOSA CELL TUMOURS

ADRENOCORTICAL TUMOURS

RENAL CELL CARCINOMA

PHEOCHROMOCYTOMA

SCHWANNOMA

OLFACTORY NEUROBLASTOMA

AMELOBLASTOMA

NEUROFIBROMA

SINONASAL SMALL ROUND BLUE CELL TUMOURS

KERATOCYSTIC ODONTOGENIC TUMOUR

CENTRAL NEUROCYTOMA (NEURONAL DIFFERENTIATION)

OLIGODENDROGLIOMA (GLIAL DIFFERENTIATION)

OTHER TUMOURS EXPRESSING CALRETININ

SOFT TISSUE TUMOURS:
-DESMOPLASTIC SMALL ROUND CELL TUMOUR
-GRANULAR CELL TUMOUR
-SYNOVIAL SARCOMA

-CARDIAC MYXOMA
-THYMIC CARCINOMA
-ADENOMATOID TUMOUR

USED IN THE DIAGNOSIS OF HIRSCHSPRUNG'S DISEASE

Special AT-rich sequence Binding Protein

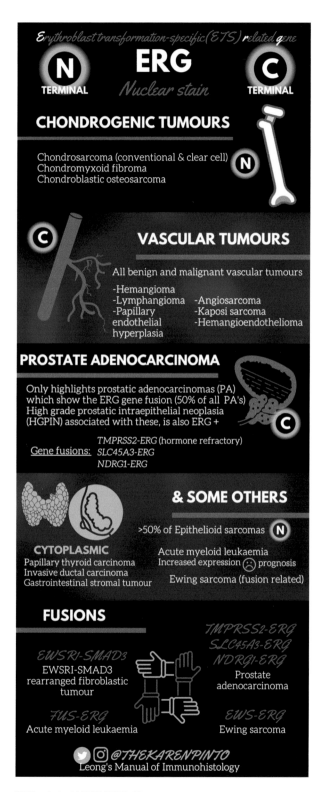

ERG

Erythroblast transformation-specific (ETS) related gene

N TERMINAL **C TERMINAL**

Nuclear stain

CHONDROGENIC TUMOURS

Chondrosarcoma (conventional & clear cell)
Chondromyxoid fibroma
Chondroblastic osteosarcoma

N

VASCULAR TUMOURS

C

All benign and malignant vascular tumours

-Hemangioma
-Lymphangioma   -Angiosarcoma
-Papillary   -Kaposi sarcoma
endothelial   -Hemangioendothelioma
hyperplasia

PROSTATE ADENOCARCINOMA

Only highlights prostatic adenocarcinomas (PA)
which show the ERG gene fusion (50% of all PA's)
High grade prostatic intraepithelial neoplasia
(HGPIN) associated with these, is also ERG +

C

Gene fusions: *TMPRSS2-ERG* (hormone refractory)
               SLC45A3-ERG
               NDRG1-ERG

& SOME OTHERS

>50% of Epithelioid sarcomas **N**

CYTOPLASMIC
Papillary thyroid carcinoma
Invasive ductal carcinoma
Gastrointestinal stromal tumour

Acute myeloid leukaemia
Increased expression ☹ prognosis

Ewing sarcoma (fusion related)

FUSIONS

EWSRI-SMAD3
EWSRI-SMAD3
rearranged fibroblastic
tumour

TMPRSS2-ERG
SLC45A3-ERG
NDRG1-ERG
Prostate
adenocarcinoma

FUS-ERG
Acute myeloid leukaemia

EWS-ERG
Ewing sarcoma

🐦 📷 *@THEKARENPINTO*
Leong's Manual of Immunohistology

SRY related HMG-BOX 10

FLI1
Friend Leukaemia Integration 1

NORMALLY EXPRESSED
- Haematopoeitic cells
- Blood vessels

ROLE
- cell proliferation
- tumourigenesis
- development of blood vessels

FLI1 negative SRBCT's
1. Small cell osteosarcoma
2. Mesenchymal chondrosarcoma
3. Blastemal predominant Wilms tumour

1 Ewing sarcoma

90%

When used in combination with other immunostains, it can help differentiate Ewing sarcoma from other small round blue cell tumours (SRBCT)

Though mainly seen with *EWSR1-FLI1*, can be seen with other fusions too

Did you know?

FLI1 + 70-100%

Of Ewing sarcoma with *EWSR1-FLI1* fusion

BUT !! Other FLI1 positive SRBCT's
- Lymphoma
- Melanoma
- Merkel cell carcinoma
- Desmoplastic small round blue cell tumour

Vascular tumours   **2**

FLI1 is expressed in all benign, intermediate and malignant vascular tumours

- Hemangioma
- Angiosarcoma
- Hemangioendothelioma
- Kaposi sarcoma
- Littoral cell angioma

Internal control

The normal blood vessels & lymphocytes within the tissue are always positive for FLI1

3 Skin tumours
- Melanoma
- Merkel cell carcinoma

And some more   **4**
- Synovial sarcoma
- Epithelioid sarcoma
- Phosphaturic mesenchymal tumour
- Solid pseudopapillary neoplasm
- Sex cord stromal tumours

🐦 📷 *@TheKarenPinto*
Leong's Manual of Immunohistology

Transducin-like enhancer of split 1

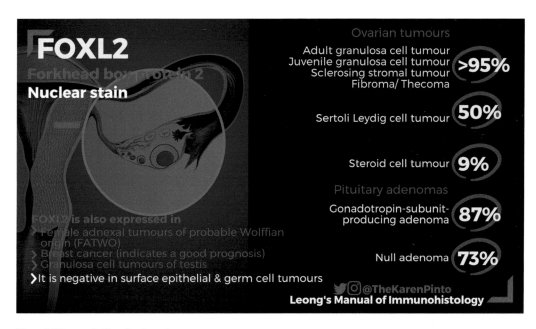

Thyroid Transcription Factor - 1

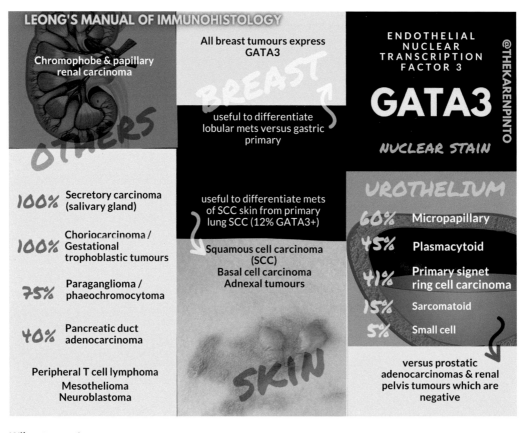

LEONG'S MANUAL OF IMMUNOHISTOLOGY

Chromophobe & papillary renal carcinoma

OTHERS

All breast tumours express GATA3

BREAST

useful to differentiate lobular mets versus gastric primary

ENDOTHELIAL NUCLEAR TRANSCRIPTION FACTOR 3

GATA3

NUCLEAR STAIN

@THEKARENPINTO

100% Secretory carcinoma (salivary gland)

100% Choriocarcinoma / Gestational trophoblastic tumours

75% Paraganglioma / phaeochromocytoma

40% Pancreatic duct adenocarcinoma

Peripheral T cell lymphoma
Mesothelioma
Neuroblastoma

useful to differentiate mets of SCC skin from primary lung SCC (12% GATA3+)

Squamous cell carcinoma (SCC)
Basal cell carcinoma
Adnexal tumours

SKIN

UROTHELIUM

60% Micropapillary

45% Plasmacytoid

41% Primary signet ring cell carcinoma

15% Sarcomatoid

5% Small cell

versus prostatic adenocarcinomas & renal pelvis tumours which are negative

Wilms tumor 1